CHOICES FOR LIVING

COPING WITH FEAR OF DYING

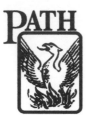

PATH IN PSYCHOLOGY
Published in Cooperation with Publications for the
Advancement of Theory and History in Psychology (PATH)

Series Editors:
David Bakan, *York University*
John M. Broughton, *Teachers College, Columbia University*
Robert W. Rieber, *John Jay College, CUNY, and Columbia University*
Howard Gruber, *University of Geneva*

CHOICES FOR LIVING

COPING WITH FEAR OF DYING

THOMAS S. LANGNER, PH.D.

Retired, Formerly
School of Public Health
and Department of Psychiatry
Columbia University
New York, New York

KLUWER ACADEMIC / PLENUM PUBLISHERS
NEW YORK, BOSTON, DORDRECHT, LONDON, MOSCOW

Library of Congress Cataloging-in-Publication Data

Choices for living: coping with fear of dying/Thomas S. Langner.
        p.   cm. — (PATH in psychology)
    Includes bibliographical references and index.
    ISBN 0-306-46607-4
        1. Fear of death.   2. Conduct of life.   I. Langner, Thomas S.   II. Series.

    RC552.F42 C46 2002
    616.85′225—dc21

                                                                        2001023688

ISBN 0-306-46607-4

© 2002 Kluwer Academic / Plenum Publishers, New York
233 Spring Street, New York, N.Y. 10013

http://www.wkap.nl

10   9   8   7   6   5   4   3   2   1

A C.I.P. record for this book is available from the Library of Congress

Printed in the United States of America

PREFACE

On January 1, 1994, I turned 70 and it suddenly dawned on me that I would not be around forever. I started to reread Ernest Becker's Pulitzer prize-winning book *The Denial of Death*. I was struck by the fact that Becker focused on killing or wielding power over others as a major mode of coping with the fear of death. Killing others created the illusion of immortality, since the killer had the power of life and death over others. This book was shortly followed by *Escape from Evil*, which dealt further with "man's need to feel powerful and to banish death."

The more I thought about it, the more I felt I should write about the whole gamut of ways in which people cope with the fear of death and dying. These rage from the most positive coping modes such as Creativity, Love, Humor, Intellectualization, and Procreation, to the most negative coping modes (those most destructive of the self and others) such as Counterphobic Behavior, Gambling, Dissociation, Repression/Denial, Suicide, Projection, and Killing. Somewhere in the middle lie Obsessional Behavior, Living Life to the Hilt, Living Better or Longer, Group Membership, Religion, and Mementos and Monuments. I call this a "moral hierarchy" of behavior used in coping with the fear of death and dying.

Many books are written about bereavement but very few are written about the fear of one's *own* death. Even the books that deal with one's own death often focus chiefly on terminal illness (Kubler-Ross's On *Death and Dying* or Nuland's *How We Die*). In contrast, this book looks at the ways in which death-fear operates on a back-burner all our lives, and how it influences the life choices we make and the paths we follow. Anticipatory bereavement and mourning are for the inevitable loss of self.

As this book went to press, disaster struck the United States, with multiple terrorist attacks launched on New York City and Washington D.C. In the wake of these events over 6,000 people are missing or dead. The media warn of the possibility of further attacks of increasingly lethal dimensions—chemical, biological, nuclear—situations which we may not be equipped to prevent or handle should they occur. Economic decline, already in evidence before the attacks, has taken a steeper slide due to the damage done by the terrorists. The airline industry and others are in a state of near collapse, causing further anxiety among the American population regarding the future. The combination of financial insecurity and fear of attacks of unknown type and magnitude have created a mood of depression in this country, which is shared to some extent by other countries around the world.

Choices For Living, although clearly not written for this specific purpose, directly addresses the emotional state in which our nation and much of the world now finds itself. In addition to elaborating on the modes of coping that may be seen as productive—creativity, love, humor, religion, procreation—it explores the maladaptive modes of suicide and killing which can be seen as responses to the same fear of death. Killing others may be seen as a means to control fear and attain immortality. Much of the terrorists' motivation is derived from that search for immortality and to stem a perceived threat to their form of Islamic society. The role of projection—attributing your feelings to your enemies—is discussed, as is the function of dehumanization, enmification , and animalization. Enemies turned into non-humans, pigs or Satans can be killed with impunity. Dissociation helps killers keep their hatred for their enemies "compartmentalized" so that they can preserve it in a pure form to fuel their lethal activities without regard to the tenets of all the major faiths, including Islam.

Wars, genocide, race prejudice and other man-made evils are discussed along with their potential multiple causative factors, and suggestions for reducing those evils are made. Coping with death fear from day to day, without paralysis and without denial, but by continuing with one's roles and occupations is strongly recommended.

Choices For Living has been written both for professionals and academics and for anyone interested in psychology, psychiatry, sociology, philosophy, or politics. It attempts to leaven theory with numerous relevant examples of current events, famous or infamous personalities, life stories, and case histories. I hope this book may also be therapeutic for readers as they face their own finitude. Writing it has surely been helpful to me in coping with my own fear of dying which, I am well aware, is a good example of intellectualization as a coping mechanism. Lastly, I hope that this book will help our people who are confronted with a clear threat to their lives. Good choices in living can counter the legitimate fears we now have.

ACKNOWLEDGMENT OF PERMISSIONS

Grateful acknowledgment is made to the following for permission to reprint previously published material:

Excerpt from *Men of Music* by W. Brockway and H. Weinstock, 1939. Copyright © 1939 By Brockway & Weinstock. Reprinted with the permission of Simon & Schuster.

An excerpt from *Facing the Music* © 1981 by Harold C. Schonberg. Reprinted by arrangement with Harold C. Schonberg and The Barbara Hogenson Agency, Inc.

Excerpt from *The Denial of Death* by Ernest Becker. Copyright © 1973 by The Free Press, a Division of Simon & Schuster, Inc. Reprinted with permission of the publisher.

Excerpts from *Revolution in Psychiatry* by Ernest Becker. Copyright © 1964 by The Free Press, a Division of Simon & Schuster, Inc. Reprinted with permission of the publisher.

Excerpt from *Escape From Evil* by Ernest Becker. Copyright © 1975 by Marie Becker. Reprinted with permission of The Free Press, a Division of Simon & Schuster, Inc.

Excerpt from *Love, Sex, Death and the Making of the Male* by Rosalind Miles. Reprinted with permission of Simon & Schuster, Inc.

Excerpt from *Attachment and Loss, Volume II: Separation: Anxiety and Anger* by John Bowlby, reprinted by permission of Basic Books, a member of Perseus Books, L.L.C. Copyright © 1973 by The Tavistock Institute of Human Relations.

Poem, "What lips my lips have kissed" by Edna St. Vincent Millay. From COLLECTED POEMS, HarperCollins, copyright © 1923, 1951 by Edna St. Vincent Millay and Norma Millay Ellis. All rights reserved. Reprinted by permission of Elizabeth Barnett, literary executor.

Excerpts from "Jacques Derrida," *The New York Times* 1/23/94, by Mitchell Stephens. By permission of the author.

Excerpt from *Identity: Youth and Crisis* by E.H. Erickson, 1969, W.W. Norton, by permission of the publisher.

Excerpts from *The New York Times*, with the permission of the publisher, as follows:
James, J., 3/19/95, "He no longer has to make points. He just makes them."
Browne, M.W., 2/11/97, "Young astronomers scan night sky and help wanted ads."
Burns, J.F., 5/14/96, "Everest takes worst toll, refusing to become stylish."
Abbott, L.K., 4/9/96, "Death Rattle," *The New York Times Book Review.*
Daley, S., 11/9/97, "Apartheid torturer testifies as evil shows its banal face."
Sims, C., 3/13/95, "Argentine tells of the dumping of captives at sea."
Butterfield, F., 2/15/96, "Insanity drove a man to kill at two clinics, jury is told."

Excerpt from "A Civics Lesson" by Benjamin R. Barber. Reprinted with permission from the 9/4/96 issue of *The Nation* magazine.

Excerpt from a book review of *The Denial of Death*, by Lloyd Demause, in *History of Childhood Quarterly*, Vol. 2, #2, (Fall, 1974) by permission of the author.

Excerpt from *By the Grace of Guile: The Role of Deception in Natural History and Human Affairs* by L. Rue, 1994, by permission of Oxford University Press.

From *The Passion of Ansel Bourne: Multiple Personality in American Culture*, by Michael G. Kenny; copyright © 1986 by the Smithsonian Institution. Used by permission of the publisher.

Extracts from *Sybil* by Flora Rheta Schreiber, copyright © 1973, H. Regnery, reproduced with permission of The McGraw-Hill Companies.

Extracts from *Alter Egos: Multiple Personalities* by D. Cohen, 1996, Constable & Robinson Publishing, Ltd., by permission of the publishers.

Extract from "Multiple posttraumatic personality disorder" by David Spiegel, in R.P. Kluft, *Clinical Perspectives on Multiple Personality Disorder*, 1993, American Psychiatric Press, by permission of the publisher.

Excerpt from *Repression and Dissociation*, by J.L. Singer (Ed.) 1990, The University of Chicago Press, by permission of the publisher.

Excerpt from *The Death of Satan: How Americans Have Lost Their Sense of Evil* by Andrew Delbanco. Copyright © 1995 by Andrew Delbanco. Reprinted by permission of Hill & Wang, a division of Farrar, Straus and Giroux, LLC.

ACKNOWLEDGMENTS

I would like to thank the people who read and commented on early drafts of the chapters of this book. John Orton. and Andrew Lazarus sent me detailed written comments that were very helpful. My mother-in-law, Norma Kassirer, read many chapters and made important suggestions about style.

Joseph Jaffe made many pertinent comments; he persuaded me to think of dissociation as a continuum and pointed to my placement of coping modes in a hierarchy as a new and important contribution. Theo Skolnick suggested links to existentialism and also made relevant observations about style. Robin Winkler also made valuable comments about style.

Others helped me with specific areas or chapters. Robert Rieber suggested the inclusion of many significant references. His discussions of the satanic, of "enmification," of the possibility of alternating states of the "true believer" and the conscious evildoer (or charlatan) existing in one person—and many other topics—were consistently invaluable.

Herbert Spiegel sat with me for three hours in his office while we discussed dissociation; much of the theoretical discussion in the dissociation chapter is based on that meeting. He suggested that I use some case histories of multiple personality disorder that were published well before *Sybil* became a best seller, and before recovered memory became a cottage industry. Dr. Rieber joined with Dr. Spiegel in criticizing the overdiagnosis of multiple personality in several articles and public lectures.

Maurice Green discussed some of the psychodynamic aspects of the book with me.

Dr. Rieber put me in touch with Eliot Werner, who was Executive Editor, Behavioral and Social Sciences, Kluwer Academic/Plenum Publishers. Without their help, this book would never have been published.

I specially want to thank Sharon Panulla, my new Sponsoring Psychology Editor, and Jennifer Stevens and Lesley Rodriguez, Production Editors, for their patience and cheerful support during the long process of producing this book.

Praise is also due Terry Kornak, who hunted down my "witches," subdued my footnotes, and made many good suggestions.

I am also grateful to Bruce Dohrenwend, Barbara Solomon, and Corlies Smith, who aided me on the path to publication. In addition, I owe gratitude to the many coworkers who assisted me in my own research, and to those on various research teams where I learned the vicissitudes of interdisciplinary studies.

Last, I wish to thank my family. My wife, Susan Kassirer, listened patiently to my theories and taught me a great deal about punctuation. Her sister, Karen Kassirer, guided me through many word-processing problems. My seven-year-old daughter Laura helped me with the Canon copier, and often sat on my lap while I was writing at the computer. My grown children by my first marriage, Lisa, Josh, Eli, Gretchen, and Belinda, heard me hold forth on my theories and often came back with alternative explanations of behavior.

The genesis of this book may derive partly from my experiences with death in my family. My parents, Herbert and Ruth, both died slow painful deaths of cancer; my sister, Clare, committed suicide at age thirty. All three of them gave me a great deal of love.

CONTENTS

CHOICES FOR LIVING

COPING WITH FEAR OF DYING

Attitudes Toward Death

Death as Part of Life

The inevitability of death, the awareness of one's own mortality, and the degree of one's concern with it have been the subjects of countless poems, songs, essays, books, and paintings. The questions of what constitutes life, the existence of an afterlife, and the very meaning of our short span on earth have engaged prophets and philosophers for as far back as we have records. Thoughts about death constitute a fair portion of the conscious thoughts of most people, but there is a great variation among different tribes, nations, and social classes. There is also tremendous individual variation in attitudes toward death, from welcoming to passive acceptance to angry fighting back.

There is the brave and accepting "Sing no sad songs for me, when I am gone" of Christina Rossetti (in Speare, p. 243). There is the heartwrenching melody and stern Biblical message of Brahms' song ("Vier Ernste Gesänge) (Brahms, 1968) See also "Alexander Kipnis sings lieder," (Sound recording), Berkeley, CA: Music and Arts, 1991, two digital sound discs, mono, 43/4 inches):

> O Tod! O Tod! Wie bitter, wie bitter bist du!

There is the defiance of Dylan Thomas:

> Do not go gentle into that good night,
> Rage, rage against the dying of the light!
> (Thomas, 1957, "Do not go gentle into that good night," p. 128 1914–1953)

The most common emotion engendered by death is fear. In Shakespeare's exquisite words:

> Claudio: Ay, but to die, and go we know not where;
> To lie in cold obstruction (*stagnation*) and to rot.
> The weariest and most loathèd worldly life
> That age, ache, penury, and imprisonment

Can lay on nature is a paradise
To what we fear of death.
(Shakespeare, 1965, Act 3, Scene I, 1623)

When this fear of death becomes extreme, it can seriously interfere with an individual's daily functioning. In front-line combat, for example, anger against the enemy can combine with fear, so that one "freezes." Loss of bladder and bowel control can occur, as described in the soldier's expressions, "I shat my brains out" or "I was pissing green." In Walter Cannon's (Cannon, 1919, 1963) famous treatise he describes how, during stress, the sympathetic nervous system takes over (adrenaline or epinephrine) and the parasympathetic (acetylcholine or norepinephrine) is subordinated. This causes physiological changes; our saliva stops flowing ("His tongue clove to the roof of his mouth") and our pupils dilate ("Her eyes blazed with anger").

> Terror is even greater than anguish. It is anger and rage so intense as to paralyze all action against the assailant. It is the fear of death incarnate... (Foxe, 1939, p. 13)

Coping with Death

Why death should be such a central concern might seem obvious to some. "Why not? It is the end of life!" Birth and death truly define life itself, the beginning and the end. When we talk about fear of death, and how we cope with it, we are taking on the description of life itself. One needn't reify Life and Death as two entities (or instincts), Thanatos and Eros, as Freud (1920) did, although the metaphor is helpful.

We spend much of our lives seeking to justify our existence, to validate our behavior, and to establish our self-esteem. We are constantly searching for ways to make our lives meaningful. These activities are crucial to our continued living, because we are (for the most part) self-examining creatures. In their absence, we could face depression, suicide, or a "living death." Our finitude hovers in the background. The way we live our lives, then, has much to do with how we cope with death. Conversely, the way we deal with death, our attitudes toward it, and our ability to face it in a reasonable way determine to a great extent how we live our lives.

In his seminal article, "Attitudes Toward Death in Some Normal and Mentally Ill Populations," Herman Feifel paraphrased Kurt Eissler:

> We are mistaken to consider death as a purely biological event. The attitudes concerning it, and its meaning for the individual, can serve as an important organizing principle in determining how he conducts himself in life. (Eissler, 1955)

This statement can serve as the keystone of this book. Our aim is to connect our everyday ways of living with our fear of death.

The fear of death is a composite of many fears: our early fears of separation, of individuality, of leaving our mother, and finally of leaving the world and being alone. Gardner Murphy, in a review chapter in Feifel's book, lists seven "attitudes toward death," six of which are fears.

1. Death is the end (no panic, no fear, acceptance).
2. Fear of losing consciousness (loss of control or mastery)
3. Fear of loneliness (separation from loved ones)
4. Fear of the unknown
5. Fear of punishment (hellfire, mutilation, disintegration)
6. Fear of what might happen to loved ones left behind, especially dependents
7. Fear of failure (unfulfilled lives, tasks left undone, regrets)

While the fear of death has many different aspects, subject to the individual's background and experience, the origins of these various dimensions of thanatophobia are obscure. The possible causes of fear of dying are discussed in the following paragraphs.

At this point, one could add indefinitely to Murphy's list, but one important addition might be helpful. *Fear of individuality* (related to the child's necessary separation from the mother) may be a small part of the fear of death. If I die as an individual, it is final. If I die as part of a group, I live on through the group. My continuity with family, state, or mankind will ease the fear, while my individuality will increase it. This is also related to subfear 3, loneliness, since the greater the degree of individuality, the greater the separation and loneliness. In his book, *Solitude*, Anthony Storr (1988) notes how the capacity to be alone is crucial to creativity.

> Learning, thinking, innovation, and maintaining contact with one's own inner world are all facilitated by solitude.

Highly creative people may not fear loneliness as much as the average man, but they seem to fear that their creative tasks will be left incomplete (subfear 7), as expressed in Keats' famous sonnet:

> When I have fears that I may cease to be
> Before my pen has gleaned my teeming brain,
> Before high-piléd books, in charactery,
> Hold like rich garners the full ripened grain ...
> (Keats, p. 221)

Keats had good reason to fear leaving his work incompleted, since he died at age 26 in 1821. In December 1818 his younger brother, Tom Keats, died after a long bout with tuberculosis. At the beginning of that year Keats wrote this sonnet, between the 22nd and 31st of January, 1818. He may well have had premonitions of his own death then, triggered by his long exposure to Tom's spitting up blood. On December 22nd of 1819 he wrote that he was "rather unwell." In January of 1820 he had a severe hemorrhage, and again in June (Keats, pp. 25–28).

The rich metaphor of his ideas as grain, and the feeling that his mind was teeming with ideas that could be gleaned or harvested, are of interest, for they show the sureness and self-confidence of a genius. Even those of us who are less gifted may have fears about leaving tasks incomplete, or wish we had a chance to live our lives over again, so that we might fulfill our goals.

Where do all these fears originate? What is the relationship of fear of death to anxiety? Is fear just more specific, while anxiety is "free-floating?" Norman O. Brown (1959), while focusing on Freud's concept of the "death instinct" (which I feel is not necessary to our understanding of the fear of death) has made the connections between anxiety and death quite simple and clear.

> ...birth...is in itself the death of a fetus as well as the birth of a baby, is also a bio-logical separation from the mother conferring biological individuality on the child. The prototype of psychic traumas (is) the experience of wanting but not being able to find the mother...Furthermore, all these separations are experienced as a threat of death: again in Freud's own words, what the ego fears in anxiety 'is in the nature of an overthrow or extinction.' ...Anxiety is a response to experiences of separateness, indi-viduality, and death.

The key concepts up to this point are ways of coping, self-esteem, the search for meaning, and anxiety. (I assume here that the fears of separation, loss of esteem, meaninglessness, and anxiety are derivatives of the "basic anxiety" which is the fear of death. But is this fear of death instinctive or learned? The loss of the mother actually does mean death for most "higher" mammals, whose young have a long period of helplessness before maturing, and are dependent on her for milk and protection.)

However, there are profound differences between humans and other mam-mals. Animals, especially primates, may share the human infant's prolonged helplessness. The peregrine falcon has to teach its young to hunt in mid-air, which takes up to two years of dependency. The major difference, then, is not this dependent period, but the development of the human brain which enables man to construct symbols through language. The consciousness of time and of the limits of his life span make man a different creature altogether.

Modern neurology has located the newly evolved regions of the brain that are specifically concerned with language.

> The neocerebellum, a thin layer of cells atop the older brain region, evolved more recently along with the prefrontal cortex, Dr. Courchesne said. Humans are the only creatures with large versions of these two brain regions and the only ones with lan-guage. Moreover, brain-imaging studies show that the neocerebellum is activated only when semantic reasoning is required. (Anon, 1994, p. C6)

As far as we know, animals do not have a prolonged or continual fear of death. They are not capable of carrying the thought of death in their minds, since they do not have the symbolic tool of words. This does not mean that when they smell a predator they have no fear. Many wild animals, such as deer or rabbits, may die of shock when trapped by a human or animal hunter. As far as we know, their fear of being killed or injured does not last beyond the moment, or until they see a similar predator. Visitors to the Galapagos Islands have noted how fearless the animals are. The boobies, the seals, the iguanas, and tortoises have no fear of humans. There are no predators, and there is no fear. You can walk up to wild animals and touch them!

The origins of the fear of death are still cloaked in mystery. Freud thought that "basic anxiety," the fear of death, was instinctive. But if it is, then why is there not phylogenetic continuity? Why didn't our animal ancestors experience it? We can't know, as animals can't talk and tell us. To compound the problem, there seems to be a growing consensus that fear of death and dying grows out of the infant's earliest experiences. Just how this happens is still open to conjecture, and involves some concepts of developmental psychology and philosophy. The genesis of the fear of dying is discussed later, in Chapter 2.

What are some of the other factors that affect or modify our fear of death? Feifel (1959b, pp. 114–130; see p. 126) states that reactions to impending death (and thus to death in general) are a:

> function of various factors, among the most important of which are 1. Psychological maturity 2. The type of coping techniques available to the individual 3. Some demographic variables such as religious orientation, age, socioeconomic status, etc. 4. The severity of the organic process (most relevant to the dying patient) and 5. The attitudes of the physician and significant others in the patient's world (again more relevant to the dying patient).

I would like to focus on items 2 and 3. I especially want to avoid becoming entangled in the problem of the dying patient, (nos. 4 and 5), since literally hundreds of good (and bad) books have been written about how people die, how to help people die, how to deal with grief, bereavement, widowhood, the loss of a child, etc. Significantly in short supply, however, are publications dealing with how people who are not in the process of dying and not near death deal with their fears of dying. How do people grieve for the eventual loss of their lives? How do they handle the inevitability of their own death?

Why another book about death? Why are books about death so topical, so popular? Although there are a large number of mechanisms that deal with the fear of death, one is especially relevant to this question. It may account for the spate of books skirting the issue of one's own death. On a (June 19/1994) N.Y. *Times* best-seller list there appeared two books on near-death experiences. Number 1 on the nonfiction list was *Embraced by the Light*, by Betty J. Eadie, "A woman's near-death experiences." Number 9 on the list was *Saved by the Light*, by Dannion Brinkley with Paul Perry, "an account of two near-death experiences by a South Carolina businessman." Following this was Number 10, *How We Die*, by Sherwin B. Nuland: "A physician and surgeon reflects on life's final chapter" (Nuland, 1993). The attraction of these books seems to be that they deal with death in a removed way. The "near-death" does not threaten us, since these people survived and "lived to tell the tale." This gives us courage. Perhaps we can survive too! Dr. Nuland discusses in detail the actual process of dying from AIDS, cancer, heart attack, Alzheimer's disease, accidents, and stroke. According to the jacket copy, the book is "... meant ... to help us rid ourselves of that fear of the terra incognita." While it may help to know the details of one's physical deterioration and death, the question of the sources of fear are not central to the book (see his Introduction, p. xvii).

The repression (or denial) of death, the suppression of one's finitude into the unconscious, is a major cause of the ills of our contemporary world, and has been the cause of many of the major man-made plagues in history. An article by Michiko Kakutani (1994, pp. C13 and C18) discusses the incredibility of American reality, and the problems it poses for novelists. Since truth is now so much stranger than fiction, how can the writer keep the interest of his television-immersed audience? She cites "Tonya and Nancy, Amy and Joey, the Menendez brothers and the Bobbits." Here we have an attack on a rival skater, statutory rape and attempted murder, fratricide and matricide, and a wife's castration (penis amputation) of an abusive husband. Add to this the probable murder of his ex-wife and her lover by football hero O. J. Simpson. Kakutani goes on to say that there are few sexual taboos left. It might also appear that there are no taboos about death, as death or its likelihood is involved in each lurid story. The attraction of these tales is incredible. More than 100 million people watched "O. J." being chased by the police on television news programs—an example of our fascination with and even preoccupation with violence and death. This is what "sells." I feel that we are so obsessed with the deaths of other people because we have repressed thoughts of our *own* death. Observing the death or near death of others helps keep the "wolf away from the door." Death is something that happens to others. "It won't and can't happen to me." The expression "There, but for the Grace of God, go I" can be taken as a warning of impending doom, but when we see or read about other people dying (especially those who are not family or friends), we are more likely to reassure ourselves of our own immortality. (Freud felt that deep down everyone feels he is immortal). The reasoning may be, "I am still in a state of grace, since I am alive, and so must be protected by God."

The relationship between our insatiable appetite for scandal, especially if it involves heroes such as athletes (O. J. Simpson), movie or TV stars (Michael Jackson, Elizabeth Taylor), or political leaders (Nixon, Clinton) is based on our need for models of achievement and power, especially those who have overcome adversity. Frank Rich (1994), in his Op Ed column in *The New York Times*, makes the very connection between the current lust for scandal and violence and the fear of death that we are focusing on.

> In a country where there is no royalty and where, post Watergate, politicians are held in almost universal contempt, celebrity is next to Godliness. Indeed, we want to believe in celebrities for the same reason we want to believe in God: their omnipotence and

> invincibility, however illusory, hold out the promise that we, too, have a crack at
> immortality … On Friday, O. J. Simpson's fame inspired a comparable rooting interest.
> If he could defy murder charges, a police pursuit, and suicidal impulses—in other
> words, defy death—there was a vicarious victory over mortality for his audience as well.

Rich notes that when the hero fails us, we grow angry at the betrayal of our hopes.

> We don't look kindly on celebrity gods who fail, forcing us to crash-land from fantasy
> back into the mire of our own mortality.

This withdrawal of our love and trust is evident in the cases of Michael Jackson (for reported sexual abuse of children), and of Richard Nixon (for his "stonewalling" about Watergate). Mahatma Ghandi, Elizabeth Taylor, St. Bartholomew, Norman Cousins, and other martyrs still retain our love. We feel that we shall "overcome" (death, illness, or misfortune) if they were able to.

Death may be the last heavily repressed area of our lives. It is possible that because sexual repression is easing, we focus more heavily on death (although in its desensitized forms, such as the death of others). The "popularity" of death in the news and in our reading may be aided by changes in our scientific knowledge, and our loss of centrality in the universe. Among others, Norman O. Brown (1959) and Ernest Becker (1973) focus on the repression of death (but disagree on the source of this repression). While repression as a method of coping with death is involved to some extent in all the other coping mechanisms, it is discussed in detail in a separate chapter. Becker's belief that repression is instinctive and necessary for dealing with life conflicts and its harsh realities seems to us more reasonable than Brown's belief that man can throw off all his repressions and eventually become free.

To the major concepts involved in this complex investigation, (coping, self-esteem, meaning, and anxiety) should be added the search for control over one's fate. It is possible to have some control over the source of meaning in one's life. However, there is no true control over one's longevity. The only control we have is in the way we live, and the mechanisms and coping behaviors we choose to deal with our fear of death and to facilitate the way we conduct our lives.

I shall rank these coping behaviors in an arbitrary hierarchy (according to my own values). These values center on how much harm a behavior does to the individual and to others, and how much help it offers in controlling death fear. The "golden rule" is a central tenet of most religions: "Do as you would be done by." This is stated somewhat negatively, with a focus on the self, but in Albert Schweitzer's "reverence for life" there is the positive aspect—namely, helping others, showing love for humanity, for the stranger. I would rank this aspect of religion at the top of the list. Unfortunately, *established* religion is almost universally a trigger for warfare and hatred. Some examples include: the battle of Muslims versus Hindus in India; the war of Christians versus Jews which still continues; the perpetual "jihad" (Holy War) of the Arab extremists and the Jewish "Kach" followers of Rabbi Kahane); and the seven Huguenot Wars (1562–98) between Protestants and Catholics in France, "marked by fanatical cruelty on both sides," (Levey, 1983, p. 712) among many others.

Although they do not coincide with my hierarchy of coping modes, we can benefit from Becker's (1973) four "levels of power and meaning, the *Personal* (which he sees as self-obsession and pure narcissism), the *Social* (focused on family, and thus somewhat limited), the *Secular* (allegiance to humanistic abstractions, such as science, history, and humanity, which transcend the self and family), and lastly the *Sacred*, or highest level, which he sees as linking the self to creation, the universe, and to God in some form. Few individuals find meaning in only one level, and those who do are probably troubled (in my opinion). As mentioned earlier, the highest level (Sacred) can become very destructive when embodied in established religion. On an individual level, it may well be at the top of the hierarchy, but there are few people in this world, perhaps an Albert Schweitzer or a Mother Teresa, who are able to develop their individual religiosity to such moral heights. More on this later.

COPING BEHAVIORS, LISTED IN ORDER OF INCREASING NEGATIVITY AND DESTRUCTIVENESS (TO THE SELF AND OTHERS)

1. *Creativity:* An immersion in creative work—art, music, writing—is in itself an obsession that crowds out death-related obsession. You "live through your creations," and in rare cases achieve a kind of immortality or the illusion of immortality.
2. *Love:* Caring for others, especially for the stranger, lifts the individual out of himself and his fears. The reciprocation of that love by others in his family, his friends, lovers, and others offers strong emotional support and diminishes death fear.
3. *Humor:* This is one of the bulwarks against the threat of death. It is not the type of humor that denigrates others, but the "laughing at fate" that is life-enhancing and perhaps life-prolonging.
4. *Intellectualization:* Writing about death and/or examining philosophical "secrets" that cannot really be revealed (such as what happens after death). Jacques Derrida's "deconstruction"* is the best example of this quest. My writing this book is a very minor example. By studying a threatening subject, such as death, one distances oneself from it. It is a very effective coping mechanism. Its downside is that, if the "distancing" becomes too great, intellectualization often becomes an escape from reality.

---

* Death is considered the ultimate secret.

5. *Procreation:* Having children is one way of living on. It should involve love and respect for the children as individuals in their own right, not as little clones of narcissistic parents. Since this misuse of Junior is so common, I would rank this approach to immortality somewhere in the middle. Having six children myself, I am also aware of the environmental threat of the population explosion. The family tree shelters only one's own, another reason for lower rank.

6. *Obsessive–compulsive behavior:* Striving for worldly success, the Protestant Ethic, originally linked to religion and a "state of grace," now focuses on health, productivity, success, wellroundedness, etc.

7. *"Living life to the hilt"* — *Living better, living longer:* Living life to the hilt can be a healthy response to the finitude of life, but when exaggerated it becomes an anodyne, keeping the feelings of deadness away. An example is the (often drunken) orgy of the soldier at his "Port of Embarkation." It is a last fling before possible death. In the movie "The Last Detail" (1973) with Jack Nicholson, a young sailor being transported to the brig (prison) is given a "night on the town" before incarceration. It is shown as a great kindness on the part of the arresting sailors.

Bachelor parties are a similar "last fling" in the eyes of the macho groom and his buddies, who see marriage as the end (death?) of his single life and his "freedom."

Perhaps *"living life fully"* could be contrasted with "living life to the hilt." The first could be considered in the normal range, the second pathological. However, we know there have been entire social movements and philosophies that embraced these lifestyles — for example, the Apollonian versus the Dionysian ("Eat, drink, and be merry, for tomorrow we die") cultures and the Greek cults.

Living life longer than others (if not in better health) is often a source of pride for the elderly. To live beyond those in one's age cohort gives a brief sense of immortality.

Living better than others or better than you lived originally (or better than your parents lived) is part of the American Dream. It has its roots in the Protestant Ethic. If you could accumulate more worldly goods (which proved you had worked hard) your chances of achieving a state of grace and entering heaven were considerably improved. Max Weber called this "worldly asceticism." Thorstein Veblen carried this idea further, showing that "conspicuous consumption" was a way of gaining stature in our society. The more wasteful the behavior, the greater the status. We have developed a "potlatch" behavior that puts the Kwakiutl ceremony of burning their possessions to shame. With the advent of the "communications highway" we are able to order things simply by touching the object when it appears on the computer screen! All of this consumption has put possessions (especially electronic gadgets) between us and death. It is obsessive behavior of a special kind.

8. *Group membership:* Becker (1973) refers to sources of meaning for the individual. Belonging to a group—the family, state, nation, club, university, sports team (or identifying with some larger group as a "reference group," even though one is not a member) can be a strong bulwark against fear of dying.

9. *Religion:* Belief in the afterlife is a form of denial, but it is one of the most effective ways of diminishing the fear of death. The belief in metamorphosis is very widespread, and also effective. I have been so strongly influenced by Freud's *Future of an Illusion* that I can't help thinking of religion as a neurosis. Religion is also a major rallying point for war and killing, a definite minus. Many people have said that "Fear created the Gods," but fear also created the belief in the afterlife, an effective bulwark against fear for much of the world's population.

10. Mementos *and Monuments:* The family photo album, an autobiography, memoirs and diaries, pyramids, endowed chairs, charitable trusts and wills are all ways of extending one's life, and one's control, beyond the grave. These range from the very humble to the most grandiose methods of coping with the fear of death.

11. *Counterphobic behavior:* Dangerous sports are one way of saying "I can't die" although they often do end in death. Hang-gliding, scuba-diving, boxing, rock and mountain climbing, surfing, acrobatics, and contact sports all involve great risk of injury and death. The counterphobe may think, "If I live through this, it will prove I'm immortal."

12. *Gambling:* This is usually considered to be another form of obsessive–compulsive behavior. In this context I prefer to group it next to counterphobic behavior. It has the quality of a defiance of fate. Although it may be self-destructive in the long run, in the short term it preserves hope.

13. *Dissociation:* Some seek oblivion because their fear of death, or a living death, is so overwhelming. Initially drugs (including alcohol) are used to obtain a "high," which brings the semblance of enjoyment and good living. It is a bromide that drug use becomes a withdrawal from life. Schizoid thinking is another way of dealing with early threats to life.

    Dissociation exhibits a continuum of severity, ranging from multiple personality (or identity) disorder through milder forms such as meditation and daydreaming. In its milder forms it can be an excellent adaptation.

14. *Repression/denial:* Repression and denial are closely related terms. Repression is defined (psychoanalytically) as "the rejection from consciousness of painful or disagreeable ideas, memories, feelings or impulses" (Flexner, 1987, p. 1635). Denial is defined (psychologically)

as "an unconscious defense mechanism used to reduce anxiety by denying thoughts, feelings, or facts that are consciously intolerable." (Flexner,
1987, p. 532). These terms seem applicable to adults, since they presumably already have rather well-formed ideas about death. Children,
however, up to about age ten, do not have *realistic* ideas about death, so
that they cannot be said to be in denial or to be repressing ideas about
death in the same way that adults do. (Maria H. Nagy, in Feifel, 1959, p.
97) (Adolescents, and some adults, who have committed suicide have
been shown to have had very immature ideas about death, and gave
clues, such as leaving notes for the delivery man for the following day.)

In *Denial of Death*, Becker discusses the "disappearance" of the
fear of death. He extensively quotes Gregory Zilboorg and Charles W.
Wahl, both of whom use the term "repression." Denial (or repression)
is seen as a mechanism necessary for psychological survival—as an
escape from the "terror" of death. "Repression takes care of the complex symbol of death for most people" (Becker, 1973, p. 20).

15. *Suicide:* While there are many types of suicide [see Durkheim's anomic
suicide (Durkheim, 1973) and the altruistic suicide, such as Hara-Kiri,
the Kamikaze pilot, or the suicide of the professional soldier who has
failed], the majority of Western suicides are a way of preempting death.
They say, in effect, "You can't fire (kill) me, I quit!"

Suicide can also be viewed as a solution to a seemingly insoluble
problem. Paradoxically, it can also be viewed as an escape from death—
a living death—which is an intolerable situation, usually caused by a
major loss in work, love, or status which is "resolved' by the suicide.

16. *Projection, killing, and the problem of evil:* A paranoid individual has
fears of all kinds, but he is terrified of being attacked by others. (It may
be that the early linkage of paranoid schizophrenia to homosexuality in
psychoanalytic thinking was the result of the extremely repressive
behavior of society toward homosexuals. Although this has not
improved 100%, as the difficulty of the previous administration in per-
suading the armed forces to accept homosexuals attests, the *content* of
paranoia may be changing as a result of social changes.)

The projection of his own aggressive and sexual impulses onto various religious and ethnic groups is a hallmark of the paranoid personality and the more severe forms of this disorder. If one fears being killed,
one may seek a potential killer to fear. Similarly, if one wants to kill,
then that wish must be projected upon others to protect the self.

Killing: Homicide and the killing of animals is another form of the
mechanism of denial. Becker (1973), in his classic book, shows that people who kill others gain a perception of control over life and death. In so
doing, they achieve a kind of illusory immortality. It was upon a recent

re-reading of *Denial of Death* that I began to think constructively about fear of dying (and about my own fear of death, as I passed my 70th birthday). It seemed to me that Becker had chosen to focus on homicide, the most destructive coping method, and that there were many more or less positive ways to confront death. I made a list of them.

The above list of coping modes or ways of dealing with death, with elaborations and some excursions from the main path, will form the framework of this book. I hope that it can also be a critique of our values and behavior, and point the way to the less destructive adaptive modes. This seems to be one means of fighting back against a world filled with incredible cruelty, condoned sadism, and with mounting interpersonal and international violence.

2

The Probable Causes of the Fear of Dying

The simplest hypothesis about fear of dying is that it is instinctive and universal. We know that some animals do not seem to fear humans, and that these animals live in areas where there are no predators. That would seem to rule out phylogenetic continuity. However, we don't really know what animals think about death, since we doubt that they can conceptualize their behavior and do not have a complex language capacity.

What about humans? While fear of death and dying seem almost universal among adults, there are many people who through their religion or meditation or other means seem to have transcended a fear of death. Some, of course, welcome it, especially those who have endured great suffering.

Children as young as three have exhibited fear of death. Of course, we don't know if this is instinctive or learned. Fear of death may exist in the preverbal child, but we have no sure way of finding out about it. We also know that children are exposed to death of family members, especially grandparents, and pets, and in scarcity cultures often observe the death of their parents at an early age. Moreover, prayers such as, "If I die before I wake, I pray the Lord my soul to take" are not exactly reassuring. There are, then, numerous opportunities for children to learn about death from an early age. (It would be of interest to see if children on farms where animals are slaughtered have a greater or lesser fear of death, and whether their concepts of death are more or less realistic than those of urban children.)

So much for the instinctive hypothesis. We can't prove or disprove it. As for the learned fear hypothesis, I would prefer to come to the simple conclusion that fear of dying is due to the inevitable momentary abandonments of the infant by the mother and/or father, and the deep threats to the child's existence that these momentary lapses pose. Given the almost total helplessness of a human infant, the absence of a caretaker to give milk, comfort, and protection really spells death. Infants who are abandoned live at most for a few days. The pangs of hunger, the discomfort of wetness from feces or urine, and the distress of temperature changes make them cry for help. When these basic needs for food and shelter are not met, even for a moment, the subsequent absence of the care-giver must produce fear.

Would that our explanation could be so simple. A long history of often conflicting theory is not necessary here, but a review of the main ideas involved is essential.

Freud posited a basic struggle between the sexual instinct (intended to pre-serve the species) and that of self-preservation (which corresponds to the pleas-ure principle and the reality principle). This conflict was believed to be the cause of repression. He then turned to love versus hate as the basic duality, but found them fused in the sadist. In his search for a final antithesis, he turned to life versus death. The life instinct was called Eros. The death instinct, called Thanatos, was clearly seen in masochism.

> Now ambivalent fusions, such as sadism... represent an extroversion of the innate death instinct, a transformation of the desire to die into the desire to kill. achieved by Eros... (Brown, 1959, p. 80)

How is the fear of death related to the "death instinct?" Again, Norman Brown has made explicit a connection that Freud did not make.

> Although Freud does not make the necessary theoretical links between anxiety and his death instinct, he does say that what the ego fears in anxiety "is in the nature of an overthrow or an extinction." It looks, therefore, as if the specifically human capacity for anxiety does reflect a revolt against death and individuality, or at least some dis-turbance in the organic unity of life and death. (Brown, 1959, p. 109)

Now fear of death may be viewed as a basic instinct of self-preservation (allied to Eros, and pitted against the death instinct, or Thanatos). However, this fear, which has been called the "basic anxiety," can be crippling, and can cause a "living death." If it is instinctive, it does not have to be learned from the expe-riences of early childhood. A critique of the tendency to derive fear or anxiety about death from experience, or to treat it as learned behavior, is given by Feifel:

> It is also relevant to observe that when anxiety about death is noted in the psychiatric literature it is often interpreted essentially as a derivative and secondary phenomenon. Freud derived his fear of death from castration anxiety and from fear of losing the love-object, i.e., anxiety about separation from the mother. There is good clinical evidence that this displacement does occur. But as Wahl (1959, in Feifel, p. 19) points out, one wonders whether this formulation also serves in part a defensive need on the part of psychiatrists themselves. (Feifel, 1959, p. 123)

(I assume that if fear of death is a basic instinct, it is not so easily treatable or preventable. However, if it is learned, it may be more in the province of psy-chiatry, especially preventive psychiatry, and may also yield more easily to treat-ment. Thus the "displacement" may really be a defense of one's own livelihood.)

Wahl states that thanatophobia, or fear of death, is a fear that is often found in children as young as three years of age. Since this antedates the Oedipus complex, it supports the idea that it is associated with separation anxiety, an earlier stage of conflict, rather than with castration anxiety.

Our first formulation of the origin of the fear of death could be put schematically as follows:

Momentary abandonments → Threat to child's existence → Fear of death

Wahl introduces several new steps in this sequence. He states that the child is exposed to various intrafamilial stresses. These produce frustration, rage, anxiety, or threat of parental loss. The child's response is a wish to banish the frustrating parent (death wish). By the Law of Talion (*Lex Talionis*) to think of an act is to do it, and equal punishment will be given to oneself (an eye for an eye). Thus the child fears that he may die, because of these hostile wishes. (Note the root "talon" in the word "retaliation." A claw can do much damage.)

Certain circumstances increase the frustration of the child.

These circumstances are usually punitive rejection of the child by unloving, vacillating, or capricious parents, strong sibling rivalry, or the actual experience of parental loss by separation or death. The first two strongly induce the formation of death wishes toward the frustrating figures (and Talion death fears for the self). (Wahhl, 1959, p. 25)

I would like to revise this formulation slightly. In a study that I and a team of colleagues conducted, approximately 2000 mothers were interviewed concerning the behavior of one of their children. Many societal and intrafamilial factors were investigated for their impact on reported child behavior (backed up by community searches of police, Welfare and school records, and direct psychiatric observation of some 300 families). Three factors describing parental behavior were especially powerful in predicting the outcome of child behaviors five years later: parental coldness, punitiveness, and lability (called "vacillation" or "capriciousness" by Wahl). Depression, antisocial behavior, withdrawal, compulsivity, and many other dimensions of emotional disorder in the child were predicted by these parental behaviors (Eisenberg, 1975, 1976; Gersten, 1974, 1976; Greene, 1973, Langner, 1969, 1970, 1974a,b, 1976; McCarthy, 1975, among others).

If we substitute these parental behavior factors in Wahl's discussion, we get a formulation something like this:

Stresses on child (cold, punitive, or labile parents) → Frustration, rage and anxiety in the child → Death wish toward frustrating parents → Fear of own death (via lex talionis)

The differences between these two versions of the genesis of the fear of death cannot easily be resolved. I prefer the spareness and economy of the first formulation. It does leave us wondering how death and abandonment become equated in the child's mind. The Wahl version (with our greater specification of harmful parental behavior based on large-scale research) makes for a clearer explanation, but introduces two new concepts—the formation of rage in the child and the death wish toward the parents—as factors generating the child's own thanatophobia. Both of these concepts are hypothetical and hard to test. In psychotherapeutic sessions patients often express feelings of rage against parents, as well as guilt over this rage. However, this adult or child scenario may not be an accurate model for the process in an infant. None of these patients are pre-verbal, and the fears discussed are believed to be developed very early, before language skills have developed.

Both Feifel (see earlier) and Wahl treat fear of abandonment (and Talion punishment) as a displacement of death fear onto the parents, or "unconscious irrational symbolic equivalences of death." They seem to take death fear as a given.

> Hence, the fear of death is in reality two things: a realistic concern that some day we shall cease to be and, secondly, a variety of other anxieties which parade under the panoply of the death fear, and these are varied in character and scope. Some of these symbolic equivalents are the fear of abandonment and the fear of Talion punishment... (Wahl, 1959, p. 28)

Rather than seeing death fear as a given, I consider its possible origins, including: (1) a biological or innate fear akin to the startle reflex and the general arousal system, (2) a realistic learned fear based on late childhood, adolescent, and adult experience; or (3) a learned fear growing from early infant experiences of (even momentary) abandonment. I opt for the third choice. Some evidence for it is found in the lack of "object constancy" in the infant. She doesn't believe that a hidden object or her mother exists or will reappear, unless in full view. Hence the ubiquitous mother–infant game of "peek-a-boo," which reassures the child that when her mother's face is covered by her hands, she still exists. After innumerable tests of this truth, the child learns to hold the image of the mother (or toy) in mind, even in the mother's temporary absence. Since this "constancy" has to be learned, the infant may initially feel abandoned the instant the mother's face is out of sight.

From the aspect of intervention or prevention, the choice of hypotheses about the genesis of the fear of death is critical. From our standpoint, which is the description of the different ways people (adults) have of dealing with this set of fears, the origins of the fears are not crucial.

3

CREATIVITY

An immersion in creative work—art, music, writing—is in itself an obsession that crowds out death-related obsession. You "live through your creations," and in rare cases achieve a kind of immortality (or the illusion of immortality). One can be "creative" in baking a pie, raising a child, teaching, running a business, or almost any activity to which one brings some new approach. I prefer to restrict the meaning of "creativity" to the arts and sciences. Otto Rank's writings on the psychodynamics of art and artist have never been improved upon, and constitute a main source for this section. Rank noted that religion was the wellspring of the arts, and that immortality was the goal of both:

> This man-made supernatural world-view forms the basis of culture, since man had to support himself increasingly with more and more powerful symbols of his need for immortalization. The most powerful instrument for the creation of his own cultural world was religion as expressed in cult ("culture"), from which sprang the fine arts, as well as architecture, drama and literature; in a word, the sum of what survives the short span of one personal life-time. (Rank, 1958, p. 64, originally published 1941)

We tend to think of the great creative artist as someone who actively seeks immortality for himself through his works. For example, Keats mourns the fact that he will die "before my pen has glean'd my teeming brain," and finally says "I stand alone, and think, till love and fame to nothingness do sink." Here is surely a person who desires fame, and seeks it through his writing. The self-assuredness of a truly great artist can be disconcerting to the average non-genius. For example, in his sonnet, "Shall I compare thee to a summer's day," Shakespeare makes clear his works will be immortal. He says to the object of his love, "But thy eternal summer shall not fade ... Nor shall Death brag thou wand'rest in his shade, When in eternal lines to Time thou growest, So long as men can breathe or eyes can see, So long lives this (his poem) and this gives life to thee." Not only does the poet become immortal, but the subject of his poem also will be immortal, owing to his "eternal lines"—as long as mankind is alive!

It is more difficult to demonstrate this same striving for immortality in the fine arts, since few of these artists have verbalized their claim to immortality. The fact that cathedrals and monasteries held most of the early paintings was attributable to the preponderance of religious art in the Middle Ages. Because the art was housed in the strongest buildings, and seen by generations of worshippers, its immortality was assured. Before that time, the various temples, and the Egyptian and Etruscan tombs, were safe repositories for painting and sculpture.

Rank makes the point, however, that the goal of early art was not to ensure an individual's immortality, but rather an affirmation of *collective* immortality.

> Art, then—at least in its beginning—was not the satisfaction of the individual artist to attain immortality for himself in his work, but the confirmation of the collective immortality-idea in the work itself as a picture of the soul. (Rank, 1932, reprinted in 1989, pp. 13–14)

Rank goes on to show how each society embodied its idea of the soul in its gods. Portraits of Anubis, Zeus, and Christ each depicted the ideal type, "the soul in concrete form." Durkheim would have said that these were "collective representations" of society. It is one's own limited society which gives one immortality at this early stage. Later on, as communication between societies increased, immortality was afforded the artist beyond the boundaries of his own culture. This change parallels the growth of individualism. The artist could now, through his own work, become immortal. He was not just a humble contributor to society...to his temple or cathedral. He achieved immortality through translations of his written works, performances of his plays and music, exhibitions in the art museums of the world.

Does the artist achieve immortality only at a great cost to himself? The stereotype of the starving consumptive artist has been seized upon by our society as an "ideal type." Self-sacrifice in the name of creation is the rule. Keats dies of consumption, Poe dies an alcoholic, Mozart dies young and penniless. Mental as well as physical illness is seen as a wellspring of creativity. Schumann's insanity and Edvard Munch's obsessions are endlessly cited as the source of their creative productivity. But in fact insanity and neuroticism often interfere with creation. Schumann's music suffered as his madness grew.

> After a rosy beginning (at age 40) Schumann got on badly with the Düsseldorfers. His conducting rapidly became notorious. He was incompetent, so lost in a dream world of his own that he could not even beat time accurately...On one occasion he went on automatically waving his baton after a composition was finished ... The Düsseldorf compositions reveal one thing all too clearly: the drying up of Schumann's inspiration ... Years before he had heard ghostly voices, but only at rare intervals. Now these auditory sensations multiplied and became painful (1853–4)...On February 6, 1954, Schumann wrote to Joachim: 'Music is silent at present. And now I must close. Night is beginning to fall'. (Brockway and Weinstock, 1939, pp. 308–311)

By the end of that month, Schumann threw himself into the Rhine, but was rescued. The next month he committed himself to a sanatorium, and a little over two years later died in the arms of his wife, Clara. Although it is possible that Schumann's inspiration would have dried up even without his insanity, it is more likely that his later compositions were written in his lucid moments, and were affected by his illness.

The Romantic poets are more frequently pictured as "tortured souls," as exemplified by Shelley, Keats, Byron, Wordsworth, and Coleridge than poets of other periods. Yet each of these men had at some time been involved in politics or the life of their times, and were not totally withdrawn or psychotic. Coleridge and Wordsworth had championed the French Revolution, and Byron lost his life fighting for Greek freedom (Marshall, 1966, p. xxiii).

We have a strong tendency to identify with people who have sacrificed themselves in the service of a cause. Perhaps this is because we ourselves fail to live up to the ideals of self-sacrifice and community service that have been taught by almost every major religion and culture. The hero who dies for his fellow man is best exemplified by the crucified Christ. His love for others and his ability to turn the other cheek are indeed rare. By starving himself, Ghandi became a hero for India's millions, and brought an end to British domination. The same self-sacrifice by (shorter term) starvation enabled the pop singer Kate Smith to raise millions for war bonds during World War II. People are convinced of sincerity when they see sacrifice. Even when this is not voluntary, as in the case of John F. Kennedy, it is sufficient to create heroic status. The slain war hero, the frail poet who dies young, and the soldier who has a "rendezvous with death" all capture our imagination and our sympathy. Those who die "before their time" (in other words, those who die young) receive our special sympathy. Some are elevated to a status perhaps beyond their actual artistic achievements because of an early or tragic death. This may be true of Sylvia Plath or Anne Sexton. Diane Arbus, although an excellent photographer, has become equally famous for her attraction to the bizarre and for her suicide. It is unlikely that Ernest Hemingway's suicide by gunshot enhanced his fame, and it is not part of his "legend." The same might be said of Isadora Duncan's death by strangling on her scarf while riding in an automobile. Perhaps the *established* artists' fame is not increased by a tragic or bizarre death. Marilyn Monroe, on the other hand, never reached her peak as an actress, and her suicide and depression have contributed greatly to the popular appeal of her life story. Vincent Van Gogh's art and his suicide went relatively unnoticed during his lifetime. Virginia Woolf was already an established writer at the time of her suicide. If anything enhanced her fame other than her writing, it was the diverse sexual activity of her social set, not her suicide.

While creativity and obsession seem closely associated, there is a world of difference between the average obsessive individual and the creative genius. The average citizen goes about his culturally dictated rounds in a blind, copy-cat way that accepts the role society has cut out for him. The creative genius carves out new paths for himself, and is often withdrawn from society or in conflict with it.

There may be some neurotic compulsivity in creative artistic production, but its goal is to produce new ways of looking at the world, not to mimic or copy what has already been done, said, painted, or composed.

The average person uses the compulsivity of everyday life to keep the Grim Reaper from the door (or from his thoughts).

> Man ... accepts the cultural programming that turns his nose where he is supposed to look ... he learns not to stand out ... to embed himself in other-power ... He doesn't have to have fears when his feet are solidly mired and his life mapped out ... All he has to do is to plunge ahead in a compulsive style of drivenness in the 'ways of the world' ... (Becker, 1973, p. 23)

The difference, then, is not necessarily in the degree of drivenness, but in the greater blindness of the average person, and the more innovative vision of the creative individual. By his concentration, the genius diminishes his fear of death, and may even gain some immortality because of his vision. Vision also implies long-range goals, while the nose-to-the grindstone attitude suggests looking downward, never at the sky.

Creativity demands a certain withdrawal from society, so that the artist may discover a new view of the world. Rank states that the conflict between self-assertion and self-surrender (the individual versus society) is just much more intense in the artist than in other humans. He then shows how the fame brought by creativity pulls the artist back toward society.

> The individual may, by his nomination to be an artist, have asserted his independence of the human community and rooted himself in self-sufficient isolation; but ultimately he is driven by the work he has autonomously produced to surrender again to that community. (Rank, 1932, reprinted in 1989, p. 409)

Earlier I mentioned the Romantic British poets, and Mozart, Munch, and Schumann as we tend to picture them today—as victims. Yet they never laid their diseases or problems out on the table, like dirty laundry.

> Painting pictures in their own blood was, metaphorically speaking, what many artists of the nineteenth century were doing. Even when they weren't mentally unsound or dying of syphilis or tuberculosis, they were preoccupied with death—their own or that of the Beloved. One's personal disease and impending death were unmentionable. (Croce, 1995, p. 89)

Not all creative people are obsessed with death, but there are some outstanding examples in fields other than poetry and literature, where it is easier to read their thoughts directly. In music, there are funeral marches and songs (particularly German *lieder*) whose text is concerned with death and loss. Through memoirs and anecdotes we sometimes get a glimpse of musician's obsessions. Theodor Reik's book about Gustav Mahler, *The Haunting Melody*, is the main source for Harold Schonberg's chapter, "Mahler's Mystic Ninth." He describes how Mahler was obsessed with Beethoven's Ninth Symphony, and with the existence of life after death during his whole lifetime. Schonberg tells the "twist of fate" story which is as chilling as "Birnam Forest Come to Dunsinane" or the fact that Duncan was a Cesarean birth, at the climax of Macbeth.

> Mahler also was frightened at the implication of finishing a Ninth Symphony. Had not Schubert, Bruckner, Beethoven himself, died before finishing a tenth? When Mahler did get to work on a Ninth Symphony, and finished it, he crossed out the number and published it as *Das Lied von der Erde*. Then, when composing his next symphony, he told his wife: 'Actually it is, of course, the Tenth, because *Das Lied von der Erde* was really the Ninth.' And, when it was near completion, he said 'Now the danger is past.' As a matter of fact, it was not past. He died a few months after finishing the work that was published as his Ninth Symphony. (Schonberg, 1981, p. 123)

Mahler was much troubled by existential fears, no doubt exacerbated by the promiscuity of his wife Alma, who had affairs with or married many of the leading intellectuals and creative leaders of Europe. Stewart Feder, a psychiatrist and musicologist, mentioned that at one point, when Alma was having an affair with Gropius, the architect, Mahler had a four hour "walk in the woods" with Sigmund Freud, who managed to relieve much of his anxiety and return him to his work! His concern with the Ninth is very similar to an "anniversary depression." There are cases of a twin suffering a heart attack on the anniversary of his twin brother's death (Engel, 1975, pp. 24–25). Frequently there are anniversary depressions when the adult reaches the same age at which the same-sex parent died.

An interesting parallel to Mahler is found in the ideas of the conductor, Sir Colin Davis. In 1995 he was 67 years old. He seemed obsessed with death. He was interviewed on a BBC program called "On the Psychiatrist's Couch" by Anthony Clare.

> ... He said that he thought every day about the fact that he was going to die. 'I don't know what else music can be about,' he said now, pushing back his wiry gray hair with a sigh, and pulling on a briar pipe that had gone cold. 'Every piece of music is a rehearsal of one's own life; it comes out of nothing and disappears into nothing. Music can speak to us in that direct way about the way we actually are. Painting has a beginning and no end, and thus gives us a sense of security. It will be there tomorrow. When a symphony goes, it's gone'. (James, 1995, p. 46)

Davis' concern with his own death and the parallel he draws between his own life and the life of a (performed) symphony is fascinating. The obsession with death is common enough among creative people, but the sense that each creation "dies" is a much more depressive view of the artist's work. Certainly Beethoven or Wagner or Mahler could not have made such a statement. The composer knows that his work lives on, and will doubtless be performed by conductors and musicians. The interpretation may die, but the published music lives on. Painting (and sculpture, architecture, and literature) likewise lives on, and is not as evanescent as Sir Davis' rendition of a symphony, or the work of other performing artists, such as actors. Even the work of actors is now preserved in movies and videotape, as is that of many great performing artists and conductors. Sir Davis' view of "the way we are," performing creatures with a beginning, a brief moment on stage, and an end, is much like Shakespeare's, a depressingly realistic view of our short (and meaningless?) lives.

Again, the bard of Avon uses the player as a metaphor, but this time to describe life itself:

> Tomorrow, and tomorrow, and tomorrow
> Creeps in this petty pace from day to day
> To the last syllable of recorded time;
> And all our yesterdays have lighted fools
> The way to dusty death. Out, out, brief candle!
> Life's but a walking shadow, a poor player
> That struts and frets his hour upon the stage,
> And then is heard no more: it is a tale
> Told by an idiot, full of sound and fury,
> Signifying nothing.
> Hamlet

This famous quotation is perhaps the greatest expression of existential anxiety in the English language. First, life drags on, it is petty (not noble), and leads only to death. Our life itself is an actor, filled with vanity and worry. Life must end, and is meaningless. The actor and the conductor, of course, are hewing to the lines or the music set down for them.

We also use the word "actor" for somebody who makes decisions and acts on them. Shakespeare leaves no doubt here that the actor is more like a puppet, a "poor player," whose part, or life's "tale," has been written by an idiot. He leaves no room for a protecting God, a cosmic plan, an afterlife, or even for immortality through one's life work. In these lines, he makes Sir Colin Davis look like an optimist. (But Shakespeare did believe his own work would be immortal, as stated earlier.)

So far, we have dealt with artistic creativity as a means of coping with the fear of dying. Great composers, writers, and painters are all capable of lifting us out of our humdrum world that "creeps in this petty pace." Even at his most depressing, Shakespeare makes the message of inevitable death palatable, understandable, and beautiful through his wonderful imagery. Great music or art can transport us beyond the humdrum yet unpredictable world. Becker summarizes the impact of great art, music, or writing:

> ...The true artist is so rare. He gives us conviction without blindness or without sameness, which is why it is said that the true artist holds up a picture of the ideal that for us should be the real. The truly esthetic object affirms human victory over the chaotic, and with it affirms human possibility... The esthetic object demonstrates that life is not in vain, by holding up tangible evidence of human creativity... Science could be esthetically consummatory as well as art. The scientist... builds man into the world and opens new vistas at the same time—as surely as does the artist. (Becker, 1964, pp. 238–239)

The creativity of great scientists cannot be in doubt. The scientist creates hypotheses, and tests them against the evidence of the outside world. He often creates technologies that are based on these hypotheses and theories, many of which have practical significance for the lives of his fellow-men. It can be argued that the atomic bomb created evil, but the exploration of the fission and fusion of the atom has also laid the groundwork for whole new fields of scientific creativity. Nuclear medicine is now used to help identify cell activity in many diseases. We have paid a great price for entering the nuclear age, and the shadow of Hiroshima and Nagasaki will hang over the United States and the rest of humanity forever. Exposure to nuclear weapons production caused an increase in leukemia. Many people have died from radiation illnesses, including those exposed at Chernobyl and the uranium miners in many countries (Wald, 1995). Despite this, we have gained a great deal, and opened up whole new fields of inquiry in the atomic age. The Chinese invented gunpowder, and used it only for fireworks for centuries before Western society employed it for killing. The misuse of scientific innovations does not diminish their positive contributions.

The great scientist creates order where there has usually been chaos. He puts together seemingly disparate facts and comes up with a synthesis. The best examples of this are Einstein's Theory of Relativity, Freud's theory of the unconscious (linking repression, dreams, slips of the tongue, humor, etc.), and Darwin's theory of natural selection (ranging from the breeding of domestic animals to the shape of finches' bills). These theories, and the evidence used to support them, are indeed esthetic creations. They gave all people a new way of looking at themselves and the world. The devotion to their work, and the tremendous effort involved, make us ask about the motivation of these giants. Freud managed to write even when he was in constant pain caused by cancer of the jaw. Darwin suffered from illness all his life after his voyage on the Beagle. His malady has been diagnosed as "Chagas disease," which is transmitted by a South American relative of the "kissing bug" (a true bug, with piercing mouth parts, a foul odor, and thickened fore wings, of the order Hemiptera). Nevertheless, he wrote on evolution, on emotions in man and animals, on coral reefs, and on earthworms, to mention a few of his works! Einstein worked on his theories while holding a routine job at a patent office. The energy poured into creation certainly acted to counteract the illness of both Darwin and Freud, and the threat of death for both of them.

What are the properties of these great creations? In science or art, they are usually of some lasting value. They are not evanescent. A theory that is disproved in ten years, or a painting that peels in five, is not worthy of the name "great." The Taj Mahal is here to stay. The Acropolis may be here for some time, too, until the acid from automobile emissions eats away the marble. Creative objects are usually unconventional in some sense. They look at what everybody else looks at, but in a new way. The "prepared mind" is always cited as an element in scientific discovery. The standard example of "serendipity" is Sir Alexander Fleming's discovery of penicillin. Over centuries, millions had looked at moldy bread. Hundreds of scientists had discarded Petri dishes with "spoiled" cultures. Only one man noticed some droplets forming that prevented his culture from growing. Picasso's "Demoiselles d'Avignon" incorporated African masks and geometry into female figures. The cubist planes were a startling new way of seeing the human face. The creative object seems to be larger than life. It transcends the natural world. Beethoven's Ninth Symphony is writ large. The chorus says all men will be brothers. It is noble, architectonic, "heavenly." J. S. Bach's "Chromatic Fantasy and Fugue" has these same awesome qualities. One can choose creative objects from many different genres. Michelangelo's sculptures—the Pieta, David, Moses, the Prigioneri, Dawn, Evening, Night and Day—are all moving and larger than life-size. Add to this the grandeur of his Sistine Chapel painting.

Leonardo da Vinci was a genius in many fields. He is best known for his massive fresco, "The Last Supper". It is badly damaged, and some day may not meet the criterion of permanence. Further back in time, the cave paintings of Lascaux in France, and Altamira in Spain, are of great magnitude. Huge caves 50 feet high are covered with large floating drawings of bison, deer, horses, and other animals in natural pigments of ocher and black. My visit to Lascaux in 1953 was truly exalting. It conjured up a world of cave-dwellers, some of whose painting has never been improved on in 30,000 years! (Unfortunately, Lascaux had to be closed to the public, because condensation from human breath was starting to affect the paintings. A full-scale replica can be visited.)

The creative object lifts the creator and the observer out of the everyday world. It gives the artist immortality, and to some extent it gives immortal life to the culture. The glory and the grandeur that was Greece will live forever. It was based on the architecture, sculpture, and philosophy of that culture, and lives on as a model for the Western world. As Shakespeare said, "It gives life to thee," meaning that the poem (or creative object) lives on after the death of the person (or culture) to whom it was dedicated. Who would remember the Russian Count Andreas Rasumovsky if Beethoven had not dedicated his three string quartets of Opus 59 to him? The Kingdom of Benin will be remembered for its bronze sculptures long after the country is forgotten. Egypt's pyramids, tombs, and statues, especially the busts of Nefertiti and Ikhnaton, have gained it an eternal life, which is just what the artists intended. The examples are endless. Artistic and scientific creativity elevate both the creator and the culture to what Rank and Becker call the "heroic" level. In sum, creativity is one of the most effective ways of diminishing the fear of death, for both the individual and the society. It "gives life," and it enhances the illusion of immortality.

4

LOVE

To write a short section on the relationship of love to death and dying is a daunting task. So many great writers and thinkers have written about love—Plato, Stendhal, Dante, C. S. Lewis, Freud, Fromm, Austen, Shakespeare, Wilde—to name a few!

To write about the relationship between love and fear of dying, it is necessary to define that elusive term, "love." This word covers so many types of relationships and attitudes that it is futile to try to discuss them all here. To mention a few, there is passionate love, romantic love, brotherly love, Christian love, parental love, and courtly love.

The elusiveness of a single definition of love is emphasized by Ellen Berschied ("Some Comments on Love's Anatomy" in Sternberg, 1988, p. 263):

> Rather, the genus love is a huge and motley collection of many different behavioral events, whose only commonalities are that they take place in a relationship with another person ... and that they have some sort of positive quality to them.

There have been myriad attempts to classify types of love. Sternberg (1988) has edited a book that describes several different methods of classifying love. Some are typologies based on factor analysis applied to questionnaire data, while others are systems based on the thought processes of a single learned individual. Since the researchers who factor-analyzed the responses to questionnaires about love made up the questionnaires, the factors that evolve must be based on a priori assumptions of the investigators. Thus their results are really not too much different from the categories of the armchair philosopher, who sits down to classify the types of love from his own experience and from the literature.

Sternberg himself in "A Triangular Theory of Love" (1986) and in *The Psychology of Love*, "Triangulating Love" (1988, pp. 119–138) starts with three components of love which he places on the points of a triangle. These are Intimacy (I), Passion (P), and Decision/Commitment (C). Combinations of these three factors yield six types of love: Liking (I), Intimacy only, as in friendship, closeness, warmth; Companionate (I+C), Intimacy + Commitment, as in a long-term

25

friendship or love in marriages that have lost physical attraction or are lacking in passion; <u>Empty Love</u> (C), Commitment to love without intimacy or passion, a stagnant relationship, love in arranged marriages; <u>Fatuous Love</u> (P+C), Passion + Commitment, the "whirlwind courtship," "Commitment is made on the basis of passion, without the stabilizing element of intimate involvement; <u>Infatuation</u> (P), Passion alone, "love at first sight," obsessional love; <u>Romantic</u> (I+P), Intimacy + Passion, "liking and physical attraction."

If all three components are present, Sternberg calls it <u>"Consummate love."</u> He says, "I believe a classification is important so that love can be understood in its multiplicity rather than as a unitary phenomenon" (1988). While this typology seems very neat, it may be somewhat restrictive.

Another classification, by John Alan Lee (in Sternberg, 1988), uses Greek names for love types. <u>Eros</u> (erotic, love at first sight, physical attraction and pleasure) corresponds to Sternberg's *infatuation*.* <u>Storge</u> (pronounced "store-gay") describes a slowly developing love between siblings or playmates, often described as affection or friendship (*liking*). <u>Ludus</u> is his name for the roving lover, flirtation (*passion, although often not a deeply felt passion, with no intimacy or commitment*). Lee's secondary types are <u>Mania</u>: obsessive, addicted love (*infatuation*); <u>Pragma</u>: pragmatic, compatible, the "arranged marriage" (*empty love, with commitment but no passion or intimacy*); <u>Agape</u>: Christian love, selfless and altruistic, love of mankind (*possibly a combination of commitment, with passion focused on God or on ideals, and compassion reserved for the less fortunate*).

C. S. Lewis (1960) came up with a simpler scheme. His types are Agape, Affection, Philias (friendship and pragmatic love), and Eros (romantic love).

There seem to be two general ways of looking at types of love. One is by listing the qualities of love. The other is by examining the people involved in the love relationship. Agape or Christian love could be called sibling love (brotherly love) or love of mankind. I have chosen both methods. One method, naming father love, mother love, or marital love, tells us *who* is involved. Yet within marriage, for instance, there can be both qualities or types of love, romantic or companionate.

Although I can find almost no direct references to the connection between fear of death and love in general, much less between fear of death and various types of love, there are at least two strategies that can be employed. First, one can eliminate the types of love that probably are *not* helpful in reducing death fear. The roving lover, the uncommitted, may be temporarily elated from each onenight stand or new relationship, but in the long run, this kind of love does not provide the emotional support that most people need.

> Adulterous relationships feed on their frustration. The fact that the beloved is not always available, and that the culmination of the love is fraught with danger, are both the thrill and the frustration, the bliss and the agony. (Goldberg, 1993, p. 191)

* The words in italics are my guesses as to the corresponding types in Sternberg's system.

Infatuation and Mania (passion without intimacy or commitment) will eventually wear out, or exhaust the infatuated lover. I associate this with unrequited love, and that is also destructive of the individual. (However, the masochist may thrive on it!)

The types of love that I think would be emotionally supportive and thus help calm one's fear of death and dying are romantic love, companionate love-friendship, pragmatic love-affection, and agape or Christian love.

Before describing the way in which these types of love might reduce fear of dying and prolong life, let me add some words of caution. First, any love relationship is bound to be limited, if not by separation or divorce, then by death of one of the participants (with the possible exception of the love of the fan for the idol). That is why love of a group (nation, family, or tribe) offers more hope of continuity and immortality. For this reason, agapic love may be more stable, since the beloved, all of mankind, is not likely to die soon. Love of one's children alone is not a permanent bulwark against death fear, especially in our society where children typically leave home after reaching maturity.*

How often in songs and poems we hear the phrase, "Our love will never die." It will, of course, when both parties are dead, and it may be hard to sustain (without rancor and sorrow) after the death of one of the partners. Romantic love, or any other kind of love, can only bestow the illusion of immortality.

In addition, there are death-encouraging aspects of love; Oscar Wilde's, "You always hurt the one you love" was made into a popular song! Unrequited love and sexual jealousy can lead to depression, suicide, or homicide. Love then does not automatically instill a sense of calm or of immortality. It does so only under certain conditions.

Jane Goldberg points out that there is a "dark side" of love, and that we must become familiar with it in order to control it and perhaps even to benefit from it. This is an elaboration of the "shadow self" approach, which has a bit of the Jungian mystique about it. She says that love of God has created death and destruction, that most murders are committed against loved ones, and that our beloved children are constantly abused (Goldberg, 1993, p. 21).

LOVE IN GENERAL

There are some aspects of love in general that may offer a bit of protection against fear of death and dying. Becker, as usual, has seen the link between love and self-esteem, which is so crucial in the fight against fear.

> If one is loved for what he is, as a unique existential object, then the crucial awareness dawns. He would not be loved if he were anything else. ...A primary endeavor of

---

* In societies where there are three-generation households, once typical of American farm families, there should be diminished death-fear owing to the continuation of close child–parent bonds, all things being equal. In addition, the illusion of immortality is more easily fostered in large families.

psychotherapy is thus accomplished by love; the individual accepts his past and his uniqueness as irrevocable, as necessarily and desirably so. (Becker, 1964, p. 242)

If the splendid existential (love) object is so real, and so much a part of the world that includes me, then I too am an irrevocable part of a meaningful world ... then life itself must be of value. (Becker, 1964, p. 246)

In other words, love, especially reciprocated love, is life affirming. Perhaps this is what is meant by the old platitude, "Love's what makes the world go 'round." Becker, like Goldberg, warns that the love object promises much, but "may give little or nothing." Reciprocation of love, then, is one key to lessening the fear of dying.

We all know about the virtues of love, which have been expressed in many ways. Yet, if I were to ask you just what advantages love adds to life, you might be hard pressed to give an answer. Here is one simple expression of love's advantages.

When we truly love, we are willing to change and we do often change. We lose weight, start exercising, forgive our enemies, accept others, love ourselves, feel alive, believe that life is worthwhile. (Bradshaw, 1992, p. 181)

If there is any advantage to being "in love," being loved, or bestowing love on someone, it is that life seems worth living. That is the first line of defense against fear of dying.

LIFE STAGES AND LOVE

Infancy and Childhood

In a previous discussion of the origins of fear of death and dying, the role of parental behavior has been stressed. The destructive effect of parental coldness, lability, and punitiveness on the child has been shown in my own research, and (under other labels) in countless studies. These parental attitudes and behaviors affect the most basic needs of the infant and child, for she needs to be fed, kept warm, and diapered when wet. Rocking and cuddling help peripheral circulation, which is not well established in the early months. Warmth, stability of parental response, and absence of punitiveness are requirements for the emotional growth of the child. Without these conditions, fear of death and dying, depression, and in severe cases wasting syndrome will result. Punitiveness is associated with later antisocial behavior.

In his writing on attachment and loss, Bowlby (as mentioned earlier) dismisses the "death instinct" theories of Freud and Melanie Klein, and sees the child's fears as having direct survival value. The child's fears are not generated by anger at the parents, which is then presumed to be reflected back via "lex talionis" to become part of the castration complex. On the contrary, Bowlby and those who follow his "attachment theory" see the child as having realistic fears (which may include direct fear of the parents), and assume that these are genetically determined.

> A tendency to react with fear to each of these common situations—presence of strangers or animals, rapid approach, darkness, loud noises, and being alone—is regarded as developing as a result of genetically determined biases that indeed result in a 'preparedness to meet real dangers.' Furthermore, it is held, such tendencies occur not only in animals but in man himself and are present not only during childhood but throughout the whole span of life. Approached in this way, fear of being separated unwillingly from an attachment figure at any phase of the life-cycle ceases to be a puzzle and, instead, becomes classifiable as an instinctive response to one of the naturally occurring clues to an increased risk of danger. (Bowlby, 1973, p. 86)

We know that fear of death and dying are present in children as young as three, and these fears may be present preverbally, but cannot be expressed in words. Hence they take the form of fear of darkness and abandonment. These are often called the "psychological equivalents" of death for the child, for whom being alone (in the dark) and being abandoned are in fact a direct threat to life.

Conscious fear of death does not frequently appear in children until the age of ten. In his discussion of the literature, Bowlby notes that Sylvia Anthony, in her study of the development of the child's ideas of death, decided that fear of death is not instinctive, but is learned.

> ... She believes that it is through the equation with separation that death acquires its emotional significance: Death is equated with departure ... To the young child death means its mother's death, not its own. (Bowlby, 1973, p. 384)

It may seem redundant to say that infants and children need parental love to protect them from the fear of death. If the threat of abandonment were the only concern, we would still see many fearful children. In fact, there are direct threats to children's lives every day, due to war, famine, disease, the "mean streets" of our city slums, and violent parents. In recent times we read headlines about the murder of children by their parents every day. The illusions of the sanctity of "mother love" have been shattered. In 1996 Governor Pataki of New York State asked for changes in the law, so that children can be taken away immediately from parents who are abusive, especially those parents who are addicted to drugs. In the past, children were kept with the mother in all but the worst cases of abuse, or the removal of the child from parental custody would take months or even years. On August 31st, 1996, four-year-old Nadine Lockwood was found starved to death by her mother. This starvation took place over a period of one year. The mother, Carla Lockwood, admitted mistreating the girl "because she did not want or love her," and confessed that she knew she was mistreating her by withholding food and medical attention (McFadden, 1996, pp. 1 and 24).

In 1995 Elisa Izquierdo was found beaten to death. She had been struck and sodomized over a two-year period, and died after her head was slammed against a cement surface. None of the other five children in her family were assaulted, and this was also true for the other six Lockwood children.

The case of Lisa Steinberg, beaten to death by her adoptive father while her adoptive mother looked on, was different only in that it occurred in a middle-class family. These cases received more publicity because of their brutal or bizarre nature.

The drowning of the two Smith boys by their mother, who strapped them into their car seats and pushed the car into a lake, also belies the instinctive quality of "mother love." Mother love is learned through receiving love from your own mother. Harlow's monkeys and Jane Goodall's good and bad primate and African hunting dog mothers attest to the wide variability of parental love (as if we didn't all know this by experience!).

The obvious absence of love, then, makes the case for love as a defense against fear of death and dying all the more vivid and convincing. Rather than an "absence of love," we might call it just plain hatred of the child in these extreme cases, usually involving the one child who is cast as the scapegoat.

Short of hatred, lack of love itself can end in death. Jane Goldberg, speaking of the "necessity of love," cites the work of Renee Spitz:

> Spitz observed and filmed 34 infants in an orphanage. Although their physical needs were adequately attended to, these children were rarely fondled, caressed, played with, or exposed to any of the other kinds of nourishing attention that loving mothers bestow on their infants. Within three months, the babies had difficulty sleeping, had shrunken, and were whimpering and trembling. Two months later, most of them had taken on the appearance of idiocy. *Within a year, twenty-seven of the thirty-four infants had died* (italics mine). (Goldberg, 1993, p. 41)

Is lack of mother love confined to single mothers, mothers in poverty, or drug-addicted mothers? Not at all. The mothers involved in the brutal child murders just described were on drugs, or had destructive relationships with abusive or rejecting men. Yet their anguish is dimly reflected in the everyday life of all parents, especially mothers. Goldberg describes in detail the difficulties of pregnancy and birth, and the fact that pregnancy deprives both parents of much of their former sex life. This increases anger at the children, or focuses anger on one target child. With the birth of their first child, the husband finds he has "traded in his wife for a mother." This often awakens the incest taboo the husband developed as a defense against sexual involvement with his own mother. Again, the result may be a loss of sexual interest and avoidance by the husband—more cause for anger. Goldberg describes how exhausted the mother gets during the early months and even years after the birth, how she longs for sleep. When the infant or child finally goes to sleep, it is a reprieve for the mother.

> There's also a much more mundane reason why parents don't often have sex. They may simply be too tired—if one parent—almost always the mother—is too exhausted from the toils of childrearing to even move her body in other than essential ways, the other parent may resent this fatigue and the children who caused it. (Goldberg, 1993, p. 137)

Interestingly, Goldberg points out how many of our beloved fairy tales have a theme of getting rid of children. A stepmother or witch in "Cinderella" and "Snow White", and the "Pied Piper of Hamelin" are seen as metaphors for the mother's infanticidal wishes.

Many of the cases of violence against children can be attributed to poor bonding. It has recently been cited that stepfathers are 40 to 100 times more likely to be involved in serious physical and sexual abuse of children than biological fathers, regardless of socioeconomic factors (Angier, 1995, quoting Dr. David Popenoe, Prof. of Sociology at Rutgers University, p. C5). There is a disturbing parallel between this behavior and that of some of the larger predators. The new male mate may try to kill off the young that are not his own, to "protect his gene pool," in the jargon of the sociobiologists.

Despite the rigors of parenting and the anger it engenders, infants give back love to their parents, and for the most part are cherished and loved. Some of the reasons for this love may be narcissistic—to continue the family name; to have the child join the family profession, business, or trade; or to "live through" the child, forcing a career that was secretly desired by the parent. Notwithstanding the hazards of parental love, most children do receive some affection, and some survive the worst imaginable childhoods. The importance of love in promoting self-esteem and reducing the child's fear of death (or its equivalent fears of the dark, being alone, strangers, and loud noises) cannot be overestimated.

Most academic studies of children focus on developed or industrialized countries, where children may be victims of parental neglect and abuse, but are less likely to be plagued by poverty and disease. Fear of death, especially in children, needs to be studied in developing countries, where even the young are constantly exposed to life-threatening events. What about war? Almost every group of humans has experienced war, and some societies live in an almost constant state of combat. Do we love our children enough to prevent wars? Love of country, clan, or tribe seems to be given preference over protecting our children from war. We let our young soldiers go into combat when they are barely out of their teens, but in many countries, children as young as seven or eight are recruited for warfare. A 1995 report of the United Nations Children's Fund, cited in a *New York Times* editorial, gives the shocking statistics:

> The Children's Fund counts 149 major wars between 1945 and 1992. In the last decade, child victims of war include 2 million killed, 4 to 5 million disabled, 12

million left homeless, 10 million psychologically traumatized, and more than 1 million orphaned or separated from their parents.

It is from a biased middle-class ethnocentric position that we can even ask the question, "Do children have a fear of death?" If we were to ask the children of Rwanda or Burundi if they feared death, the results might be very different from those in studies conducted in Europe and the United States. The age of conscious fear of death and dying might be much lower when children see their parents and siblings gunned down or hacked to death with machetes. Likewise, children of our urban slums are constantly exposed to death by gunshot, stabbing, and beating.

Love for their children has not succeeded in keeping parents from supporting wars. In fact, a frequent rationale for starting a war is the defense of their children, or securing the future of their children. Love of country and love of God seem to take precedence over love of children, and these two "loves" are the major excuses for starting wars. Often war is really based on the search for power by political groups who do not represent parents in general. The fact that acceptance of war belies our professed love for our children does not diminish the importance of everyday love, caring, and support given by so many parents to their children. The frequent betrayals , abandonments, or assaults on children by their caretakers and the resulting depressions and antisocial behavior are mounting evidence of the importance of parental love in preventing fear of dying and its equivalents. (Antisocial behavior, especially in preadolescent children, is a way of expression depression, and depression is often based on anger.)

Sibling and Peer Group Love

In a way, there can be no purer love than the love of siblings. Sternberg (1988) calls this "Companionate," a combination of Intimacy and Commitment, but with no Passion. John Lee (in Sternberg, 1988, pp. 38–67) would call this "Storge." It is often described as affection or friendship, and it is distinctive in that it lacks passion. C. S. Lewis (1960) would call it Affection, and reserves another term, "Philias," for friendship or pragmatic love, in which rewards are expected from the other person.

One would think that "brotherly love" would be associated with brothers, but it is typically classified under the heading of agapic, or Christian love. It refers to love of mankind in general, and specifically love of the stranger, the non-family member, the outsider. More about this type of love later.

There is some anecdotal and research-based evidence for the supportive role of siblings. In large families, siblings often form a peer group of their own. This group may even be in opposition to the parents. Leonard Bernstein, the composer and conductor, and his brother and sister formed such a peer group, and even developed a secret language that their parents could not understand. This was a defense against an authoritarian father, who said he wouldn't spend a dime for Lenny to have music lessons, since he would just grow up to play in a klezmer (small Jewish folk-music) band! His mother had to sneak him money for piano lessons.

Peer orientation is not always best for children. Often peer-oriented children, especially boys, tend to exhibit antisocial behavior, as they model on older brothers or gang leaders. One of the best predictors of juvenile delinquency in our longitudinal study was the arrest of an older brother. This is probably more prevalent in lower socioeconomic groups, where street norms prevail. The contribution of peer norms to delinquency was best discussed by Albert Cohen (1955). To gain the approval of their gang members, delinquents would steal. They often stole worthless objects, since their primary goal was to gain recognition and love from their buddies. Parent-oriented children (and to some extent only children, who have no siblings to model on) are less likely to get into trouble, and if they do, are less likely to be arrested owing to the protection of their families. Smaller families also tend to be wealthier, so "singletons" are more frequently found in higher socioeconomic levels.

Our studies showed very little in the way of increasing child and adolescent psychopathology with increasing (higher) socioeconomic status. There was one marked exception. Reports of sibling rivalry increased as socioeconomic status increased! This fits in with the possibility that large poor families have sibling peer groups, whereas rich kids struggle with each other for parental affection and worldly goods.

In many countries, team sports have become a positive peer experience, especially for adolescent males. This has become a male cult, and is fostered by the parents of "Little League" baseball up through college and later through professional sports. The pressures on young athletes to win for their community can be tremendous, as depicted so poignantly in the film "The Last Picture Show." Nevertheless, these early male-bonding experiences are significant for the perennial grads who long for the halcyon days of youth. There is an "enduring" quality that suggests that the old wish for immortality is still strong.

> ... Everything else in our lives comes and goes. Baseball endures. Baseball was a better love than my first love. It is an older friend than my oldest friend. This is one goddam beautiful game. (Miles, 1991, p. 127)

Choosing a profession that involves a peer group like that of adolescence may well be a way of stopping the clock and coping with the fear of dying.

> For many men, possibly even a majority, the tragedy of growing old can descend before they have even completed the process of growing up. Pop stars like Mick Jagger, Bill Wyman, Eric Clapton and Elton John...are not the only Peter Pans of modern society. Professional athletes too have perfected a way of life which allows them to refuse to grow up, but remain instead in the golden world where every boy could enjoy the thrill of the game ... (Miles, 1991, p. 202)

While there have recently been a few female bonding movies, such as "Thelma and Louise," they can hardly hold their own against the numerous

Westerns, war movies, and classics such as "Butch Cassidy and the Sundance Kid." Can an occasional "Little Women" balance the overwhelming output of stories about male companions, from the Legend of King Arthur and the Knights of the Round Table to *Huckleberry Finn, From Here to Eternity,* and *The Naked and the Dead?* It is not without regret that I must admit that women are generally more mature, and cling less to their adolescence than do men, at least in the United States. Their forward-looking focus on having a family and raising children is in sharp contrast to the often maudlin nostalgia of the Peter Pan male, who is glued to the football game on television, and will still argue that his alma mater was "the best in the whole damn country."

This bonding does give men the illusion of continuity. Being part of the "team" seems less lonely than being on one's own. It is the strength of the group, of society, which Durkheim first described, that gives men (and women) their strength in the fight against death and physical deterioration.

Why then do women seem to need much less of this peer "bonding"? One guess is that they have generated their immortality with their own bodies. We don't need Margaret Mead to counter Freud's "penis envy" with a male "womb envy," but the physical bearing and care of children give women a real edge in the race for immortality.

To look briefly at the "dark side" of sibling and peer love, the story of Cain and Abel is as relevant today as it was thousands of years ago. There is rivalry between peers of both sexes. A lawsuit was recently filed by the parents of two girls who both wanted to be valedictorians, and had perfect grade-point averages. The competition for dominance in male gangs has been documented. In one case, no boy was allowed to bowl a higher score than the gang leader, and they unconsciously failed to exceed his score (Whyte, 1955). In the movie "Heathers," girls create a vicious pecking order in high school. In a content analysis of mainland Chinese comic books in which I was involved while working for the U.S. State Department's "Voice of America," a most popular theme was "My sister stole my boyfriend." Siblings and peers, like all the sources of love, have the potential for good or evil. They can be supportive and diminish fear of dying and death-related anxieties, or they can make life a living hell for their victims.

LOVE BETWEEN ADULTS

Romantic Love

The topic of romantic love could easily fill this book, and there are thousands of references to it. Romantic love is one of the most sustaining of all the types of love, and although it is illusory, it helps to maintain the illusion of immortality, which is half the battle against fear of dying. Millions of love songs and poems throughout the ages have proclaimed that "our love will never die."

Berscheid reports that more than 80 percent of college men and women say that they will not consider marrying a person they are not in love with. She distinguishes between "I love you," and "I'm in love with you" (in Sternberg, 1988, p. 368). Being "in love" signifies the presence of romantic love. She suggests that the term "romantic love" be looked on as a fairly long-term state of the "in love" individual. It is a combination of behaviors and emotions, and not all the emotions are positive. They encompass fear, anger, sexual desire and depression (in Sternberg, 1988, p. 371). Of romantic love, or Eros, Berscheid says:

> The definitive behavioral events in this class … have to do with sexual desire; its other seemingly distinctive qualities … its short life, the ability of the loved one to dominate the person's fantasy, the idealization of the loved other, (and) desire for possession and exclusivity. (in Sternberg, 1988, p. 364)

The feeling states of romantic love are governed by the reciprocity of the loved one. If she loves him back, he is elated. If he spurns her, she is depressed to the depths. This lability, this state of being whipsawed between joy and sorrow, is typical of people "in love."

> We are never so defenseless against suffering as when we love, never so forlornly unhappy as when we have lost our love object or its love. (Sigmund Freud) (Train, 1993, p. 49)

> With you there is life and joy and peace and all good things … away from you there is turmoil and anguish and blank despair. (Bertrand Russell in a letter to Lady Ottoline Morrell) (Train, 1993, p. 49)

Romantic love, like all the other "ideal types" of love, is hard to define, and tends to blur into other types. In the sense that Max Weber used the term "ideal type" there is no person who fits the type exactly. The ideal type is only a construct, which is supposed to help in one's thinking. Berschied, although she thinks her answer is inadequate, says romantic love is "about 90% sexual desire not sated" (in Sternberg, 1988, p. 373). This would suggest that romantic love occurs primarily in unrequited love, which is patently untrue. It does seem as if romantic love tends to change from the premarital period through the middle and later decades of marriage toward affectionate love. Sternberg's Romantic love involves Intimacy and Passion, without Commitment.

Companionate Love

Sternberg's view of Companionate love (which would come later in marriage or any long-term relationship) involves Intimacy and Commitment, but no longer any Passion. Does it make Romantic love terribly mundane to say that its passion is usually subject to extinction over time? (Experimental psychologists found out long ago that tastes and smells and other stimuli are subject to extinction.) That would make our Romantic love objects mere sexual stimuli that inevitably dwindle in strength. On the positive side, we can say that Commitment steps in as Passion bows out. Thomas Moore's famous poem (and song) fervently denies that passion fades away with the inevitable aging of our sweetheart:

> Believe me, if all those endearing young charms,
> Which I gaze on so fondly today,
> Were to change by tomorrow, and fleet in my arms,
> Like fairy gifts fading away,
> Thou wouldst still be ador'd, as this moment thou art,
> Let thy loveliness fade as it will,
> And around the dear ruin each wish of my heart
> Would entwine itself verdantly still.
> (Thomas Moore 1779–1852) (Marshall, 1967, p. 171)

This poem is a truly great and moving description of Companionate love and makes a promise that commitment and intimacy will never fade. A second verse says "No, the heart that has truly lov'd never forgets, But as truly loves on to the close, …" I do wonder, though, if any woman of any century would like to think of herself as eventually becoming a "dear ruin."

Perhaps it is easier to give a prose description of Companionate love, rather than rely on a triangular model or a poem. According to Walter Lippmann:

> … when a man and woman are successfully in love, their whole activity is energized and victorious. They walk better, their digestion improves, they think more clearly, the secret worries drop away, the world is fresh and interesting, and they can do more than they dreamed that they could do. In love of this kind *sexual intimacy is not the dead end of desire as it is in romantic or promiscuous love*, but periodic affirmation of the inward delight of desire pervading an active life" [italics mine]. (in Train, 1993, p. 47)

This Affectionate or Companionate love is often called "mature love." It probably started with Romantic love (Intimacy + Passion) and the Passion dropped out (gradually, we hope) and was replaced with Commitment.

While there is more Sturm und Drang in Romantic love, I think it is just as capable of sustaining self-esteem and diminishing fear as Companionate love. It has the quality of an obsession. The face, voice, smile, eyes, and body of the beloved are constantly in view in the "mind's eye." This acts as an anodyne or drug that tends to keep thoughts of death at bay. The down side of this obsession is that as soon as the beloved grows cool or distant, depression and even suicidal or homicidal thoughts can develop. As long as there is reciprocity, then, Romantic love can serve as a bulwark against death fears. Affectionate or Companionate love, by definition, includes reciprocity and long-term commitment.

In the Middle Ages, passionate love was considered a demonic possession. Aldous Huxley wrote that before Rousseau, the passionate love of Paris for Helen (leading to the Trojan War), Dido for Aneas, and Paolo and Francesca for each other were looked on as "disastrous maladies." Rousseau and the Romantic Movement turned this demonic possession into the highest form of love (Aldous Huxley quoted in Train, 1993, pp. 24–25).

The sexual basis of Romantic love sometimes gives it a bad name. The heritage of the Middle Ages is still with us, as described in detail by Adolf Gugenbühl-Craig:

> For a long time Christian theologians could recognize sexuality only in connection with reproduction. They experienced the erotic as something demonic and uncanny, as something that had to be fought against or neutralized. All of these medieval theologians were certainly intelligent and differentiated people, in honest search for truth and understanding. That they experienced sexuality as demonic, therefore, cannot be so easily discounted. They were expressing something quite true. (in Zweig, 1991, p. 98)

After this, the author shows how sexuality is demonized in our times. He cites the view of some of the most extreme women's liberationists that sex is mainly a political weapon used to suppress women. Another example is the belief that viewing the primal scene has disastrous effects on children. The exclusion of any sexual activity between patients and their spouses or loved ones in hospitals and in many prisons is another instance of censure, as is the practice of forbidding athletes to have sex before competition or for the duration of contests such as the Olympics. I could add to this the current criticism of out-of-wedlock pregnancies, combined with the attempt to deny contraception or abortions to teenagers, in the fear that it would encourage greater sexual activity. A hue and cry came from the "family values" contingent of the Republican Party, when "Murphy Brown," played by Candice Bergen on U.S. television, gave birth as a single mother. The Vice President at that time, Dan Quayle, made a large issue of how TV was undermining the morals of our teenagers.

The lack of control involved in Romantic love, its obsessional quality, and its basic sexuality make it a threat to this day, even though we give lip service to marrying only for romantic reasons. Because it still has demonic connotations does not make it any less of a defense against death fear than the more stable and less passionate forms of love. The obsessive character in fact may help to stabilize Romantic love, for it is the basis for that "blindness" to the loved one's faults that adds to the longevity of the relationship.

An opposing view is held by Goldberg. Because it is based on illusion, she sees it as fragile (and for our purposes thus less helpful in dealing with death fear).

> Romantic love is blind because it thrives on fantasy and illusion; it looks inwardly at one's own hopes and desires rather than at the reality of who the other person is ... But such an imaginative love is fragile ... When we discover the complete, unvarnished truth about our beloved—their imperfections and their all-too-human traits ... we feel betrayed by both our lover and our love. (Goldberg, 1993, p. 177)

This view ignores the importance of illusion and fantasy in the preservation of ourselves, however. Religious belief is a prime example of the sustaining effect of illusion, particularly the belief in the afterlife.

In Eugene O'Neill's *The Iceman Cometh*, the drunks say to Hickey, the drummer (psychoanalyst) who forced them to face reality and give up their pipe dreams, "You've spoiled the likker." Stripping away all illusion can take the juice out of life. Moreover, the way in which the lover handles the revelation of the "truth" about the beloved is very much a function of personality. Years ago I served on a review committee for the National Institute of Mental Health. After a long work day, a woman psychologist who had made many contributions to the day's discussion and I decided to have supper together. We were both married, and talked at length about our marriages. She said that though she had found many faults in her husband as time went on, she continued to discover endearing and wonderful qualities in him as well, qualities that were a complete surprise to her. She felt these balanced the faults and shortcomings that she had detected. I was struck by the wisdom and maturity of her view, and by her realistic acceptance of her husband. It was not *just* acceptance of him "warts and all," but a delight in discovering wonderful new secrets about him.

Liking

Liking, according to Sternberg, consists of intimacy, without commitment or passion. It is the love found in friendship. Companionate love lacks only passion. Lewis calls this *Philias*.

Does the importance of friendship for reduction of anxiety and death fear need belaboring? It is common knowledge that people who have a network of friends are apt to be less fearful, and are generally happier. The number of friends reported by adults and by mothers reporting for their children correlated directly with mental health in both the Midtown Study of adults and our study of Manhattan's children. There are numerous studies, especially in sociometric research, showing a correlation between mental health and extended friendship networks. Since anxiety, fear, and anger are the basis of depression and antisocial behavior and most major categories of mental disorder, it is not beyond reason to assume that having a greater number of friends was in part responsible for the reduction of these emotions.

Love That Fosters Death Fear

Empty Love This is commitment without intimacy or passion, the "Pragma" of Lee's classification. It is the pragmatic compatible love, the arranged marriage. It is difficult to find examples of this type of love, since we are so accustomed to some intimacy or passion in our relationships. If you know of a woman or man who is just "hanging in there," trapped in a relationship she or he doesn't really like, this may be "empty love." It does not act to reduce death fear; in fact it may exacerbate it. Arranged marriages are rare in our current society, but all over the world there are millions of child brides who are committed by their parents to what we would consider a loveless life. The royal marriages of the past are of this type. They were arranged for purely political purposes. Stefan Zweig described the unhappiness of Marie Antoinette upon being wed to Louis XVI. For years she was unable to become pregnant because Louis had phimosis, a constriction of the foreskin, which interfered with erection and ejaculation. After he was operated on, she became pregnant, but had already taken a lover. This might be called "involuntary commitment," since most members of royal families, until recently, went along with the choices their parents and ministers made for them.

Fatuous Love and Infatuation   It's difficult to make distinctions between these two types. Sternberg calls Passion + Commitment with no intimacy "Fatuous," and Passion alone, without Intimacy or Commitment, "Infatuation." One dictionary (Flexner, 1987) defines infatuation as a "foolish or all-absorbing passion." Fatuous is defined as "foolish, inane," or secondarily as "unreal or illusory." Let's look at some examples. John Hinckley was clearly infatuated with the actress Jodie Foster. To get her attention, he shot then-President Ronald Reagan. He now claims he has regained his mental health, and wants to be released. His passion was certainly foolish and all-absorbing, but he didn't show anything like long-term commitment. Many millions of people have been infatuated with movie stars. Marilyn Monroe and Elvis Presley are still worshipped, and Presley fan clubs still exist. Aren't these long-term fans fatuous, since they show passion and commitment over the long term? At face value, passion without the slightest chance of intimacy seems incapable of reducing death fear and giving emotional support to its practitioners. Yet even empty love, fatuous love, and infatuation can offer some emotional support. The supportive role of fantasy and illusion should not be dismissed. What seems to us like inane love can sustain a person over a lifetime. To the observer, there may be a large element of masochism involved, but to the infatuated lover, his distant (and usually unresponsive) love object is the saving grace of his life.

You don't have to be a borderline psychotic (Hinckley) or a killer to be infatuated and foolishly in love. Take the example of Cyrano de Bergerac,* who writes passionate love letters for his soldier-companion. The letters are addressed to the companion's lover, whom Cyrano distantly worships. He conceals his secret love of her for a lifetime. At least Priscilla had the wisdom to say to John Alden, "Why don't you speak for yourself, John." If she hadn't spoken up, John might have kept on pleading the case of Myles Standish, and might then have become an example of Fatuous love.

---

* Cyrano is the self-sacrificing hero of a verse play written in 1897 by Edmond Rostand. His character was based on a French soldier, swordsman, and writer who lived from 1619 to 1655. Aside from his infatuation, the character is noted for his sensitivity about his very long nose, which often gets him into swordfights.

Promiscuous Love   I find that Sternberg's types don't quite cover all the important kinds of love and lovers. One of these we could call Promiscuous. Lee (in Sternberg, 1988) uses the term *Ludus* for the roving, flirtatious, and uncommitted lover. While there is a strong sexual drive in this type of love, there is no passion in the usual sense of the word. The most famous rake was Don Juan, and sexual addiction (Don Juanism) takes its name from him. The French detective novelist, Georges Simenon, wrote prodigiously. Between novels, he had sexual encounters with thousands of women, mainly prostitutes. He was also given to vomiting after the completion of each novel. He is clearly a case of sexual addiction as well as promiscuity. Not all promiscuous lovers are so clearly under a compulsion to be "sexual athletes."

A more recent example of extreme promiscuity is "Magic" Johnson. By his own admission, he had thousands of heterosexual contacts with fans who were attracted to him as the top star of U.S. basketball. He made a public statement about his promiscuity, and attributed his contracting AIDS to this activity. Athletes and movie stars are in a position to become sex addicts, since they have so many infatuated fans.

The promiscuous man (or woman) is not protected against death fear to the degree that the romantic or the companionate lover is. The more extreme the behavior, the greater the suffering of the roving lover.

> … the wives, mothers and girlfriends of compulsive Casanovas are not the only victims of these entanglements. Despite the admiring notion of the man who … 'gets plenty' as super-macho … there is a mass of evidence to show that in illicit amours, whether they go right or wrong, men bleed too. 'The problem with adultery is that it is inherently a self-punishing self-defeating exercise,' says Dr. Gessler. … 'adultery is a fantasy flight to find the real mother, the woman who will offer him unconditional all-embracing love, who will provide the nourishment he desires, who will serve his bodily needs as instantly, adoringly, as he dreams she must have done in his primal heyday.' (Miles, 1991, p. 191)

While adultery is not synonymous with promiscuity, it represents a step in that direction. Obviously, not all rovers are seeking a mother in vain. Many men use women as a tranquilizer, or to boost their self-esteem. It is unfortunate that we inherited the term "object-relations" from Freud, because the treatment of the "loved one" <u>as an object</u> distinguishes the immature and promiscuous lover from the other types. The promiscuous lover certainly treats women as objects, and doesn't see them as individuals.*

Rosalind Miles sums up the dilemma of the promiscuous lover quite neatly:

> Living in mortal fear of defenselessness and abandonment, promiscuous and unfaithful men are nevertheless compelled to reenact the ritual motions of rapprochement,

---

* Freud's use of the word "object" is in the sense of objective or aim, as in "the object of my affections." Treating someone "as an object" uses the word as synonymous with "a thing," something lifeless.

intimacy and severance. Constant copulation, as a defense against defenselessness, condemns the philanderer to a continuous replay of his feelings of vulnerability and loss, inferiority and powerlessness... (Miles, 1991, p. 195)

As perverse as it may seem to the observer, promiscuity serves as a defense against death fear (defenselessness and abandonment), although its compulsive quality and its social risks make it a painful and often dangerous coping mode. Its health risks were great before the days of antibiotics. Syphilis was one of the deadliest killers. After a brief hiatus, AIDS took its place as a new plague, threatening the hard-won sexual freedom of the twentieth century. Not all AIDS victims are promiscuous, and women, especially in developing countries, are most likely to become infected by their husbands.

Brotherly Love   Brotherly love seems to be a better term than Christian love, for surely there are Muslims, Buddhists, Jews, and Taoists, among others, who love their fellow men. This is the selfless love that puts the needs of the outsider, the stranger, the other, before the needs of one's own self, family, nation, or religion. Albert Schweitzer, the physician, organist, and philosopher, said that "reverence for life" or "affirmation of life" was the "fundamental principle of morality." This reverence for life, for one's neighbor, involves sacrifice.

Take the question of man's duty to his neighbor. The ethic cannot be fully carried out, without involving the possibility of complete sacrifice of self. (Albert Schweitzer, quoted in *The New York Times Magazine*, Jan. 9, 1995, in Seldes, 1967, p. 328)

This "reverence for life" really means reverence for the life of others, and explicitly demands sacrifice. In this, it reflects the Crucifixion, and the Christian faith of Dr. Schweitzer.

Reverence for life ...does not allow the scholar to live for his science alone, even if he is very useful to the community in so doing. It does not permit the artist to exist only for his art, even if he gives inspiration to many by its means. It refuses to let the business man imagine that he fulfills all legitimate demands in the course of his business activities. It demands from all that they should sacrifice a portion of their own lives for others. (Seldes, 1967)

Otto Rank pointed out that creative people (and this could include the business man as well as the scholar and artist) make a sacrifice in return for their success.

If we look back at the modern artist-type as we know it, even in biographical form, since Renaissance days, there can be no doubt that the great works of art were bought at the cost of ordinary living. (Rank, 1932, reprinted in 1989, pp. 428–429)

Rank viewed supreme art and full experience (of life) to be "two incommensurable magnitudes." One must be sacrificed for the other. This is just as true for great achievement in other occupations. Perhaps there is an inevitable sacrifice of the pleasures of ordinary living for all who succeed, although their success seems to be more motivated by self-concern or even narcissism at first glance.

Compassion (whose synonyms are sympathy, commiseration, mercy, tenderness, heart, and clemency) is a major element in Brotherly love. It involves not just the feeling of sympathy for the less fortunate, but also the desire to alleviate their suffering. The importance of compassion was beautifully expressed by Bertrand Russell, whose political radicalism was based upon it.

> The thing I mean … is love, Christian love, or compassion. If you feel this, you have a motive for existence, a guide for action, a reason for courage, an imperative necessity for intellectual honesty. (in Seldes, 1967, p. 620)

The most extreme position on Brotherly love was taken by Erich Fromm. Ignoring the qualities of the loved one, he would have us love all of mankind.

> In essence, all human beings are identical. We are all part of One; we are One. This being so, it should not make any difference whom we love. (Fromm, 1955, quoted in Branden, 1981, p. 215)

This position, in fact the view that Brotherly love is of a higher order than Romantic love or Companionate love, has come in for bitter criticism. The issue can be fudged by simply redefining love to fit one's philosophy. John Schaar has shown how Fromm fused two incompatible views of love. First is the idea that love is universal. "Love of one person implies love of man as such." Second is the exclusive quality of erotic (read Romantic) love; "… erotic love is by its very nature exclusive and not universal."

> Fromm will not tolerate exclusiveness: the magic circle of love must be opened. So in the end he denies the essential exclusiveness of erotic love and fuses it with universal love.
> 　(Fromm says) Erotic love is exclusive, but it loves in the other person all of mankind, all that is alive. It is exclusive only in the sense that I can fuse myself fully and intensely with one person only. Erotic love excludes the love for others only in the sense of erotic fusion, full commitment in all aspects of life—but not in the sense of deep brotherly love. (Schaar, 1961)

If we use the term "Brotherly love," and keep its main qualities of sympathy and compassion separate from the passion and intimacy of Romantic (erotic) love, the conflict created by using the term "love" to cover all kinds of positive relationships is partly solved. Schaar, apparently arguing for the exclusivity of erotic love, castigates Fromm for diluting the meaning of the term "love."

> Fromm makes love synonymous with sympathetic relations among men. This, of course, is one of the characteristics of our day, which has agreed to make love mean affection, loyalty, care, and concern, as it usually does, for example, in the state of matrimony.* This strips love of the aura of mystery and enchantment which has always surrounded it … (Fromm) … confuses love with its consequences. Many things, such

---

* This would seem to support the idea I suggested earlier, that Companionate love gradually replaces Romantic love in the later stages of marriage.

as the care, responsibility, respect and knowledge which Fromm speaks of, grow from
love, but they are not love itself. (Schaar, 1961)

The same criticism of Fromm's idea of love as universal is articulated by
Nathaniel Branden: Again he seems to be talking about Romantic love (for that
is the subject of his book), while Fromm is promoting Brotherly love.

Love by its very nature entails a process of selection, of discrimination. Love is our
response to that which represents our highest values. Love is a response to distinctive
characteristics possessed by some human beings, but not all. Otherwise, what would
be the tribute of love? (Branden, 1981, p. 214)

Ridiculing Fromm's idea that since we are all part of mankind, love of one
is equal to love of all, Branden says:

If we were to ask our lover why he or she cared for us, consider what our reaction
would be if told 'Who shouldn't I love you? All human beings are identical.
Therefore, it doesn't make any difference whom I love. So it might as well be you.'
(Branden, 1981, p. 213)

Other than the issue of universal versus particular criteria for choosing a
lover, an even more basic criticism of Brotherly love (as love of the highest order)
is that human beings, by their nature, are just not capable of such a pure and perfect love. Schaar, talking of the mystery of love, says that few can ever attain it.

Most men never truly love another nor are they truly loved by another on this earth.
We can accept that sadness or we can with Fromm try to conceal it by equating sympathy with love. (Schaar, 1961, p. 129)

Long before Fromm had written about love, Freud inveighed against the idea
of brotherly love and love of mankind. In discussing how society binds the members of a community to each other, he says that restrictions on sexual life produce
"aim-inhibited libido," which fosters the development of friendship. He examines
the commandment "Thou shalt love thy neighbor as thyself," and considers it
unnatural, and an obligation which involves a sacrifice. (This is the very point that
Albert Schweitzer is trying to make—Christian love does involve self-sacrifice.)

Freud first raises the issue of particular (rather than universal) criteria for
choosing to love someone.

If I love someone, he must be worthy of it in some way or other … But if he is a
stranger to me and cannot attract me by any value he has in himself or any significance he may have already acquired in my emotional life, it will be hard for me to
love him. I shall even be doing wrong if I do, for my love is valued as a privilege by
all those belonging to me; it is an injustice to them if I put a stranger on a level with
them … [Freud, 1929, in Civilization, War and Death, edited by John Rickman,
Psychoanalytical Epitomes, No. 4, The Hogarth Press, New Enlarged Edition, 1953
(orig. 1939), p. 50]

He then launches into the more basic question of whether humans are even
capable of such an exalted type of love. Here his view of man as having aggressive

and sexual drives that he can barely control leads him to believe that one cannot love one's neighbor, much less one's enemy.

> And there is a second commandment that seems to me even more incomprehensible, and arouses still stronger opposition in me. It is 'Love thine enemies' ... (The truth is) that men are not gentle, friendly creatures wishing for love, who simply defend themselves if they are attacked, but that a powerful measure of desire for aggression has to be reckoned as part of their instinctual endowment. The result is that their neighbor is to them not only a possible helper or sexual object, but also a temptation to them to gratify their aggressiveness on him, to exploit his capacity for work without recompense, to use him sexually without his consent, to seize his possessions, to humiliate him, to cause him pain, to torture and to kill him. *Homo homine lupus* [Man is a wolf to man] (derived from Plautus, Asinaria II, iv, 88) ... This cruelty ... reveals men as savage beasts to whom the thought of sparing their own kind is alien ... (Freud, 1929, op., cit. pp. 50–51)

Finally, Freud sums up his view of Brotherly love (loving neighbors, enemies, and strangers) as a reaction-formation (a behavioral tendency developed in direct opposition to a repressed impulse—that is, the impulse to kill, rape, etc.). Love of the neighbor or of mankind is looked on as "aim inhibited." In aim inhibition, the natural object is considered to be someone of the opposite sex, but societal prohibitions and commandments inhibit this sexual drive, and channel it into a more generalized kind of love, one that is asexual.

> Culture has to call up every possible reinforcement in order to erect barriers against the aggressive instincts of men and hold their manifestations in check by reaction-formations in men's minds. Hence its system of methods by which mankind is to be driven to identifications and aim-inhibited love relationships; hence the restrictions on sexual life; and hence, too, an ideal command to love one's neighbor as oneself, which is really justified by the fact that nothing is so completely at variance with original human nature as this. (Freud, 1929, op. cit., p. 51)

Clearly, Brotherly love is an ideal or model for behavior that humans find difficult to attain. The ideal is a goal toward which we can strive. Robert Browning said "A man's reach should exceed his grasp, or what's a heaven for?" Romantic and Companionable love are also ideals, but are more easily attained. The Biblical injunction to "Love thy neighbor as thyself" holds the key to the dilemma of Brotherly love. Very few people really love themselves. To the degree that you feel guilt, shame, and anger at yourself, to that extent are you incapable of loving your neighbor, the stranger, or mankind. The achievement of some degree of self-love and self-acceptance is a prerequisite for developing Brotherly love. No wonder, then, that so few people are really capable of loving mankind, the stranger, or even their neighbor.

Most religions support the Golden Rule—"Do as you would be done by." The tenets of Christianity rose from Judaism and are echoed in all the great religions. Most men strive toward ideal behavior as defined by their culture, but those ideals are usually in conflict with the "shadow self," the unconscious, sexual and aggressive instincts, or the collective demons inside the human animal. Some writers attest to that:

> The Christian ideal has not been tried and found wanting. It has been found difficult, and left untried (G. K. Chesterton, "What's Wrong with the World," quoted in Seldes, 1967, p. 147)

> How very hard it is to be a Christian (Robert Browning "Easter Day," quoted in Seldes, 1967, p. 146)

> There is no possibility of anyone realizing the Christian ideals. For human beings simply cannot, in the nature of things, be superhuman. (Aldous Huxley "Cardiff, What Great Men Think of Religion," in Seldes, 1967, p. 149)

The love of God, and the belief in the afterlife, have sustained millions of people facing immediate death, and hundreds of millions more who faced eventual death. Religion is treated in a later chapter as a mode of coping with fear of death and dying. Brotherly and Christian love may involve sacrifice in caring for others and putting the stranger before oneself and one's family. This sacrifice is often paid back by heightened feelings of self-esteem and the pleasure of giving. Brotherly love, then, does have a positive and immediate function in warding off anxiety and fear. In the long run, Brotherly love may save us all from Armageddon, from the pitting of every man against his fellow man. The progress we make in establishing world peace; in abolishing nuclear, biological, and chemical weapons; in outlawing land mines that maim millions; and in assuaging poverty , hunger, and sickness around the world may seem completely altruistic. In fact, it is not only "brotherly," but also self-preserving. When we help others in this way, we help ourselves both directly and indirectly. We also reduce the terrible fear of the death of mankind that has gripped our world since the advent of the nuclear age.

SPECIAL EVIDENCE OF LOVE'S POWER

There is evidence of the power of love to allay fear of death and dying, to prolong life, to revive those who are unconscious, to prevent suicide, and to affect the physical growth of children. It isn't necessarily any one type of love, but is worth mentioning. There is so little proof, and so little experimental research (partly because of the unacceptability of providing loving support to an experimental group and withholding it from a control group), that for now we must rely on scattered and sometimes anecdotal evidence.

There is growing evidence for the role of love in promoting longevity. The importance of loving care and emotional support when dealing with terminally ill patients has been stressed by Elizabeth Kübler-Ross (1969) and Bernie Siegel

(1986). Not only does love from the medical staff and family increase the chances of recovery, but returning home to a pet after a heart attack reduces the risk of dying.

> There has also been clinical evidence, reported in Public Health Reports (July-August 1980) that pet ownership can add significantly to the probability of survival in heart attack patients after discharge from a coronary care unit—although the reason for this has not been determined. (Nieburg, 1982, p. xv)

Part of the reason for this increased survival is found in the very same introductory section of Nieburg's book.

> In his book <u>Pets and Human Development</u>, the psychologist Boris Levenson suggests that pets can help human beings from infancy to old age solve developmental problems by *providing affection, instilling a sense of competence through* the experience of *nurturing* and by *relieving loneliness* (italics mine). (Nieburg, 1982, p. xiv)

I later mention Lisa Foster, the wife of Vincent Foster (U.S. President Bill Clinton's personal attorney until Foster's suicide) as an example of how compulsivity sometimes fails to protect against suicide and death fear. It is clear that the love of her children, not her compulsive workaholic attitude toward churchgoing, the PTA, and other organizations, was the key to her psychological survival.

> I wanted to die after he died ... I couldn't stand the idea of my children having to go through it (suicide) more than once. It's just the most awful thing in the world, and I can't let them think that I'd do it too. I mean, somehow, I've got to stay alive, for them. (Boyer, 1995, p. 62)

This sense of responsibility for another living being, animal or human, seems to be a common thread tying the heart attack patients to the survivors in families of suicides. Giving love protects against death, death fear, and suicide, as well as, or even better than, receiving love.

There is more evidence for the critical role that love plays in promoting the survival of the very ill. This is true in the case of unconscious patients, who may appear to be out of touch with their loved ones. Not so. In 1996 a woman was severely beaten in Central Park in New York City. For several days she lay in a coma, and nurses tried to take the place of her family, who could not attend since she carried no identification. They rubbed her back and talked to her.

> I tell most families yes, definitely speak to the patient on an adult level, and try to eke out minimal responses, said Dr. Seymour Gendelman, director of clinical neurology at Mount Sinai Medical Center. Experts said there is no definitive proof, but a great deal of anecdotal evidence suggests comatose patients recover better with loved ones at their side. (Furse, 1996)

Later on I will make reference to the fact that Durkheim (1897) (and now many others) have found that married men have a much lower rate of suicide than unmarried, divorced, or widowed men. There is much to be said for this fact as evidence that love acts as a bolster against death fear and suicidal thoughts or acts. However, the fact that married women (at least in Durkheim's France) did not have a lower suicide rate than their unmarried peers seems to question whether love or some other factor protects married men. Someone suggested that men just don't know how to take care of themselves, and are thus more dependent on their wives. Durkheim thought that unmarried men were more subject to sexual anomie—the unlimited and uncontrolled expression of sexuality, which I called "promiscuity"—than women. This is less true in modern times in most Western countries, since estimates of adulterous wives range from 25 to 40 percent in Britain and the United States. Durkheim's conclusion was that men profited more from marriage, as an anchor for their anomic drives, than did women. This is probably true to this day, as a European survey disclosed.

> Not surprisingly, men in general can suffer intensely from a marriage breakup, and measurably more than women on almost every criterion available. A European Economic Community survey of 1989 found that over 50 percent of divorced men regretted losing their partner, as against less than 25 percent of the women. Divorced men, especially those who remain unmarried, display soaring rates of cerebral and coronary thrombosis, cancer, career breakdown, mental distress, insanity and suicide. (Miles, 1991, p. 231)

We all have an intuitive sense that love or lack of it (as in the case of Spitz's orphans) can have a profound effect on health. Lack of love can clearly be a cause of wasting and death in infants. Less well known is a possible connection between love and physical growth. My assumption is that lack of love or some distortion of parental love (coldness, punitiveness, lability, etc.) causes increased anxiety in children (over and above their hereditary levels of fear of the dark, loud noises, and strangers). This greater anxiety in turn has recently been found to be related to growth and adult height.

> The study...found that adolescent and pre-adolescent girls who were overly anxious grew up to be roughly one to two inches shorter, on average, than other girls...Previous research showed that children and adults of both sexes with anxiety or depression have lower-than-normal amounts of growth hormone, the chemical that stimulates the growth of muscle and bone in children and teen-agers. (Gilbert, 1996)*

These results held up even when socioeconomic status was controlled. (Wealthier people are taller, at least in the United States.) Most telling was the fact that the strongest relationship between anxiety and height was found in girls of ages 11 to 20 when *separation anxiety* (italics mine) was diagnosed. "They were 1.7 inches shorter than the girls in whom no emotional problems had been found." I initially said that fear of death and dying is learned, and derives mainly from separation anxiety. Overt separation anxiety is obviously not as common in 11- to 20-year-olds as it is in infants. Here we have girls who have retained and perhaps heightened their original fears. I would guess that they were exceptionally fearful

* Exact date is uncertain. The study was published in a June issue of *Pediatrics*. The lead author is Dr. Daniel S. Pine, a child psychiatrist at the N.Y. State Psychiatric Institute and Columbia University of New York.

of death and dying. That difference in height may also have negative survival value. It is a truism that emotional and physical illness go hand in hand. Maybe shorter girls are aware of their social disadvantage. They can be rejected by peers. Bullying and teasing are common among teen agers, and the victims may have good reason to become anxious. Thus the original separation anxiety may be reinforced by later peer-group experiences.

Love, in Closing

There can be no doubt that most forms of love can act to reduce the fear of death and dying. Even the most masochistic forms of love, love of a sadist or totally unrequited love, can give some hope and meaning to a life. Each expert who writes on love has his favorite kind, and this is usually a reflection of his own personality makeup. Erich Fromm exalted brotherly love above all other kinds.

Alan Soble (whose book, *The Structure of Love*, was by far the most difficult among all the books I have read in preparing this chapter) defines two traditions; the erosic (sexual, courtly, and romantic love) and the agapic (Christian-neighbor love and God's love for humans.)

> Personal love, some have argued, can succeed (or be genuine) only if it is 'agapized,' that is, transformed by agape into a second-view ("agapic") love...Does personal love need a dose of agape?...Does conceiving of personal love in terms foreign to the eros tradition provide a better understanding of it? My eventual conclusion is 'no'. (Soble, 1990, p. 4)

Soble, then, clearly favors erosic love; the sexual and the romantic. Norman Brown and Walt Whitman exalted unfettered sexual expression as the highest value. They felt everyone should be free to sound his "barbaric yawp" from the rooftops. Casanova and the Marquis de Sade had their own preferences. Many marriage manuals criticize romantic love as immature and fragile, while elevating "mature' companionate love to the highest position. *In my view, each of these loves may be appropriate to a particular individual, in a particular historical time and place, and at a particular stage of life.* Courtly love (for example, the love of Lancelot and Guinevere behind King Arthur's back, or the tragic love of Tristan and Isolde, with its "Liebestodt") is certainly dated, in its ideas of chivalry, moral purity, and unconsummated love as an ideal. Courtly love was probably functional and appropriate in its time. Consummation usually ended in guilt or death.

> Courtly love was idealized to the extent that it remained unconsummated. The value of the love relationship was justified by the ennoblement of the lover, who was motivated to perform virtuous and courageous acts to win the love of his ideal; for the woman, it was justified by the fact that she was the source of such ennoblement. Unfulfilled and unsatisfied desire fueled the striving and the passion; few relationships were portrayed as surviving consummation. (Branden, 1981, p. 24)

The love of Peter Abelard (1079–1142), the French philosopher, and his student, Heloise, survived his castration by thugs hired by her uncle. He then became a monk, and she became an abbess. Although separated, they wrote to each other until death ended the relationship. It is hard to imagine such lifelong commitment in the face of the incredible obstacles found in our modern world. In that place and time, it seems more appropriate, though still an exceptional love.

Aside from the question of whether there is one supreme kind of love, or a hierarchy of love, a central problem about love still puzzles me. Is love logical or psychological? Is it based on reason, on qualities of the beloved that make him or her "special"? Do people make rational choices in their mates? Or is love totally "blind," as the expression goes? Is it completely illogical? Are the qualities in the beloved that people claim are the reasons for choosing this one person as a mate really constructions of the chooser? Worse yet, are these qualities so overdetermined by repetition compulsion, by the unresolved problems of childhood, that hidden properties in the beloved are the real determinants of choice? If we see someone "marrying for money" or for power, we think we have a clear-cut case of logical (if not socially desirable) choice. Yet underneath this choice may be an attachment to a tyrannical father, or a need to diminish fears stemming from extreme childhood poverty. Was this choice motivated by simple greed, or by some early victimization?

Stendhal said the beloved was really the creation of the lover,* a view I personally favor. Beauty (or virtue or wit or wisdom) is in the eye of the beholder. This looks at love as essentially romantic and irrational. I have previously stressed the importance of illusion, and how necessary it is to mankind's survival. I will repeat it, especially in the chapter on religion. Freud referred to religion as an illusion, but said it was probably a necessary one. In the same breath, he pleaded for logic and reason, hoping it would eventually prevail.

Previously I quoted authors who said that no one can really know another person well, and no one can really love another completely. This may be considered the "dark side" of love. But these same two facts (if they are indeed facts) may also be looked upon as the bright side of love, by a process called "cognitive restructuring." Our lack of mutual knowledge allows us to construct and rearrange the image of our beloved in a positive way, often in the face of contradictory information and experience.

> Illusions are the key to a happy unconscious life. 'The idea that we understand one another,' Mr. Bollas writes, is 'largely illusory.' But that doesn't mean we are hopelessly isolated. It just means that 'because we do not comprehend one another...we are therefore free to invent one another...We are free to misperceive.' (Boxer, 1995, p. 40)†

---

* [Stendhal, 1949 (first published in 1822)]. His real name was Marie Henri Beyle. On Love (De L' Amour, 1822) is a psychological analysis of love long before Freud or Fromm. He also wrote two great novels, The Red and the Black, and The Charterhouse of Parma. His heroes were probably the first to exhibit upward mobility "as we know it."

† The quotation is from Christopher Bollas, a British psychoanalyst, and is contained in a review of two of his books, Cracking Up and Being a Character.

We all know people who have maintained a positive image of a lover despite obnoxious or even life-threatening behavior on the part of their "sweetheart." Almost every day we read about a woman who failed to get an order of protection from her husband or boyfriend, and when beaten up several times did not press charges. Granted, the police protection often fails, and a murder results. While we can't blame the victim for the savagery of the spurned or malicious male, there is often a reluctance to prosecute, and a desire to give him "just one more chance." This cycle of beatings and female forgiveness is almost a bromide in cases of alcoholism and drug abuse combined with domestic violence.

Is this the product of poor education, of poverty, or of the implanting in girls of norms of submission and dependence? I think not. There are literary examples of *men* who have suffered horribly at the hands of their sweethearts. Somerset Maugham's *Of Human Bondage* comes to mind. The indignities heaped on Professor Unrath by Lola-Lola, the cabaret singer (played by Marlene Dietrich) in the movie, The Blue Angel (1930) are not to be believed. She eventually ruins his life. Perhaps the beatings administered by women to men are more subtle and less likely to end in death.

If lack of intelligence plays a major part in creating an image of one's lover that contradicts reality, then how could Hannah Arendt, above all a brilliant philosopher, have continued to see her mentor and lover, Martin Heidegger, as a God? At 18, Arendt was Heidegger's pupil when their on-again–off-again affair started. She was Jewish, and he became a Nazi. He blocked or ended the careers of many Jews and anti-Nazis in his role of rector of the University of Freiburg. She whitewashed his Nazi activities, and called him the "king of the empire of thought."

> In (Arendt's) view, genius excuses everything—male chauvinism, hypocrisy, anti-Semitism, totalitarianism. Since the separation of intellect from responsibility has recently had a sinister history, one might read the love story of Arendt and Heidegger as a warning about the dangers of elevating men into gods ... If there is an object lesson in (their) love, it might be not only that the worship of genius is dangerous but that even the most all-encompassing passion, looked at from the outside, seems like folly. (Steiner, 1995, p. 41)

To the outside observer this may seem a totally irrational love on the part of Arendt. Her view of Heidegger was a massive reconstruction and illusion, built by a woman of genius. Her intelligence didn't keep her from distorting her lover's real attributes. However, looked at from her point of view of the actor (not the observer) her reconstruction had a primary function: to save her pride and her self-esteem. She had let him walk all over her. She had been a vulnerable student admiring the great professor. She had stood by while he persecuted the Jews (in his own academic way). To preserve her ego, she elevated him to Godlike status. Even her idea of the slaughter of the Jews as the product of the "banality of evil" (in discussing Eichmann, who gave the orders but didn't do the actual killing of six million Jews, Gypsies, and political prisoners) now seems like a whitewash of the Holocaust and of her connection to Heidegger. "Banality" is really a glaring diminutive when used to describe such horror. A later chapter discusses the concept of evil, and how killing is one mode of coping with death-fear and of attaining an illusion of immortality. Killing another human is never banal. Evil is evil, and can't be watered down.

Arendt's illusion probably saved her from the guilt, depression, and self-hatred she would have felt if she had allowed herself to see Heidegger for the contemptible Nazi that he was. We have to look at the motivation of lovers, and ask why they hang in there when to us it looks like sheer masochism. For Arendt, her loved one made her career, and taught her what he knew of philosophy. He was always the master, she the student and slave. Was this based only on masochism? I think not.

As is true in so many cases, if we look "under the hood," we can find an explanation and motive for the seemingly insane love. Loving a person for your own purposes is surely more common than loving him or her in order to promote their welfare. If you love someone primarily to satisfy your own needs (a narcissistic love) then you are more likely to develop an illusory picture of them. If you love them for their own sake, for what you can give to them, then your view of them tends to be more realistic.

Analyzing the types of love and how they relate to fear of death and dying misses the mystery, the commitment, the great joy, the poignancy, and the sorrow of love. Here is a well-known quote from the Bible that goes beyond analysis to the heart of why committed love gives us strength when we have it, and leaves us in sadness and fear when we have lost it. Ruth's love for her mother-in-law, Naomi, despite Naomi's bad luck, is in contrast to that of her sister-in-law, Orpah, who returns to her people in Moab. These same words could apply to a committed love between a man and a woman.

> And Ruth said, 'Intreat me not to leave thee, or to return from following after thee: for whither thou goest, I will go, and where thou lodgest, I will lodge: thy people shall be my people, and thy God my God: Where thou diest, will I die, and there will I be buried: the Lord do so to me, and more also, if aught but death part thee and me.'
> (Ruth I:16–17, *The Holy Bible*, King James verson)

And finally, the poem "What Lips My Lips Have Kissed" by Edna St. Vincent Millay (1941, from *The Harp Weaver*) expresses the loss of past loves in the summer of life, and the approach of winter (aging and death).

> What lips my lips have kissed, and where, and why,
> I have forgotten, and what arms have lain
> Under my head till morning; but the rain
> Is full of ghosts tonight, that tap and sign
> Upon the glass and listen for reply,
> And in my heart there stirs a quiet pain
> For unremembered lads that not again
> Will turn to me at midnight with a cry.

Thus in the winter stands the lonely tree,
Nor knows what birds have vanished one by one,
Yet knows its boughs more silent than before:
I cannot say what loves have come and gone,
I only know that summer sang in me
A little while, that in me sings no more.

5

HUMOR

We said before that humor is one of the bulwarks against the threat of death. It is not the kind of humor that denigrates others, but that makes fun of death. "Laughing at fate" is life enhancing and perhaps life prolonging. I would classify humor about death into some crude categories. (Each joke or remark may draw on several of these categories.) There is humor that:

1. Diminishes or belittles death, and our concern about it (our existential anxiety).
2. Belittles life, so that losing life becomes less threatening.
3. Pokes fun at our striving for immortality or illusion of the afterlife, and points out our forms of denial.
4. Invokes laughter as a form of therapy.
5. Gallows humor: Makes fun of the illusion of choice as to the time, place, and method of dying. Stresses the inevitability of death.

Freud believed that evidence for the unconscious was found in the material of dreams and humor. Repressed material broke through the usual censorship during sleep, in slips of the tongue, and in jokes (Freud, 1916, 1917). For this reason, so many jokes deal with death, sexuality, aggression, and taboo topics. It is interesting, however, that it was difficult for me to find good jokes about death. Bad jokes abound. For example, "Why is an undertaker the most trustworthy person around? Because he's the last person in the world who'll ever let you down." Another example of a weak joke is "Nothing's certain except death and taxes, and I wish they would come in that order." Everyone has heard cute sayings of small children at funerals. I had a neighbor, old Jack, who was laid out in a tuxedo at his wake. A five-year-old boy looked him over, and asked, "Why do they waste a good suit on him, when he's just going to turn into manure?" For more of the same, see the collection of good, bad, and indifferent jokes in John White's 1988 book, *A Practical Guide to Death and Dying*.

The first type of death humor, *which belittles or diminishes death*, is the most common. There is often a clear contempt for death. It may also make fun of our concern with death, our existential fears, and our quest for meaning. The great humorists are our best source. Mark Twain, for example, cabled from Europe to the Associated Press, "The report of my death was an exaggeration" (Cohen, 1978, N47, p. 401, N23). Woody Allen seems to have made more good jokes about death than anyone else. In one of his films, "Sleeper," the hero is frozen and defrosted in another century. Allen is reputed to have arranged for his own preservation by means of cryonics (the deep freezing of human bodies at death for preservation and possible revival in the future). Because he is a master of using humor to defuse fear of death, I must quote him at length.

In *Getting Even* (1971), a collection of Allen essays, the playlet, "Death Knocks," is a classic. It makes fun of the Bergman movie in which the hero plays chess with Death. It is also a put-down of the Death-figure. Death comes to "take" (another euphemism) Nat Ackerman, but Nat beats Death at gin rummy, and gets one more day to live. He calls his friend Moe.

> Hello, Moe? Me. Listen, I don't know if somebody's playing a joke, or what, but Death was just here. We played a little gin. No, *Death*. In person. Or somebody who claims to be Death. But Moe, he's such a *schlep!*

Another Allen put-down of existential fear is a sequence which ridicules our obsession with man's loneliness in a meaningless universe, pokes fun at suicide, and says 'Let's get on with life and sex while we have time," is from "Play It Again, Sam" (Allen, 1993, p. 183). This is a modern way of saying "Gather ye rosebuds while ye may."

> Allan: (The first name of the character) 'That's quite a lovely Jackson Pollock, isn't it?'
> Woman: 'Yes it is.'
> Allan: 'What does it say to you?'
> Woman:'It restates the negativeness of the universe, the hideous lonely emptiness of existence. Nothingness. The predicament of Man forced to live in a barren, Godless eternity, like a tiny flame flickering in an immense void with nothing but waste, horror and degradation forming a useless bleak straitjacket in a black absurd cosmos.'
> Allan: 'What are you doing Saturday night?'
> Woman: 'Committing suicide.'
> Allan: 'What about Friday night?'

Allen again makes fun of death (and of immortality) by being excessively concrete about work time and clothing after death.

> What is it about death that bothers me so much? Probably the hours. Melnick says the soul is immortal and lives on after the body drops away, but if my soul exists without my body I am convinced that all my clothes will be loose-fitting. (Allen, 1993, p. 245)*

---

* By permission of the author. Credits for these quotations and several shorter ones are given in the permissions acknowledgements section.

Another man named Allen (Ethan Allen) showed his contempt for death in a mixture of humor and anger. His physician said to him "General, I fear the angels are waiting for you." Allen replied: "Waiting, are they? Waiting, are they? Well, goddamn 'em, let 'em wait!" (Seldes, 1967, p. 251). Montaigne said "Of all the benefits which virtue confers on us, the contempt of death is one of the greatest" (Seldes, 1967, p. 254). In fact, since most people consider themselves virtuous, regardless of what evil they have done in life, they can hold death in contempt, unless they are convinced of the existence of an afterlife and judgment. The previous examples show contempt for death, and belittle it.

A second type of joke or remark belittles life. I interpret this as a way of avoiding the threat of death. If life is hard and unbearable, death may be welcome. That is the gist of what Mark Twain said.

> Whoever has lived long enough to find out what life is, knows how deep a debt of gratitude we owe to Adam, the first great benefactor of our race. He brought death into the world. (Seldes, 1967, p. 255)

Samuel Clemens was blessed with many rewards during his life, but he had a mentally ill daughter, and his young secretary ran off with a great deal of the old man's money. Mr. Clemens found out "what life is," but it was a far better life than that of the average man of his time. He had recognition and fame. His put-down of life seems to me a way of diminishing the loss one might feel when contemplating impending death. Loss of a "hard life" is not such a great loss after all. This is one example of cognitive restructuring, a mechanism frequently used when facing the unpleasant. The Biblical Beatitudes are often cited as examples of the "sweet lemon" restructuring. ("Blessed are the meek: for they shall inherit the earth, Matthew 5:5, Blessed are the poor in sprit, for theirs is the kingdom of heaven, Matthew 5:3). The meek and the downtrodden will get their reward in the afterlife, so their suffering in life will be rewarded, and death, by the same token, cannot be all that unwelcome. The "sour grapes" restructuring is more in line with the put-down of life. The fox in the fables of Aesop and Fontaine can't reach the grapes. To compensate, he says they are sour anyhow. If you view your life as sour, you haven't lost so much when you die—just some rotten grapes.

Seeing life as a joke, farce, or comedy is also a sour grape technique. While some death-bed remarks are not really jokes in the ordinary sense, they make a joke out of life itself, and thus make parting easier. Francois Rabelais' last words were "I am going to seek a great perhaps. Draw the curtain; the farce is played out" (Seldes, 1967, p. 254). On his death-bed, Beethoven said "Applaud, friends, the comedy is over" (Seldes, 1967, p. 609). The metaphor of the self as a player on the stage is similar to the familiar quote of Shakespeare, though not as biting as "a tale told by an idiot... signifying nothing." If life is a farce or comedy, we may take leave of it with less sorrow. These three men were accomplished and famous, and they had more meaningful lives than 99 per cent of any who ever lived. For them life became a farce only when it was just about to end.

The third type of humor makes fun of our denials, our illusions of immortality, our hanging on when all hope of life is lost. One of my favorites is the story of the Scot who is dying. He asks his friend Sandy, "Will ye be pouring a bit of whiskey on me grave each morning when I'm gone?" Sandy replies "Sure, but you don't mind if I strain it through me kidneys first?" Sandy is saying that when you're dead, you're dead, period.*

Many "medical jokes" in which doctors tell the patient bad news ridicule our massive denial of death. For example:

> A doctor says to his patient, "Sit down. I've got bad news for you."
> "O.K. Doc, what is it?" "You have incurable cancer." "Oh, my God!" "Not only that, you also have Alzheimer's disease."
> "Oh, thank God! I thought it was something serious, like cancer!"†

How we all like to bargain with death, as in Woody Allen's "Death Knocks." We quibble over the way we die, or the time we'll die, but death is always inevitable. Everyone dies sooner or later, in some manner or other.

My cousin by marriage, Bob Kaufman (now deceased), had an endless supply of jokes. He attributed it to the many hours his fellow-musicians sat in the orchestra pit, waiting to play. To pass the time, they swapped jokes. One of Bob's stories is to my mind a classic death joke, crude but to the point.

> Two men were traveling in Africa, but lost their way, and ended up being captured by a previously unknown tribe. The chief of this tribe had been educated at Oxford (which enabled him to talk English fluently). He told the younger of the two men, "You have two choices; death or Babaluga." The younger man thought to himself, "I'm young. I don't want to die." He said "I choose Babaluga." The next morning two sturdy warriors came to get him. They tied him to a tree, and 200 warriors of the tribe "buggered" (sodomized) him till he was dead. The chief came back to the older man, and said he also had the two choices, death or Babaluga. The older man thought "I am old. Why should I suffer through something like this Babaluga?" He said "I prefer death." The chief motioned to the two warriors, pointed to the captive, and said "Death—by Babaluga."

This horrifying joke operates on many levels. It says that you can't bargain with death. Second, death is inevitable. Third, death is degrading. Sex and violence are blended. The fear of bodily disintegration after death is sometimes greater than the fear of losing life. In this joke, the body disintegrates during life. The illusion of choice has that same "twist of fate" that we find in Macbeth. The three witches say "Macbeth shall never vanquished be until Great Birnam wood to high Dunsinane hill shall come against him." Ironically, Macduff's men use branches as camouflage. The witches also say that "No man of woman born" can harm Macbeth, but Macduff was a Cesarean birth, and Macbeth is doomed. We all know that inevitability is the essence of tragedy, but it is often the basis of comedy. Everyone inevitably suffers his "death by Babaluga."

---

* This story was told to me by Alexander Leighton, a psychiatrist and anthropologist. He told me his own background was Scotch-Irish.

† This joke was told to me by my cousin Bob Kaufman.

The persistence of humans in the face of bodily destruction, and the medicalization of sports reporting, are parodied by Woody Allen in a story about a southpaw pitcher.

> Kirby Kyle had a great future, but he lost a leg hunting rabbits. "He had one leg, but he had something more important. He had heart"...Another accident cost him an arm. Then he lost his sight while duck hunting, but he pitched by "instinct and heart"... "The following year Kirby Kyle was run over by a truck and killed. The following season he won eighteen games in the big league in the sky." (Allen, 1993, p. 166, from "Radio Days")

This tale makes fun of sports writing that is so concerned with players continuing the game, even though they are badly injured. We admire actors who, despite illness, say "The show must go on." Peg-Leg Bates was an famous amputee who tap-danced on his stumps. In the battle of Chevy Chase, a hero named Widdrington fought upon his stumps.

> ... needs must I wayle
> As one in doleful dumpes;
> For when his leggs were smitten off
> He fought upon his stumpes.
> (Percy, 1905, p. ix)

Our heroes never die. In the movie "Viva Zapata," after Zapata dies, someone says "I can see him riding his white horse in the sky." In the song "Joe Hill," Joe, a labor union organizer and martyr, says "I never died." Kirby Kyle is another of those immortal heroes, though he is entirely fictional.

Allen makes further fun of our denial of the fear of death, and our belief in immortality:

> *Kleinman:* It's not that I'm afraid of dying. I just don't want to be there when it happens. (Allen, 1993, p. 249)

> I don't want to achieve immortality through my work, I want to achieve it through not dying. (Allen, 1993, p. 250)

> I don't believe in an afterlife, although I am bringing a change of underwear. (Allen, 1993, p. 258, from "Conversations with Helmholtz")

Truly, Woody Allen has done all of us a great service, he has pointed out our own fears, and made us laugh.

Humor has been known to have therapeutic value for centuries, but it was the treatment regimen of Norman Cousins, told he had only a short time to live, that astounded the world. Cousins, then the editor of the *Saturday Review of Literature,* and a well-known literary figure, rented all the Marx Brothers movies, and projected them over and over again. He laughed himself into health, and wrote about it (Cousins, 1979). After that, he became active in public health. Positive attitudes and laughter seem to boost the immune system. There is evidence that T cells necessary to fight infection are produced in greater numbers when the individual's mood is positive. Neurotransmitters are at higher levels during laughter and pleasurable activity. Serotonin seems the key chemical involved, and now the wonderful effects of humor are beginning to be understood in chemical as well as philosophical terms.

Gallows humor is a standard form, and as its name implies, is the humor of those about to die an inescapable death, often inflicted by others. Weisman (1986, p. 41) says that "one does not usually laugh at a funeral or in church" because some subjects and circumstances "make laughter seem scandalous." While this is very true, there are innumerable jokes about funerals and churches, about corpses, about buying absolution, or lying about recent sins. In an otherwise excellent book, Weisman misses the point that humor is especially about those very solemn subjects of death and religion and morality. He even says so himself, but chooses to focus on the social events of funerals and churchgoing, rather than on the times when one is not in the public eye, when the jokes will fly. He says he has never heard a joke about Auschwitz. Well, here's one example of *Galgenhumor*.

> Hans and Fritz, Gestapo guards at Auschwitz, are chatting. Hans says, "Fritz, it's amazing the way you've picked up all those Yiddish words from the Jewish prisoners. How do you ever manage to remember them all?" Fritz replies with a grin, pointing to his forehead, "I keep it all up here, in my *tokus*" (rear end).

The Jews, who are about to die, have the "last laugh." That is gallows humor!

A less inspired joke appeared in a *New Yorker* cartoon. A man is standing before a firing squad. The Captain of the squad offers him a last cigarette, a common courtesy in such cases. He smiles, but rejects the offer. "No thanks, I'm tapering off."

These jokes and anecdotes are not a random sample, so they are not representative of humor about death. They do illustrate the point that humor is one of the best medicines for diminishing the fear of death and dying. The various types of restructuring that humor affords have been illustrated: belittling or scorning death; belittling life so that death is less of a loss or even welcome; making fun of our denial of death and our belief (conscious or unconscious) in our own immortality and our illusion of choice; humor as therapy influencing the immune system; and gallows humor. While humor can often be aggressive and destructive, in the case of death humor it is generally benign and high on my list of acceptable coping modes. "Laughing it off" has been one of the best medicines, especially when faced with the inevitable. Studies have shown that direct methods of coping, such as confrontation and "talking the problem out," are best in situations arising in the family or in friendships. These direct methods typically failed on the job. The boss was just as likely to fire you as to listen to your complaints. You don't "talk it over" with boss death, contrary to what Woody Allen suggests in "Death Knocks." Humor is an indirect mechanism, and is very effective when your back is against the wall, and you hear the commands "Ready, Aim! ... "

6

INTELLECTUALIZATION

My writing this book is a good example of intellectualization as an anxiety reducing mechanism. On my 70th birthday it dawned on me (with greater impact than usual) that I would not live forever. I had written about coping modes before, but as I have said, the trigger for applying a range of coping modes to the fear of death was Becker's book, *The Denial of Death* (1973). Why was one coping mode, denial, any more important than many others that came to mind? The idea for this book seemed to spring into my mind. Actually, this type of epiphany, or "aha experience" as Freud called it, is probably the result of many years of thinking about both death and coping, but during those years I had not put the ingredients together. I also had a sort of "anniversary reaction" on my 70th birthday, because I remembered that both my father and his brother died at age 73. Was this written in my genes? Did I have only three years to live? If so, why not contribute something of value? In my own grandiose way, I picked a monumental subject (in more ways than one). Who would pick such a difficult subject, and one that is so troublesome to so many people? My motivation to examine this subject had to be strong. I was coping with my fears by distancing myself from them—through intellectualization. I was holding death at arm's length and examining it, as Hamlet holds the skull of Yorick, the jester. There is also a sense of power in being able to discuss a threat in objective terms.

A secondary benefit of this coping mode is that one gathers a great deal of information. This does not lessen anxiety for all people. Some prefer to accept whatever an authority figure tells them. They don't want the details of what's wrong with them, nor do they wish to hear the prognosis. When I go to the doctor, I read up on the problem, and ask a lot of questions, which sometimes annoys the physician. In the same way, I have read books and articles and searched for information about death and dying. Am I better prepared to die? I hope I don't find out too soon. In the meantime, I am so busy writing this book that I have little time to sit and agonize about dying.

Intellectualization is closely related to creativity and obsessive–compulsive behavior. When we say "He (or she) is an intellectual" we imply in a positive way that the person is creative—a thinker. On the down side, we may also imply some compulsivity. This is not an unusual association, since it takes a great deal of concentration and effort to produce a major work of any kind. The anti-intellectual sees this as snobbism, as withdrawal, as different and threatening to his values, and indeed intellectuality does involve all of those qualities to some extent. As mentioned earlier, the creative person must withdraw from society to view life from a new perspective, and his values may directly confront those of his own culture. Not all intellectuals are creative, however, and the obsessive parroting of facts, figures, and statistics can become a meaningless exercise in distancing oneself from any expression of emotion, or a way of avoiding reality.

When I say that intellectualization is a positive mode of coping with death fear, I define it as seeking information about death and dying in a reasonable way, without having it become an obsession that precludes all other activity and normal human relationships. Almost any activity or coping mode can become compulsive. This overdetermined quality is not limited to intellectualization. One can be obsessive about politics, religion, sex, money, gambling, killing, eating, or health. The list is endless.

Intellectualization is at its height in two related fields of endeavor; philosophy and theology. While many philosophers have attacked religion, there is a strong resemblance between the two disciplines. It has been noted that Freud attacked religion as an illusion, but then created his own religion, psychoanalysis, with himself as God and Jung, Rank, Adler, and Ferenczi, among others, as disciples. Any system of ideas that is highly developed shares some of the qualities of religious and philosophical systems. Marxism, Fascism, Socialism, and Democracy are political philosophies that inspire a religious-like fervor for many peoples of the world. Feifel observed that death is a central issue in some important current religions and philosophies: "existentialism and its striking preoccupation with dread and death; Christianity, where the meaning of life is brought to full expression in its termination" (Feifel, 1959, p. 115).

Philosophers, although there are exceptions, have tended to see the dark side of life. Hobbes is famous for his negative view of the state of nature:

> No arts; no letters; no society; and which is worst of all, continual fear and danger of violent death; and the life of man, solitary, poor, nasty, brutish, and short. (Thomas Hobbes) (Cohen, 1978, p. 190; from *Leviathan*, Part i, Ch 13, 1651)

My grounding in philosophy and religion is weak, so I will not attempt to review all the philosophers who paved the way to existentialism, such as Heidegger, Sartre, and others. I have picked a philosopher whose work constitutes an extreme example of the intimate connection between philosophy and death. Jacques Derrida is famous for creating the method of analysis known as "deconstruction." The deconstruction of a text or work of art consists of picking it apart, to find ways in which it is really saying something else than it pretends to say, or fails to make the points it is trying to establish. This is not really very different from "looking under the hood of the car," as Freud did—to not mistake the fenders for the motor. The point of deconstruction is to:

> experience the impossibility of anyone writing or saying (or painting) something that is perfectly clear, the impossibility of constructing a theory or method of inquiry that will answer all questions or the impossibility of fully comprehending weighty matters, like death. (Stephens, 1994, p. 22)

How did Derrida come to make death a central part of his philosophy? We can only make a crude guess, and justly be accused of psychologizing. Yet the path to these ideas (as traumatic as it seems to have been) in no way negates the ideas themselves. Becker, as usual, has insight into this path. He says:

> If there were any doubt that self-esteem is the dominant motive of man there would be one sure way to dispel it, and that would be by showing that when people do not have self-esteem they cannot act. They break down ... When the inner newsreel begins to run consistently negative images of one's worth, the person gives up (Becker, 1962, 1971, p. 75)

What happens to self-esteem when awareness of death, of one's vulnerability, finitude, and helplessness in the face of natural and social forces breaks through the shield of repression? The "movies" and "newsreels" of Derrida are an example of what may happen.

> It is true that I am obsessed with death. I am at every minute attentive to the possibility that in the following hour I will be dead, and the person I am with will say, 'I was just in the room with him, and now he is dead.' This film is constantly in front of my eye. Each time I drive back home, which is about once a day, I watch my car getting into an accident, as if I am in a movie theater, and I hear them say, 'He just left the crossroad, and then he ...' I can't avoid watching. (Stephens, 1994)

Perhaps Derrida's early losses sensitized him to his own helplessness in the face of death. His first experience with death was around age ten, when a younger brother died. An older brother had died in infancy, and his mother showed extreme anxiety whenever Jacques was ill. He failed examinations and had a nervous collapse before graduating from college. He did not defend his doctoral dissertation until age 50, when he was already famous. He refused to be photographed for publication until the year before. This behavior was rationalized in terms of "secrets" and a reaction against the establishment. It seems to speak of poor self-esteem. The ultimate secret or question is death, and there is no answer to it. Stephens, in summing up his view of Derrida, says:

> The more personal of Derrida's mental movies about mortality cause him, he says 'deep anxiety.' It would be unfair to suggest that all of deconstruction, with its many permutations, is a response to that anxiety, but it has certainly helped motivate Derrida's own explanations of the tangled and contradictory. (Stephens, 1994, p. 25)

Is it an exaggeration to say that the philosophy or attitude or method of decon-truction is at least in part an intellectualization of Derrida's fear of death? He himself would deny that the connection is exaggerated.

> All my writing is on death ... If I don't reach the place where I can be reconciled with death, then I will have failed. If I have one goal, it is to accept death and dying. (Stephens, 1994, p. 25)

This man's early concern with death might have been completely crippling. He did founder at times. His ability to intellectualize his fear of death enabled him to have a career in philosophy, and must certainly have improved his self-esteem. His ideas on "impossible secrets" seem to reflect the impossibility of knowing about death and the existence of an afterlife. Death is the greatest secret of all, for no one who has died can tell us about it. The recent best-sellers dealing with dying and rebirth, mentioned before, attest to the public's great interest in the possibility of a reprieve. The story of the Resurrection is not limited to Christianity. It is a very popular theme. Every year there is a "Bridie Murphy" who has been reincarnated, or an amnesiac who regains his memory (is reborn).

I have chosen what may seem like an extreme individual to illustrate the use of intellectualization in warding off death fear, yet the people at the extremes help us to understand the motivation of those in the middle. Moreover, philoso-phers, theologists, and intellectuals are usually more expressive and are often able to write and speak fluently. Poets are intellectuals, and they are able to con-dense and sharpen the ideas and feelings that the average person finds hard to express.

Critics of intellectuals point out their obscurantism, their convoluted think-ing, their frequent withdrawal from society, their "ivory tower" outlook. Spiro Agnew, once Vice President of the United States, was famous for his criticism of "nattering nabobs" and "pointy-headed intellectuals." In addition to these criticisms, the issue of pedantry is often raised with regard to intellectuals and academia.

> The antithesis of laughing it off is tedious, unplayful, lugubrious pedantry. Such heavy and humorless dehumanization makes a joke of itself. When a pedant picks over unimportant details, explains the obvious, uses up too much time, it is like a dog wor-rying a bone: much effort, little nourishment. Wit would dispense with the subject in a flash. (Weisman, 1986, p. 42)

It is often difficult to assess the validity of these criticisms. Much of what intellectuals produce is complex and finely argued. It is often lacking in humor because of the subject matter—death, for example. It is "serious" writing or speech. Intellectuals raise issues that are disturbing, and they are attacked by the right for their radicalism, and by the left for their focus on ideas rather than action. (Derrida has been accused by both sides.)

While many intellectuals are activists, the majority have traditionally hoped that the pen was mightier than the sword, and that their writing would take the place of physical or political action. They have tended to stand by and tell others what they should do or how they should live. This ability to create "inner action" is more typical of the intellectual than it is of the average man. Becker points out that language permits man exclusively to generate inner action, often leading to inaction.

> Of all animals ... he is the best equipped for action in the external world ... Of all animals, paradoxically, he is at the same time alone in being able to stop external action completely, and to keep activity going in controlled inner thought processes alone. Thus the same mechanism that enables him to find an external world more rich than any other animal, permits him to lose the capacity to act in it (Becker, 1964, p. 73)

This down-side of intellectualization is a valid criticism if the individual is facing a problem about which he can reasonably intervene. One's own eventual death, or immediate death, is usually not open to intervention. There are palliatives, some preventive measures, but by and large, death is implacable; the figures of the Grim Reaper or the Juggernaut come to mind.

Hamlet is famous for having his resolution (to kill the King) "sicklied o'er with the pale cast of thought," an enterprise that "lose(s) the name of action." Language and "inner action" play their part in this most famous quotation.

> To be or not to be: that is the question. Whether 'tis nobler in the mind to suffer the slings and arrows of outrageous fortune, or to take arms against a sea of troubles, and by opposing end them? (Hamlet, III.i.56) (Cohen, 1978, p. 316, N29)

Hamlet can intervene by killing the King. He does face the possibility of death if he goes ahead with his plan, but he clearly has two alternatives: action or inaction. Hamlet has been used as an example of the conflicted intellectual, so obsessed with thought that he cannot act. The conflict between thought and action has never been better expressed, in my opinion, than in this famous monologue.

We intellectualize about death because we have no choice (except for some other mechanisms which are mostly substitutes for direct action.) In later discussions of homicide and suicide, which certainly involve direct action, the target is not death itself, but some victim or one's own self.

Because of our lack of choice, we use cognitive restructuring of various kinds in our attempt to solve the problem. This consists of various "inner actions," by which we redefine death, and change our attitudes toward it.

"Philosophy is the practise or rehearsal of death," said Plato (White, 1988; on p. 165, White quotes from the *Phaedo*). Death is the central issue of both philosophy and religion. Cosmology and ethics take second place. I've shown how much a part it plays in the creative arts. The distancing of intellectualization allows us some perspective. It takes away some of the sting, and reduces the threat. In later life people often have an epiphany, in which their whole life falls into perspective. This is a part of the religious experience too. It is a type of conversion. Younger people are also converts, but their conversions of course are usually not concerned with their own imminent death. (The "foxhole religious conversion" during war comes to mind. The ghetto youth as well as the soldier in combat is constantly concerned with imminent death.) There may be a family crisis, a sexual problem, ostracism by peers, or other events that bring on such conversions—both religious and philosophical. These events are experienced as mini-deaths, with severe depression, and in some cases they are relieved by the conversion. This is the "death and rebirth" phenomenon. There is much talk now of reinventing the self. Conservatives see this as changing color too often to match the background—as spinelessness—as a lack of values. Liberals see it as freedom to change and grow. The exaggerated version of this view is that any trauma, such as a death of a loved one or a divorce, is an opportunity for psychological growth, and should be welcomed. This is surely the age of the "sweet lemon," which has been preached by religions for centuries, and by watered-down, popularized psychoanalysis for the latter part of this century. The weight of evidence from research, including my own, would indicate that the cumulative effect of negative life events is mounting mental illness, especially depression and antisocial behavior. I think the "sweet-lemon" rigid optimists deserve the same fate as the philosopher Pangloss in Voltaire's *Candide*, who said "All is for the best in this best of all possible worlds." He repeated this maxim, and when he was thrown into the ocean, they threw a boot at him. He drowned, still repeating his silly mantra.

In sum, while intellectualization has its deficits, it is one of the best devices for defusing the fear of death and dying. It appears in many forms, such as religion, philosophy, and science. It is a mechanism and a coping mode that has produced some of the greatest works of mankind.

7

PROCREATION

The benefits of procreation in the fight against fear of death are so obvious that it is easy to belabor the point. If there is one indisputable way in which mankind has gained the illusion of immortality, it is through having children. Political speeches abound with references to "our forefathers," to the "values of our ancestors," and to our "glorious history of generations." The words *generation* and *progeny* come from the same Latin word, *generare* (to beget). A sense of continuity is produced through having children that is probably unmatched by any other personal act. I was struck by the biographies of my classmates at our 50th Harvard reunion a few years ago. Many of them described their children and wives at length, and played down their own careers as secondary. This was not due to any lack of success on their parts, for many had become distinguished in their own fields of endeavor.

The human obsession with the line of descent has been the subject of much literature. Richard the Third orders the children who are heirs to the throne to be killed. French fathers in the stories of Daudet and Merimee are continually worrying about whether this child is "really theirs" or the progeny of a secret visitor.

Arthur Schnitzler wrote of a man obsessed with his wife's giving birth to a black baby. How could this have happened? Was it her exposure to some statuary in the garden during the pregnancy?

Kings and queens have always been pressured to have offspring, especially male offspring, and the queens are watched carefully to see that no illicit liaison might produce a "pretender" to the throne. During her labor, Marie Antoinette was watched by a large group of court officials, to make sure that nobody substituted a baby not in the royal line.

The Bible, especially the Old Testament, is full of stories about fathers and sons. Abraham wants a child, but Sarah is thought too old to bear it. He has a child named Ishmael by Hagar, a servant, and Sarah promptly sees that mother and son are banished, even though she herself had suggested to Abraham that he sleep with Hagar (Genesis 16:3). Through God's intervention, Sarah at age 90 and Abraham at age 100 conceived a child, and she bore Isaac (Genesis 17:17 and 17:19). On the same day that Isaac was weaned, and the weaning was celebrated with a great feast, Sarah acted against Hagar and Ishmael.

> And Sarah saw the son of Hagar, the Egyptian, which she had born unto Abraham, mocking. Wherefore she said unto Abraham, Cast out this bondswoman and her son: for the son of this bondswoman shall not be heir with my son, even with Isaac. (Genesis 21:9 and 21:10)

God tells Abraham to heed Sarah, and Hagar and Ishmael are banished to the desert wilderness of Beersheba. This story illustrates several points about procreation. First, God promises all parties that he will "make a nation" of their sons. All three are guaranteed that they are the progenitors of nations. This is their claim to immortality. Second, Sarah protects her own biological line in two ways. By banishing Hagar she cuts off the possibility of more children from this source. She also makes sure that the line of inheritance is clear, and that Ishmael shall not be Abraham's heir. While human behavior has not improved much in thousands of years, it at least might be possible today for Hagar to get child support! Third, the importance of an heir (especially a male heir in biblical times) is illustrated. God had to intervene so that Abraham would have a line of descendants.

The topic of wills and testaments is discussed later, but these instruments, in the effects they have on the survivors, are another mechanism by which the power of the dead person is prolonged, as his or her wishes are fulfilled. This is also seen in the grooming and appointment of successors in business, academia, and other organizations.

In modern times it is not often that a couple has the assurance that their children will form a nation or a dynasty. However, the succession of kings had been assured for centuries. The royal families of most of Europe are related by planned intermarriage. When bones of the murdered Czar Peter and his family were discovered, DNA was matched to the blood of Prince Philip of England and others for identification. (These are literally "blood lines.") Many of these marriages were undertaken for political ends. Some were used to secure treaties between two formerly warring countries.

We often speak of "dynasties" in the United States, although we have no official royalty. The Roosevelts, the Kennedys, the Cabots, and the Lodges have all had generations of political leaders, and the first two have been the constant object of media attention. Early studies compared the backward Jukes and Kallikaks (fictitious names of two branches of a family involved in a study of feeblemindedness and antisocial behavior) with the eminent Edwards family of Boston, which sired judges, doctors, and other professionals. The emphasis was on genetics, rather than on social learning and economic advantage or disadvantage. The Bach family in Germany could be considered a dynasty, since beside Johann Sebastian, there were close to 50 descendants of Hans Bach who were composers and musicians!

Having children can confer or consolidate political, economic, or creative power. The production of large families is, by itself, no longer a guarantee of economic success in the United States. When this was an almost totally agrarian society, a landowner would ask an itinerant farmer, "How many hands do you have?" The more children there were, the greater the productivity, and the larger the cropper's share. With the advent of agribusiness, and the virtual disappearance of the small farm, children have become a liability or an expense, rather than a financial asset. They are now valued for their love and companionship, and for their contribution to genetic immortality. They cannot even be counted on to support parents who have reached old age. The government, through Social Security, and corporations, through pensions and annuities, must now serve this function.

With contraception readily available, it is a wonder that young couples have children in this day and age. What is their motivation? The most obvious is sexual satisfaction. The increasing percentage of children born out of wedlock testifies to this. The age at first sexual intercourse has been drifting downward. Probably owing to better nutrition, the age at menarche, or first menstruation, is also lower. Illegitimate births have increased in the majority white population as well as among minorities. For the mothers of many of these children, there is certainly satisfaction from their bonding with their babies, and fulfilling their traditional and biological role of reproduction and mothering. The disadvantages of single motherhood have been repeatedly stressed, especially by the political right wing, which would do away with Welfare. (AFDC, or Aid to Families with Dependent Children.) Yet many unmarried financially secure white and black women have decided to give birth or adopt babies, in order to fulfill their maternal desires. This gives the lie to the contention that young women are having illegitimate babies only to receive larger Welfare payments.

More evidence of maternal and paternal drives is the extreme effort barren parents make to become pregnant or adopt a child. Artificial insemination is an expensive procedure, whether in vivo or in vitro (done in a test tube). The various tests for father's and mother's fertility are expensive, and the effort to become pregnant may be prolonged and depressing. Despite all this, thousands of parents persist until they have a baby by some method. The adoption process is slow, and again very expensive. Black-market white babies cost in the tens of thousands of dollars. Babies are imported from the Philippines, and from Romania, among other countries that are poverty stricken. These babies again are expensive to adopt, and are often physically or psychologically damaged due to their isolation in orphanages.

The fulfillment of parental roles in conformity with the cultural norms is certainly a motivating force. Parents sometimes ask, "When am I going to be a grandparent?" Social pressure may come from the peer group. ("All my girlfriends have babies, and that's all they talk about.") Grandparents' visiting and adoptive rights have become an issue recently in cases where one of the parents dies, or there is a divorce, or a parent is drug addicted or mentally ill.

Our focus is on one major motivation for having children, in addition to the emotional gains through shared love, the fulfillment of parental role demands, sexual gratification, and increasing economic or political power. The sense of continuity, the "dynasty complex," the feeling that something of one's own flesh and blood will live on after one's death, is an underlying motivation in procreation. The achievement of a type of immortality, by creating children, by continuing one's gene pool (as the sociobiologists would say), is a bulwark against the fear of death. One exists "perpetually" through one's children and the generations that follow. This biological continuity is a poor substitute for not dying, but it is probably a better choice than immortality through creativity (as I defined it), since styles and taste in literature, painting, and even science may change rapidly. But there is no assurance that one's offspring will continue to reproduce.

The obsession with male children in cultures such as the Chinese and the traditional Jewish may have to do with either the system of inheritance or the maintenance of the family name, as well as cultural bias against women. The English system of primogeniture gave the entire inheritance to the firstborn son. In Ireland, the custom was to give the farm to the favorite son, which accounted for a great deal of sibling rivalry and postponed marriage (Arensberg, 1940). The traditional Chinese custom was to divide land equally among all children ("per stirpes," in our legal language). This resulted in the division of land into such narrow strips that they were often impossible to cultivate. Since the recent limitation of one child per couple in China, reports of female infanticide have been frequent. The new laws are more easily enforceable in the city than in the countryside, but the desire to have more than one child is apparently still strong, according to reports of widespread evasion of the law.

With the divorce rate hovering around 50 percent in the United States, the access to abortion and contraception is denied or made burdensome by right wing pressure on the Bush administration, the birth rates may shoot up again. Use of reproduction as a bridge to immortality must eventually be diminished. This coping mode may become less and less effective in protecting against death fears. The birth rate has also been falling, although there are strong social-class differences in the decline. If access to abortion is denied, the birth rates may shoot up again. This will increase the number of unwanted children substantially. How that may affect feelings of immortality is anyone's guess. My own thoughts on this are that the unwanted child just increases the unwed mother's (and father's) fear of death and deprivation. You are less likely to achieve a sense of pride in family and continuity from a child's birth when you really wanted an abortion and couldn't get one.

In a crowded world, there is a growing stigma attached to large families. The idea of Zero Population Growth is spreading. The environmental movement has until recently been limited to developed countries, and to the wealthier classes in those countries. As we approach eight to ten billion in world population, and

the dire predictions of Armageddon and worldwide starvation approach realization, most countries may impose a limit of one child per couple, as in China.
The achievement of immortality through one's children will then become less
attractive as a psychological option in the fight against death. Pride in succession
will become a cardinal sin, and no one will say "Go forth and multiply."

8

Obsessive–Compulsive Behavior

Repetitive, ceremonial, and compulsive behaviors have long been known to be defenses against anxiety. A typical example is compulsive hand washing (to control anxiety over some sexual or aggressive trespass, such as Lady Macbeth's "Out, out, damned spot!"). Another is found in the child's control of aggressive thoughts by avoiding the cracks in the sidewalk "Step on a crack, break your mother's back." Counting to ten is a repetitive behavior invoked to avoid cursing or violent behavior. Head banging and rocking in children, called "repetitive motor behavior," is another expression of compulsive behavior, and is an attempt to control inner conflict and relieve tension.

Repetition, especially in its most noncompulsive form, is part of what life is all about. We have to eat, work, and sleep, or else we die. Freud said that "Beauty, cleanliness and order are among the requirements of civilization." Of order he said:

> Order is a kind of repetition-compulsion by which it is ordained once for all when, where and how a thing shall be done so that on similar occasion doubt and hesitation shall be avoided. The benefits of order are incontestable: it enables us to use space and time to the best advantage, while saving expenditure of mental energy. (Freud, 1929, p. 40)

These functions (eating, working, etc.) can ideally go on without the addicted and pressured feelings of "compulsion." Modern society, unfortunately, is far from ideal in this respect, and people in "primitive" societies and developing or deprived societies are far from unpressured. When we see people who cannot help but repeat a behavior or are plagued by an idea that interferes with their role functioning, we think of the label "obsessional neurosis" or "obsessive–compulsive behavior." The "neurotic personality" at one time was the most dominant in "developed" societies. Erik Erickson, in talking about anal training and development of independence in the young child, reflects the clinical viewpoint of the 1960s when he discusses the "compulsive type."

…the machine age has provided the ideal of a mechanically trained, faultlessly functioning, and always clean, punctual, and deodorized body. In addition, it has been more or less superstitiously assumed that early and rigorous training is absolutely necessary for the kind of personality which will function efficiently in a mechanized world in which time is money. Thus the child becomes a machine which must be set and tuned. Our clinical work suggests that the neurotics of our time include the *compulsive type*, who is stingy, retentive, and meticulous in matters of affection, time, and money as well as in the management of his bowels. (Erickson, 1968, p. 108)

There has been a shift in the type of patient seen by psychotherapists from the conversion hysteric (often a paralysis of a limb, associated with sexual repression) of the 1800s and early 1900s to the compulsive type, and from the 1970s to the borderline (preschizophrenic) and narcissistic personality disorders.

In Freud's time, hysteria and obsessional neurosis carried to extremes the personality traits associated with the capitalist order at an earlier stage in its development—acquisitiveness, fanatical devotion to work, and a fierce repression of sexuality. In our time (1979) the pre-schizophrenic, borderline, or personality disorders have attracted increasing attention, along with schizophrenia itself. (Lasch, 1979)

While it is dangerous to jump from impressions of clinical patients to generalizations about the character structure of a whole society, it is a shortcut that social scientists often use. If there were not such a dearth of in-depth studies of the personalities of representative cross sections of the population, these leaps would not be necessary. However, such epidemiological studies of the general (treated *and* untreated) population are expensive, and may become scarcer than ever in the present era of cutbacks in long-term family research funding.

I might venture a guess that the obsessive–compulsive and well-enculturated individual has become so commonplace in our society that he or she is no longer seen as a "sore thumb." Erich Fromm coined the term "the culturally patterned defect." If you have such a defect, you do not suffer exclusion or ostracism because of your symptoms. You are surrounded by people who exhibit the same type of behavior, and thus you do not seek therapy. The punctual workaholic is not only accepted by our society, but is also rewarded by it. It is only when the behavior is extreme that it interferes with enjoyment and with relationships with people. It fits in well with the bureaucratic society, and with the business world. Kenneth Burke pointed out that it may fit in too well, so that people are "fit in an unfit fitness" (Burke, 1954). This raises the issue of the "sick society," which is dysfunctional for its citizens.

Regardless of its drawbacks, compulsivity is a major mechanism in the fight against fear of death and dying. When it is focused on work, it may lead to great productivity, although it can interfere with the freedom to create new methods and approaches to problems. There is a free associative aspect to both creative science and art that doesn't thrive in the compulsive personality. "Ideally," the compulsive individual is not obsessed with death directly. The compulsive behavior is a substitute for and escape from thoughts about death.*

There are many partially related terms for the obsessive–compulsive coping mechanism, making for some confusion. Some of these terms, such as "alienation," which has been discussed at great length, overlap only slightly. Others, such as "automatism," "the mirror self" (George Herbert Mead, 1962), and "pathological narcissism" (Lasch, 1979), share some of the characteristics of compulsivity. Conformity to the values and behavior of the group was central to David Riesman's "other-directed type" (Riesman, 1950). The other-directed person's "radar" was always searching for signals from others. America was moving away from individuality and "inner direction," symbolized by the gyroscope. A spate of labels for the American character appeared.

> William H. Whyte's "organization man," Erich Fromm's "market-oriented personality," Karen Horney's "neurotic personality of our time," and studies of American national character by Margaret Mead and Geoffrey Gorer all captured essential aspects of the new man; his eagerness to get along well with others; his need to organize even his private life in accordance with the requirements of large organizations; his attempt to sell himself as if his own personality were a commodity with an assignable market value; his neurotic need for affection, reassurance and oral gratification; the corruptibility of his values (Lasch, 1979, p. 123)

The common thread in these types is the compulsive conformity to the society and to the demands of others. Lasch (1979) tried to use the clinical syndrome of pathological narcissism as a description of the changing American character. [This can be a dangerous procedure, as evidenced by many books. As a good example, take *Is Germany Incurable?*, by Richard Brickner (1943), which applied the symptoms of clinical paranoia to German culture. The leap from individual to group is common, but sometimes strained.] Lasch's description of narcissistic traits overlaps that of the compulsive–conformist type in only one area: "dependence on the vicarious warmth provided by others" (Lasch, 1979, p. 75). Rather than having a fear of dependence, a trait of the narcissist, the conformist shows a fear of independence. There is a whole list of traits that are not part of the compulsive–conformist type.

---

* Obsession with death itself (not controlled by compulsivity or other defense mechanisms) can mean many things (e.g., in the dying patient) but in the healthy person, it is often a cover-up, a means of avoidance.

> It is very enlightening to find people who are constantly thinking of the past or death…Fear of death or sickness is a typical characteristic of people who are seeking an excuse to avoid all duties and obligations. They loudly proclaim that all is vanity, that life is woefully brief and that no one can know what will happen. As we have seen, such individuals avoid all tests because their pride prevents them from submitting to a trial that would disclose their real worth. [Adler, 1927 (original publ), reprinted 1994]

Compulsivity is easy to see in the routine and time-keeping of most people's lives. These traits are at an extreme in U.S. culture. Lewis Mumford stresses the "temporal regularity" of modern machine civilization. Regularity, which "arbitrarily rules over human functions ... reduces existence to mere time-serving." He likens such a life to a "prison house" (Mumford, 1934, p. 115).

The term "alienation" is used to cover a multitude of syndromes. It is too broad to describe the conformist-routinized coping mode that I see as a major method of controlling fear of death. In their introduction to a volume of essays on alienation, the Josephsons want to limit the term "alienation" to mean "an individual feeling or state of dissociation from self, from others, and from the world at large" (Josephson, 1962, p. 13). They point out that the term has been used

> ... to refer to an extraordinary variety of psycho-social disorders, including loss of self, anxiety states, anomie, despair, depersonalization, rootlessness, apathy, social disorganization, loneliness, atomization, powerlessness, meaninglessness, isolation, pessimism, and the loss of beliefs or values. (Josephson, 1962, p. 13)

This use of "alienation" as dissociation is in some ways the opposite of our use of obsessive–compulsive, which stresses routine and conformity to society, not dissociation from it. Thus alienation is discussed further under the mechanism of dissociation.

The real world is chaotic, and the most threatening possibility in this chaos is death. It is "normal" to try to control and impose order on the physical and social world. This is the goal of Becker's "well-enculturated actor":

> At the other extreme from the schizophrenic (*the dissociated is again the opposite of the obsessive–conformist, italics mine*) is the well-enculturated actor. The external world is harnessed for use: objects are treated by their use-aspects, put in their place, subdued, subserved to the intentions of the human agent. Everything is ordered. The once chaotic world is seen through rose-colored cultural glasses. By means of sure answers to common human problems, behavior is decisive, objects are created and enslaved.

> But it is not only objects that are enslaved. The fully performing cultural actor is enthralled by his own world view. His very fluid mastery becomes a rigidity of habit of the smug. As he wears his well-beaten cultural path through the world of things man keeps his nose to the ground and passes that world by, for the most part. (Becker, 1964, p. 235)

In our culture this man is "normal." But is he healthy? While he fits in with the cultural norms, his rigidity and his "nose to the ground" (also his "nose to the grindstone," via the work ethic), keep him in a state of enslavement. He is safe in his routine, but he has lost the freshness of the artistic vision. Through routine he has achieved apparent safety from death and chaos, but this steals away any creativity he may have had. It is a bargain, made at a great sacrifice. The majority of people in U.S. culture are like the younger children in Piaget's experiments, who said that you can play marbles only one way—the way they were taught ("moral realism") Why? Because that's the way marbles have always been played. Following the cultural rules rigidly is the mark of the compulsive type.

Becker's description (though applied to "man" in general!) is the clearest and most poetic of any I have read:

> Man cuts out for himself a manageable world. He throws himself into action uncritically, unthinkingly. He accepts the cultural programming that turns his nose where he is supposed to look. He doesn't have to have fears when his feet are solidly mired and his life mapped out in a ready-made maze. All he has to do is plunge ahead in a *compulsive style of drivenness* (italics mine) in the 'ways of the world' that the child learns and in which he lives later as a kind of grim equanimity—the 'strange power of living in the moment and ignoring and forgetting'—as James put it. (Becker, 1973, p. 23)

This description fits so many of our cultural types—the "workaholic," the striving politician-bureaucrat who shuns real decisions, the conformist "good-wife-and-mother" who may find her life a sham as she looks back. The work roles, the routines of the office, the factory, and of child-rearing and home-making, act as a "social corset" holding us together. The fear of death suddenly breaks through when there is a loss of a loved one through death or divorce, or the loss of a job that seemed secure.

The story of Lisa Foster, the wife of Vincent Foster, who was President Clinton's attorney, is illustrative. She was always a good wife and mother, churchgoing and sociable. She denied her husband's depression. When he committed suicide in Washington, D.C. (apparently in response to the stress of the political life) her whole world collapsed. Her faith in God disappeared. She raged against God and society. She considered suicide. (Luckily, she sought therapy and later remarried.)

> I hated everything. I was mad as hell. You can't pray, because you don't know what you're praying for. You're mad as hell at God, and so you don't know what to say. You don't want to say 'Help me,' because you think He's screwed you. If I got one card about Jesus, I must have gotten a thousand. Well, where was Jesus when I needed him? I don't know why God did this to me. You know, we're supposed to be the children of God—I wouldn't do something like this to one of my children. (Boyer, 1995, p. 62)

All the defenses of routine and compulsivity fall away at such a time of loss. Love itself is a great protector against death fear, but when a loved one is lost, the lover is more vulnerable than ever. Thus love may be one of the riskier defenses. (See Chapter 4 of this book.) Lisa's religion also did not sustain her in this crisis. She saw her years of being a good wife and mother ("enculturated") as wasted or useless, and was furious.

How many thousands of news stories tell of a man who went berserk after his wife or girlfriend left him (O. J. Simpson?) or after he lost his job? Suicide or murder often follows. What is surprising is that we don't read of more of these events. The social corset has burst, and rage and fear are uncontrolled. The sacrifices made to become a conformist now seem wasted. The loss of identity, self-esteem, and life goals complete the personality disintegration. It is not only celebrities that go berserk. Every day there is another tragedy.

A man (Juan Liriano, 43) recently released from prison, enraged after a fight with his girlfriend, opened fire inside their apartment in Corona, Queens, early yesterday, killing their six-year-old daughter and the woman's two teen-age daughters before fatally shooting himself. The gunfire erupted following an argument between the couple about their relationship. He was insecure and jealous toward Migdalia Sosa, whom residents described as pretty and attractive. (Holloway, 1995, p. 43–44)

The recent case of Susan Smith, who strapped her two young boys in their seat belts and drowned them in a lake, was also triggered by a loss of a potential lover, one who was wealthy and could have supported her in style. He wrote her a letter, saying that he couldn't take on the responsibility of two young children, and wanted to break off the relationship. Shortly after that, she tearfully reported them kidnapped on television, and set off a frantic search for a phantom black kidnapper. She confessed to the murder after the police found discrepancies in her story.

These cases, especially that of Lisa Foster, point out the fragility of obsessive enculturation as a defense. Juan Liriano was perhaps the least enculturated of these three, yet he had been out of prison for two months, and was holding a job in a relative's grocery store.

Obsessive striving (especially in the work sphere) can act as an anodyne in several ways, helping to reduce the fear of death:

1. "I have no time to fear death. I'm too busy. My mind is so full of details that there is no room for fear of death."
2. "I will be remembered for my success. That is how I can gain a bit of immortality."
3. "I am a good person because I work hard, and I will achieve a state of grace, go to heaven, and probably get a good obituary" (the Protestant Ethic). I can buy and consume goods, to show that I am worthy (Thorstein Veblen's "conspicuous consumption").

Becker sees that repression (of the fear of death) can be a positive force. It uses life energy creatively (i.e., puts it into work, striving, etc.).

I mean that fears are naturally absorbed by expansive organismic striving. On the most elemental level the organism works actively against its own fragility by seeking to expand and perpetuate itself in living experience; instead of shrinking, it moves toward more life. Also, it does one thing at a time, avoiding needless distractions from *all-absorbing activity*; (italics mine). In this way, it would seem, fear of death can be carefully ignored or actually absorbed in the life-expanding processes. (Becker, 1973, p. 21)

This all-absorbing activity can be viewed as positive, or when it interferes with functioning, as in other life settings, as the negative side of this coping mechanism. For example, the workaholic might succeed in business, academia, or in writing novels, but he or she might neglect spouse, children, and friends. Most of the great creative figures have been immersed in their work to the detriment of other role functions. Would we consider that immersion negative or pathological? Our culture has valued "well-roundedness" more than most other cultures, so we tend to judge rather harshly those people who clearly excel in one functional area while slighting others.

How are we to reconcile Becker's positive view of "all-absorbing activity" with his phrase "compulsive style of drivenness" (quoted above)? I think it is in part a matter of degree. "Drivenness" implies the inability to decrease or give up the activity. "All-absorbing" does not suggest a strong addiction to the activity. Perhaps the difference can be found when a sudden change in life, such as retirement, takes away the activity by which the person is held together against fears of dying and annihilation. The reactions that ensue (a pleasant retirement taken up with hobbies or new interests, as opposed to a disastrous retirement with depression and the early advent of physical illness) can actually indicate the degree to which work was "driven" (compulsive) or not.

I remember how my father retired from his partnership in his patent-law firm "to make room for the younger men." Actually, it was mandatory, owing to an agreement between the senior partners. Within months he was in a tearful depression. I sent him to a friend, co-author and colleague, Dr. Stanley T. Michael Stanley, a psychiatrist, who suggested that he immediately go back to work in his office as a "dollar-a-year man." Dad became an advisor to the younger lawyers. He was no threat to the partners, since he took none of their money, and had no real power. His depression lifted, and he enjoyed his life's work almost to his death. Leaving his work had been like a death to him, since the strenuous routine was his "corset." His strong reaction to retiring demonstrated that he was a workaholic, and that he was under compulsion to work. His work was more than "all-absorbing." It was the linchpin of his functioning.

If this obsession with work (or any activity that can consume time and energy and occupy the mind) really serves a terror-containing function, then moments of quiet contemplation should be very threatening to these frenetic types (another litmus test of compulsivity). We have all heard stories about the Chief Executive Officer (CEO) of some large corporation who becomes extremely restless during his vacation and can't wait to get back to the office. Is this because he is having an affair with his secretary? Not usually. It is because he can't stand the horrible thoughts he has about death and loss that come into his mind while he's sitting on the beach. If he has a fishing, hunting, or hiking vacation, he can remain active, and banish the fear of death. (By killing he gains even more power over death.) How many of our U.S. presidents have been hunters, fishermen, sailors, or travelers! These travels typically involve dangerous adventures (the white water rafting of Clinton, fishing and boating of Bush, sailing of Kennedy, and the African safaris of Theodore Roosevelt). The compulsively hyperactive man remains so on vacation, for this is his main source of inner control. It is what he enjoys both for its own sake and because it keeps him together.

A forced convalescence after an illness has caused much anxiety for these compulsively active individuals. They may have to face themselves for the first time. The example of Franklin D. Roosevelt comes to mind again. He was an active sailor whose life changed dramatically after his paralysis. (The role of blood sports and athletics in the upper classes of Europe and later in the Americas should not be overlooked. These are the training grounds for power and dominance over others. The "playing fields of Eton" have been cited as the school of British empire.)

John Kennedy, despite constant pain due to his back injury, still engaged in a high level of political, physical, and sexual activity. His brush with near-death by drowning while in the U.S. Navy, after his PT boat, No. 109, was sunk, may have made him very sensitive to the fragility of his life and body. Much of his activity may have been compensatory. His injury and convalescence did not radically change his lifestyle, perhaps because he wasn't severely paralyzed (as was the case with Franklin Roosevelt). His drivenness may have stemmed in part from the injury experience, and of course in part from the Kennedy parents' great expectations.

What is the function of the obsessive behavior? How does it function in the neurotic? How is the obsessional neurotic different from the common "compulsive style of drivenness"? Freud thought that the symptoms of neurosis were "substitutive gratification for unfulfilled sexual wishes" (Freud, 1929, p. 71). He looked on neurotic symptoms as a compromise formation between the instinct (or drive) and the demands of society (as internalized, by means of the introjection of the parents). "When an instinctual trend undergoes repression, its libidinal elements are transformed into symptoms, and its aggressive components into a sense of guilt" (Freud, 1929) (i.e., the aggressive components are turned back onto the self through the super-ego).

Becker takes a more modern view of symptom formation. He discusses the role that symptoms such as obsessions, compulsions, and phobias play in the dynamics of the psychiatric patient. The extreme neurotic is used as an exaggerated example of the dynamics of the average man (an assumption that is not always warranted). Becker quotes Roy Waldman:

> Thus, neurotic symptoms serve to reduce and narrow—to magically transform the world so that he may be distracted from his concerns of death, guilt, and meaninglessness. The neurotic preoccupied with his symptom is led to believe that his central task is one of confrontation with his particular obsession or phobia. In a sense his neurosis allows him to take control of his destiny—to transform the whole of life's meaning into the simplified meaning emanating from his self-created world.... (Becker, 1973, p. 181, quoting Waldman, 1971, pp. 123–124)

This states the essence of our idea about the reductive role of metaphor, and the "poetic" quality of symptoms. Over and above the distraction provided by the symptom, it reduces the multiple problems that face each individual to one simple problem. In this way it is economical.

The difference between the obsessional neurotic (who might have symptoms such as excessive hand washing, or elaborate routines for bedtime or eating) and the workaholic CEO is that the neurotic's "symptom choice" has interfered with his ability to function in a culturally approved manner. The CEO's symptom, workaholism, is "ego-syntonic"—that is, he likes it. It also "fits" the culture, and he is rewarded for it. The neurotic's hand washing, in contrast, leaves his hands raw, and keeps him in the men's room so long that he may lose his job. If severe enough, he may not even be able to travel to work. In another case, eating habits may be so bizarre as to be objectionable to friends and family, and interfere with role functioning in the home setting. In addition, the neurotic doesn't *like* his symptom. It is "ego-dyssyntonic." That's why he goes to a therapist, while the CEO scorns therapy until there is a severe crisis or loss.

The "simplification of meaning" is not by any means confined to neurotic individuals. Every person seizes on some theme, some event, some motto or symptom that he or she feels will encapsulate and simplify the meaning of his or her life. Of course, humor relies on exaggeration, so the following joke refers to a man with an extreme obsession. He is referred to a psychiatrist, who asks him, "Why are you here?" He says, "My friends told me to see you, because I think I'm dead." The doctor says, "Do you agree with me that dead men don't bleed?" The patient says he agrees. At that moment the doctor grabs a scalpel and jabs it into the patient's finger. Blood drips to the floor. "Well, what do you think now?" "Hmm, I guess dead men *do* bleed!"

The common element is the inability of the individual to break the habit (compulsion) or change the belief (obsession). How similar this is to drug addiction and alcoholism, which is discussed later under Dissociation. We all know how difficult it is to persuade someone whose opinion differs from ours. These deeply ingrained ideas and beliefs are defended unto the grave. Rigidity is not confined to neurotic individuals. I had intended to write more about these "fiercely defended ideas," but found that such a discussion of scientific quarrels and the "culture wars" would fill another book!

These themes and ideas and values die hard, if ever, because they are so central to the continuing functioning of the individual, even though they may seem superficial. To me they are a *shorthand* way of explaining the complexities of life—an often desperate attempt to understand what has happened. It is simpler to say "My father seduced me" or "My mother was cold and unloving," than to examine the details of the relationships. One can blame genetics: "I had a psychotic uncle, so maybe it runs in the family" or a symptom: "My hands are dirty, so I have to wash all the time." It is like a character in a murder mystery saying, "The butler did it!"

Epiphanies

Most people can tell you about an epiphany ("a sudden intuitive perception or insight into the reality or meaning of something, usually initiated by some simple, homely, or commonplace occurrence or experience") (Flexner, 1987, p. 653)* that changed their lives. These were moments that gave them shining insight into their lives, and events that gave their lives meaning and new direction. To my mind, these epiphanies or revelations are often a shorthand—a metaphor—for a process that had been going on for a long time. The epiphany and the neurotic symptom (obsession, compulsion, or phobia) are all partly metaphors. They have the quality of poetry, using condensation, allusion, and approaching the issues indirectly and symbolically. They sharpen, distort, and encapsulate, making it simple to remember. They are like puns—a condensed way of explaining life, by running motives together, just as one forces disparate words together in a pun. Freud showed how dreams, slips of the tongue, and humor (especially puns) shared all these characteristics found in the symptoms. They were his evidence for the existence of the unconscious.

Epiphanies may be the result of specialized thought or research. They are the sudden "breakthroughs" or insights not only into one's own life and motivation, but also into an artistic, philosophic, or scientific problem. Some of the epiphanies that occur after long thought come under the heading of "serendipity." In these cases luck combined with a prepared mind has produced some of the great scientific discoveries. The case most frequently cited is the discovery of penicillin, by Sir Alexander Fleming.

The structure of the benzene ring supposedly came to Friedrich August Kekulé (1829–1896) in a dream (a true epiphany!). He dreamt that he saw six snakes biting each other's tails, to form a ring. This suggested six carbon atoms in a hexagonal ring, with alternating single and double bonds joining them. This was the key to organic chemistry. Yet another time he said he dreamt that six maidens were dancing with their arms locked. He later denied that he had a dream. No doubt he had thought about this structure for years. The "epiphany" probably emerged from the sorting out of competing models, and not something that came out of the blue. Again, the snakes may be a metaphor that sums up all the deep thinking that Kekulé, a leading German chemist, must have done over a considerable period. The poetic quality of the image is fascinating for its ability to convey the structure so dramatically. That the joined snakes are an image from the subconscious mind, sounding like a dream or a myth, makes it akin to the obsessive symptom, but with a great difference. The image is inspired and

---

* Note the biblical origin, in the Christian festival of Epiphany, celebrating the manifestation of Christ in the persons of the Magi.

original. Moreover, it enhances the scientist's functioning, rather than impairing it, as in the case of the neurotic. This scientist brought order to the chaos of the molecular world. The benzene ring became the building block of the field of organic chemistry, and opened up new understanding of physiology and life itself! It made possible the synthesis of thousands of lifesaving drugs used in medicine today.

"Recovered memories" are a type of epiphany. The "aha-experience" of patients in psychotherapy who just recall that someone sexually abused them has become a U.S. cottage industry. It is not that there aren't thousands or even millions of physically and sexually abused children. These abuses also cut across social class lines, so that abuse occurs in wealthy as well as poor families. However, there is money to be made, not only by therapists, who may sometimes induce these memories. District attorneys prosecute parents, teachers, and other caretakers who have been accused of child abuse. Defense lawyers fight back, proclaiming the innocence of their clients. They sue the accusers—usually a child or young adult—and act to protect an unjustly accused molester. Many "molesters" have been acquitted after harrowing trials and years of struggle and defamation. A young woman teacher has just been acquitted of all charges. A father, an ex-policeman, accused by his two daughters of sexual abuse, lost his wife, his job, and all his money fighting back. The girls fantasized that he belonged to a Satanic cult, and that he and several fellow policemen had raped them. He has now sued the police psychologist and others who encouraged the fantasies.

Although there are great numbers of actual seductions of children, the turning tide of acquittals of accused parents suggests that many patients use "seduction" or "sexual abuse" as a metaphor for the various other types of abuse to which they have been subjected by parents—namely physical and verbal punishment, coldness, and extreme emotional lability (alternating between rage and loving behavior). These were the major factors in emotional disorder in our longitudinal study of 2000 children.*

The basic problem is that real and fantasy seduction exist side by side, and it is hard to determine the truth. If patients do fantasize about having sex with their opposite-sex parent, as Freud posited in the Oedipus (and Electra) complex, when and how often does this fantasy become true? Only longitudinal observational family studies focusing on children from birth on can begin to get a handle on this knotty problem. These are the most expensive studies to conduct, and one research team is unlikely to live long enough to complete the work. In addition, given the current "family values" rhetoric of the right wing of the Republican party, such studies of incest would be a direct threat. Who would

---

* Langner, T. S. (1969, 1970, 1974, 1976); Gersten, J. C. (1974, 1976); Eisenberg, J. G. (1976); McCarthy, E. D. (1975); Greene, E. L. (1973).

want to fund studies that would besmirch the American Family with talk of incest? Out of sight is out of mind.

Jeffrey Masson has accused the psychoanalysts of ignoring the reality of sexual abuse of children. He may be an intellectual "gigolo," as depicted by Janet Malcolm in her *New Yorker* articles, and the book based on them (Malcolm, 1983). He sued her for libel, and won. Lately she located her lost interview notes, and will probably counter-sue. Despite the theatrics on both sides, Masson has raised a real issue: that Freud may have ignored the reality of sexual abuse and labeled it fantasy (wish-fulfillment on the part of the child) because calling it real would have brought the medical (and governmental) establishment down on his head. It might have killed the young psychoanalytic movement completely.

That Freud would consciously make such a choice is doubtful. However, Zvi Lothane, a psychoanalyst, has written a book describing the ordeal of Dr. Sabina Spielrein (Lothane, 1992). As an adolescent, Spielrein had severe neurotic symptoms. Her parents took her to Carl Jung, who had a clinic in Zurich. Jung seduced his patient. Her mother discovered this, and complained bitterly to Freud. Freud played down the problem and did not intervene with Jung. Later Freud invited Spielrein to come and train with him as an analyst, and she did brilliantly. Lothane points out that Freud desperately wanted psychoanalysis to spread outside Germany, and to involve some non-Jewish psychiatrists. Jung (being Gentile, and living in Switzerland) fitted the bill, and confronting him might have curtailed the spread of psychoanalysis. The point is that Freud, consciously or unconsciously, would have done almost anything to promote his theory and his new form of psychotherapy. Avoiding the accusation that many Germans seduced their children, and avoiding the fact that Jung seduced his patient (which would have given psychoanalysis a bad name) seem to be smart choices made to protect a medical and intellectual movement in its infancy.

My own studies have shown, in the previously listed journal publications by myself and a team of co-workers that a majority of children in a cross-sectional New York City sample are abused physically and/or emotionally by parents. This is by the mother's report, and it is surprising that the mothers admit to such abuses. Severe physical punishment is still not considered cruel and unacceptable. In contrast, in almost no cases did mothers report sexual abuse by the father or a male figure. This is not only socially disapproved, but is also criminal behavior. Nevertheless, mothers described in detail spanking (often with an object in hand), hitting, food deprivation, burning, and many other punishments. Apparently none of these parental behaviors was seen as socially undesirable, except by some highly educated parents, many of whom probably lied when such questions came up. In short, "sexual abuse" reported by children, or adults looking back at their childhood, may sometimes be a metaphor for all the parental coldness, lability, and physical punishment the child has experienced.

The questions of how often and under what circumstances and within which social groups remain important matters for research to unravel.

Three examples of what we might call a "political epiphany" again point out the metaphorical nature of the single traumatic experience the individual selects as the turning point, the "aha." Three men who belong to E Pluribus Unum, an extreme right-wing political group, see the U.S. Government as the enemy, taking away their constitutional freedoms, and preparing America for a takeover by the United Nations (sic!). They believe that the Government itself bombed its own building in Oklahoma City, killing children as well as adults, so that it could justify greater surveillance of right-wing groups. Some said (in a remarkable example of paranoid distortion) that the actual bomber, Timothy J. McVeigh, was a Federal agent! Each of the three men interviewed said he had an experience that changed his political opinions radically to the right (an epiphany, though none of the three used this word).

> Many of the people in this dissident movement have something else in common: a single, profound experience that helped forge the prism through which they see a world of conspiracies and corrupt government. (Janofsky, 1995)

The events that they say triggered their scared and hateful views do not sound convincing to me.

> For Mr. Monroe, the turning point was the Kennedy assassination in 1963. For James Johnson, a utility company lineman who is black, it was a clash with white police officers more than 30 years ago. For Steven May, the owner of a small roofing company, it was a sexual harassment case that ended in the dismissal of the complaint against him but that cost him $4000 in legal fees.

In fact, these "turning points" are just easy markers to symbolize the long road to such extremely paranoid ideas. Mr. May actually says that 30 years ago he campaigned for the Republican presidential candidate Barry Goldwater. His conservative ideology was obviously brewing for a long time. Mr. Monroe said his distrust of government started at age 11, when his grandfather told him, "If they shot Kennedy, they can shoot anybody." Yet years later, as an adult, he learned from a friend that a "global secret government was ready to take over the United States." A vague distrust in childhood blossomed into a very specific ideology much later in his life.

Mr. Johnson was eight years old when two police officers "jumped out of their car and threw me up against the wall." He determined to rely on himself, not the government, to improve his life. He says we will soon be "taxed into involuntary servitude. This country is headed toward enslavement." The paradox of a black man being active in a racist organization brings his logic into question. His fear of enslavement (by the government) may be quirkily related to his being black. For a people who were enslaved, this might be an appropriate fear. However, it seems inappropriate for him to parrot right-wing ideology about being *taxed* into slavery! There is no reason to doubt that blacks, even from an early age, have been beaten up by white police. There is recent evidence that this behavior is far from diminishing. The beating of Rodney King by a group of white Los Angeles policemen was captured on videotape. Riots followed. During the trial of O. J. Simpson, a Los Angeles police detective, Mark Fuhrmann, was a witness for the prosecution. Later on, tape recordings were produced by the defense, showing that he used racial slurs and epithets almost constantly during interviews with a writer who wanted realistic police material for a television script. He said that "the only good nigger is a dead nigger." We can easily believe that Mr. Johnson was bullied or even injured by the two policemen as a child. However, his experience as a black person in Buffalo, N.Y., both before and after the incident at age eight, must have been very negative. He sums up his early experience at home, in school, and on the streets with one incident, the cops. They are another metaphor, a shorthand, for all the misery before and after the incident. They are not a fantasy, but I doubt very much that this one incident alone was responsible for his joining a group that hates his own kind, and for adopting such an extreme and idiosyncratic ideology. (He is apparently not in a high tax bracket!)

Apart from the havoc wrought upon our society by such extreme political groups, what is saddest of all is the need to explain a bewildering and complex world largely in terms of one incident (or one symptom, as in the neurotic). The bombing in Oklahoma City (in which 168 people were killed), and the shoot-out at Ruby Ridge, Idaho (in which the wife and son of Randy Weaver, a militant anti-tax racist, were killed by Treasury Department sharpshooters) are shocking, complex, and puzzling events. Along with the incident in which 80 people were killed in a conflict between Treasury agents and the Branch Davidians near Waco, Texas, these conflicts between the United States and right-wing militants or dissidents involve some tragic mistakes on the part of the government.

An inflamed response has come from the militant right, from the National Rifle Association, and the Patriots' Movement. The paranoid ideas of these groups, and of the three men interviewed, seem such a feeble, confused, and topsy-turvy response to the problems of racism, sexism, unemployment, poor education, the health-care shortage, the housing shortage, the child-care shortage, poor parenting, and other grave dilemmas facing this country. The United Nations, Blacks, Catholics, Jews, and "government bureaucrats" are again a warped shorthand for all the ills of our society.* Claude Raines, the Police Inspector in the movie "Casablanca," summed it up in his famous line, "Round up the usual suspects." (This quote works both ways, because the Inspector was an authority figure, supposedly dedicated to upholding the law. He said this with a smirk or grin, indicating

* These are clearly examples of projection onto target groups. Projection is discussed later as a separate mechanism, along with prejudice, demonization, evil, and Satan.

that it was just a gesture by the police, and wouldn't actually result in an arrest.) So both the authorities and the radicals have their "usual suspects." The radicals of the left suspect bankers, Jews, Catholics, colonialists, and the bourgeoisie, while on the right the United Nations, Jews, blacks, Catholics, and Treasury (government) agents are the villains. Remarkably, the Jews can be seen as "international bankers" or penurious penny-pinching misers. Being Jewish myself, I wouldn't mind being rich like the former, and would hate to be the latter.

ORDERLINESS

Elizabeth Kübler-Ross said that many dying patients want to set things in order before they die. We could add that most of us want to make order out of the chaos of the world and of our own affairs long before we are on our death beds. This is a normal wish, but when it becomes extreme as in the obsessive–compulsive, everything has to be neat, clean, and orderly. *Craig's Wife*, a novel later made into a movie, portrays a woman who won't let her husband tip his cigarette ashes into an ashtray without rushing to wash it out. He finally leaves her. Of course, she also tries to control him through her obsession with cleanliness.

A little compulsivity is necessary for survival in the modern world. We eat, work, and make love by the clock. Our desks have to be neat, and our files logical, or we can't function. We pay bills and taxes, and must keep some records of what we've paid or still owe. A majority of us bank our money, and get statements or have a passbook. We need a certain degree of organization and neatness in our lives. Today computers and the Internet are supposed to help us with this organization. Very often we find that our hard disks crash, that our programs have bugs, and that it is hard to get on line and to stay on line.

REPETITION

Repetition is the essence of the compulsive neurotic (the excessive hand washer) and also of Becker's "well-enculturated actor" (the average or "normal" person in our culture). Lichtenstein, in an early article, takes a look at the basic meaning of repetition.

> Repetition is an attempt or a tendency to transcend the irreversibility of the flow of time. (Lictenstein, 1977, 1983, p. 28)

He quotes Heraclitus: "Nobody is capable of diving into the same river twice" (Lichtenstein, 1977, 1983, p. 27). Despite this truth, the obsessive–compulsive and the well-enculturated individual keep on diving, hoping that this activity will make the river hold still.

TIME

Lichtenstein says that to give events and customs duration (immortality) they must be repeated. Holidays, birthdays, parades, and inaugurations must be repeated each year (or every four years) to keep these customs (and the societies and values that go with them) "alive." This repetition in turn keeps the individual feeling "alive." Perhaps some of the apparent immortality of his society will rub off on him. (I say *apparent*, for we should not forget the transient nature of the "Thousand Year Deutsches Reich," 1933–1945, the British Empire, the Roman Empire, and the ephemeral kingdom of Alexander the Great). Hence the power of group membership (discussed later).

Repetition, compulsivity, ceremonial behavior, and obsessions are all ways of stopping time. Why would anyone want to stop time? First, it makes it possible to enjoy now what one may not be able to enjoy later, when old age or death set in. The motto here is, "Gather ye rosebuds while ye may." Second, time-stopping keeps death away that much longer. There is an actual sense of time going more slowly, so life (though it may be more routine) seems longer.

The "rosebud" theme and death are linked in nursery rhymes. For example:

Ring-a-ring-a-rosie
Pocket full of posies.
Ashes, ashes, we all fall down.

This is probably a corruption of the folk-rhyme "Gather ye rosebuds." and the common burial prayer:

We therefore commit his (her) body to the ground;
Earth to earth, ashes to ashes, dust to dust;
in sure and certain hope of the Resurrection to
eternal life. (Cohen, 1978, p. 272, from "Committal" The Book of Common Prayer)

That very young children should already be thinking about death, although in seemingly once-removed games, rhymes, and songs, is not very astonishing. They are being readied for death from the cradle on! There are two obvious examples of early introduction of the concept of death by parents and caretakers. First, there is the bedtime prayer:

Now I lay me down to sleep.
I pray the Lord my soul to keep.
If I die before I wake
I pray the Lord my soul to take.

Reinforcing the association between sleep and death is far from an example of good parenting. A second gem which can exacerbate fear of death is "Rock-a-bye, baby," perhaps the commonest lullaby in the English-speaking world.

Rock-a-bye, baby, in the tree top.
When the wind blows, the cradle will rock.

> When the bough breaks, the cradle will fall,
> And down will come cradle, baby, and all.

The "gathering rosebuds" theme is a common metaphor for the pleasures of youth. Robert Herrick's (1591–1674) version is the most famous. Note the juxtaposition of Time and Death, which is an intrinsic part of the "rosebuds" theme.

> Gather ye rosebuds while ye may,
> Old Time is still a-flying;
> And this same flower that smiles today,
> Tomorrow will be dying.
> (Cohen, 1978, p. 189, N9, from Herrick's
> "To Virgins, to Make Much of Time)

It seems as if our concept of time would be very different if we lived forever. Death makes us aware of time. It leads to calendars, and to counting the years and the decades. We divide the life span into segments—infancy, childhood, the teens, young adulthood, middle age, old age (and now, "very old age") Each of these milestones can become a millstone, if we focus on approaching death. Because of the decimal system, and our ten fingers, many of us have a crisis as each new decade approaches. Physical markers contribute to our time sense: crawling, sitting, toddling, walking, loss of baby teeth, the advent of puberty, the appearance of a girl's breasts, a boy's first shave, the menarche, the first gray hairs, the menopause, and various physical changes due to aging. The physical and emotional changes belonging to each stage are immortalized in Shakespeare's "seven ages of man" (Cohen, 1978, p.311, N14).*

In sum, compulsivity and obsessions offer a "social corset" that helps to keep death fear at bay, but often at a steep price in individual freedom and creativity. These same compulsions and obsessions can sometimes result in great contributions to society for some exceptional individuals. Most people, however, who are deeply enculturated cannot be inventive because they cannot see the world anew. They are too much part of their society. Hence the implicit conflict between creativity and compulsivity (conformity, other-directedness, drivenness, rigidity, etc.)

---

* "All the worlds's a stage …"—the infant, the whining school-boy, the lover, the soldier, the justice, the pantaloon, and second childhood.

Living Life to the Hilt, Living Better, Living Longer

Living to the hilt, although it has its down side like all other coping modes, seems one of the more pleasant ways of dealing with death fear. "Hilt" is defined as "the handle of a sword or dagger," and "to the hilt" as "to the maximum extent or degree, completely, fully." It is hard to find agreement on what "living fully" means. For some it may be the intellectual life, for some the life of the creative artist, and for others, making money. I have defined it specifically to avoid these definitions, and limit its meaning to a life of hedonism, of sexual, gastronomic, and other indulgence. The Dionysian ideal, "Eat, drink and be merry, for tomorrow we die" is its core philosophy. The pursuit of happiness is even written into Jefferson's draft of the Declaration of Independence. This pursuit, when carried to today's extremes, has led to conspicuous consumption without limits.

Living to the hilt could be called a revolt against repression. The strictures of society are ignored. Adults as well as adolescents live in a state of rebellion. (Rebellion implies a compulsion to behave against societal norms.) The pure Dionysian would be "recklessly uninhibited, unrestrained, undisciplined, frenzied, orgiastic" (Flexner, 1987).

There is a tradition of Dionysianism in America. One of its greatest exponents was Walt Whitman, who said, "If any thing is sacred the human body is sacred" (Cohen, 1978, p. 415, quoted from Walt Whitman, "I sing the body electric").

Norman Brown felt that death fear was due primarily to repression, which stood in the way of happiness.

> But if repression were overcome and man could enjoy the life proper to his species, the regressive fixation to the past would dissolve; the restless quest for novelty would be reabsorbed into the desire for pleasurable repetition; the desire to Become would be reabsorbed into the desire to Be. (Brown, 1959)

In terror lest society dissolve in an explosion of pleasure-seeking without concern for the welfare of others, Becker criticizes Brown's advocacy of abolishing repression.

> It (Norman Brown's *Life Against Death*) is prized not for its shattering revelations on death and anality, but for its wholly non-sequitur conclusions: for its plea for the unrepressed life, the resurrection of the body as the seat of primary pleasure, the abolition of shame and guilt. Brown concludes that mankind can only transcend the terrible toll that the fear of death takes if it *lives the body fully* and does not allow an *unlived life* (italics mine) to poison existence, to sap pleasure, and to leave a residue of regret. (Becker, 1973, pp. 260–261)

The newer the stimulus, the greater its power. This is attributable in part to the process of extinction set up in our nervous system. People who have suffered heart attacks are told that intercourse with their spouses will not be life-threatening, but the stimulus of a new partner may kill them. Newness is a big sell in our culture. "New Ivory Soap," new breakfast cereals, and new dress styles are touted as better than the old products. This spills over into sex as well as marketing, which seems to suggest sexual or economic anomie. The desire for something new—our ideas of living to the hilt, or fully—may be a fantasy of one long orgy with one partner, or a continuous orgy with many partners. It is probable that extinction will take care of the first case, and exhaustion eventually take care of the second. "Shop till you drop" is a consumer's war cry, actually used in some advertising.

In many cultures there are special times when inhibitions and repressions are lifted and free expression is allowed and encouraged. These are usually joyous festivals, such as carnivals (*carne levare,* or lifting of meat, which takes place before Lent). They are like safety valves for the expression of all that has been suppressed the rest of the year.

The "bachelor party" (a dying ritual) was a last fling for the bridegroom-to-be. It usually involved pornographic movies, strip teases, nude dancing, and uninhibited sex. All this was a way of saying farewell to the relatively uninhibited single life, and hello to the (supposedly) restrictive bonds of marriage. This male apprehension of marriage is probably at least as old as the institution of marriage itself. It was well expressed by that master of dry wit, Samuel Johnson:

> Sir, it is so far from being natural for a man and woman to live in a state of marriage, that we find all the motives that they have for remaining in that connection, and the restraints which civilized society imposes to prevent separation, are hardly sufficient to keep them together. (Cohen, 1978, p. 208, N25, quoting Samuel Johnson in Boswell's *Life of Johnson*)

There are other days or periods when inhibitions are thrown off. Leap year is supposed to allow women a more aggressive role in initiating sex. Following the cartoon characters in "Little Abner," teenagers in the 1930s and 1940s were allowing girls to choose partners on "Daisy Mae Day." The "women's choice" is found in many tribal ceremonies. I was chosen by women (no invitation could be declined) during the Bear Dance of the Southern Ute Indians. This was one of the more pleasurable aspects of doing field work for my doctorate in Colorado. This role reversal of "women's choice" has often been practiced in folk dancing. "Living it up" has been part of the scene at least since the Dionysian festivals. In early America, the pioneers had their wild times as they moved West. "Sweet Betsy from Pike" apparently knew how to let off steam after a hard day's traveling:

> Out on the desert one bright starry night,
> They broke out the whiskey and Betsy got tight,
> She whooped and she hollered, and danced 'cross the plain,
> And she showed her bare arse to the whole wagon train.

After the high times of the "forty-niner" (the 1849 "Gold Rush") era there were other relatively uninhibited periods. Prohibition spurred a great deal of drinking. The "roaring twenties" were associated with sex, alcohol (booze), and physical violence. F. Scott Fitzgerald and Ernest Hemingway were two of the icons of the day, along with Al Capone and Dutch Schultz. In the 1930s to 1960s, the Hollywood "Rat Pack" was known for its high living, drinking, and fist fights, and Haight-Ashbury and Woodstock were known for drugs and orgiastic concerts lasting days. Jack Kerouac's novel, *On the Road*, celebrated multiple sex partners, alcohol, and drugs.

> Moriarty, a good-natured and slap-happy reform-school alumnus, is pathologically given to aimless travel, women, car stealing, reefers, bop jazz, liquor and pseudo-intellectual talk, as though life were just one long joy-ride that can't be stopped. (Dempsey, 1996)

This living to the hilt was taken up by only a small portion of the society at any one time, but it was attractive to the majority, who fed vicariously on the titillating details.

There seems to have been a recent shift from the Dionysian to what Ruth Benedict called the Apollonian ethos (well-balanced, poised, and disciplined behavior). With our concern for longevity growing more acute each year, we are less likely to eat (watch that cholesterol and animal fat!) or drink (alcohol destroys the brain cells—take no more than one drink a day to protect against heart attacks!). We are left with being merry. If this consists in part of sex, we must watch out for AIDS, venereal disease, and sexual addiction!

In reality, we have entered a new Victorian period, something akin to the "secular asceticism" of Max Weber. It is no longer driven by the desire to appear industrious in the eyes of God. It is focused on acquiring more worldly goods, and living longer and better. The "live to the hilt" people are probably distinct from the "living longer and better" group. They want to "burn their candles at both ends," as Edna St. Vincent Millay said:

> My candle burns at both ends;
> It shall not last the night;

But, ah, my foes, and oh, my friends—
It gives a lovely light.
(Figs from Thistles, "First Fig")
(Cohen, 1978, p. 251, N13)

The coping mode of "living to the hilt" may be supportive for a while, but "It will not last the night." The lovely light that comes from burning the candle at both ends is bound to go out soon—twice as fast as a candle that burns at one end. If living to the hilt is defined as an orgiastic life, then it has the same drawbacks as Promiscuous Love (Chapter 4). The lulls between affairs, flings, and one-night stands become more depressing with time and age. It becomes more difficult with time to keep the wolf (death) from the door.

If drugs and alcohol are part of the definition of "living to the hilt," then there is temporary relief from dread and anxiety, but progressively larger doses are needed to be effective. The neurological damage incurred eventually affects all relationships, and the ability to work or to love another person. The drugs become the goal, the center, and a downward economic and emotional spiral usually ensues.

If by "living to the hilt" we mean not hedonism (the seeking of pleasure for its own sake) but dedication to some purpose—creativity, the support of and love for another person (a spouse, children, a lover), or immersing oneself in some religious or political faith—then there is more of a chance for control of death fear. But that is another definition of "living to the hilt" or "living fully," which is covered in the separate chapters on creativity, religion, and love. This dedication to what is sometimes called a "higher purpose" does not preclude enjoyment.

LIVING LONGER AND LIVING BETTER

Living longer and better are closely intertwined, so I will treat them together. They are not your typical ego defense mechanisms, but they are goals that involve particular lifestyles, and we can link them to certain personality types or lifestyles. They seem broader than defense mechanisms, and it may be better to call them coping modes. Living longer is obviously based on a concern with death and dying. The search for life extension is just a watered down version of the search for immortality. Procedures to reverse signs of aging— liposuction, erasing wrinkles, tummy tucks, hair dying—are feeble attempts at stretching out youthful life, or at least a certain lifestyle. There is nothing fundamentally wrong with wanting to look attractive to others. But an obsession with one's looks, with the signs of aging, and with slight loss of memory will not really slow down the aging process, and may even exacerbate fear of dying.

Medicine, in its fight to reduce both mortality and morbidity, has succeeded in more than doubling the life span, and this is a monumental achievement.

However, living longer does not necessarily mean living better. Modern medicine has attempted to prolong the life span, but after the development of vaccines and the introduction of antibiotics, there has not been much further improvement of the life span in Western cultures. (The improvement in developing countries has been astounding, but this is because the death rate has historically been very high in such continents as Africa and parts of Asia and in countries such as Somalia and Bangladesh.)

Michael Norman (1996) divides old age into two periods. The first, from 65 to 85, runs from retirement to the onset of physical decline. In the second period are the "oldest old," those over 85. This period "is marked by what gerontologists call the 'dreadful D's'—decline, deterioration, dependency, death." He points out that our cultural values emphasize independence, mastery, and youth. Given the inability of the oldest old to be independent, some have suggested that the elderly should focus on religion, family, or some unit larger than themselves that would offer them transcendence. Norman shows that it is expecting too much of the elderly to come up with a meaning for their lives on their own, without cultural supports. This is especially true in a society that is no longer traditional, but rather transitional, where people of all ages are searching for meaning.

Scientific research has found there are three hormones that are candidates for reversing the effects of aging. According to Nicholas Wade (1996) these are pituitary growth hormone, DHEA (an adrenal hormone), and melatonin (a pineal hormone). Unfortunately, all of these hormones have serious side effects. Melatonin, because it is not a drug, is not monitored by the FDA, and its formulations can contain impurities (as in the case of imported L-tryptophan, which killed several people in the early 1990s before it was banned). Quoting the view that "the body is genetically programmed to last a certain time and then fall to pieces all at once" (like Emerson's "One Horse Shay"),* Wade submits that a single pill is unlikely to stop aging, and that seeking a cure for aging is a "fruitless quest." There is as yet no magic elixir, no "Fountain of Youth" such as Juan Ponce de Leon envisioned.

A slightly more hopeful view is given by Malcolm Gladwell (Gladwell, 1996, p. 59). He first asks, "If we are now on the verge of adding new years to human life, what kind of years will we be adding"? We may be able to cut down on morbidity as well as mortality, or we may breed a nation of oldsters who are half blind, toothless, deaf, crippled people who cannot live independently. New discoveries about how the body's cells are timed might lead to some greater life extension.

---

* The Shay, or Chaise, was a horse-drawn carriage. In the poem, each part was made exactly as strong as the next, so that when it aged, it collapsed all at once.

Fibroblasts are "repair kits" for the skin. They make collegenase to repair sun damage or cuts. Inside each fibroblast is a telomere, a kind of "timing device." Every time a fibroblast divides and the chromosomes form two new cells, the telomere gets a bit shorter. After about 50 divisions, the cells can no longer divide—the telomere "timer" has cut off cell reproduction. "The length of your telomeres may be a better indicator of how 'old' you are than the number of years you have lived" (Gladwell, 1996, p. 61). (If you bake yourself in the sun , you will look very old by forty or fifty.) The idea of cellular clocks is now a hot issue in biology.

Of course, the hope of the life extensionists is that there will be some way of controlling cellular clocks (which turn cell division *off*) so that they will continue to run but not cause the cell proliferation that is cancer. The popular interest in the quest for immortality is shown by a headline in 1994: "Immortality Enzyme Is Discovered." The telomeres in cancer cells are protected and even renewed by the enzyme telomerase, hence the "immortality enzyme" label.

Will eliminating cancer or heart disease, the two big killers, extend the life span? On average, eliminating cancer would give a typical American only about three extra years of life expectancy. Gladwell points out that the average 70-year-old American woman has a life expectancy of 85 years, 12 of which will be active, and 3 of which will be inactive (bedridden, incapable of independent living). Curing cancer, would give her an extra 14 months of life, but only half of those months will be active. Other illnesses will crop up: diabetes, arthritis, Alzheimer's, Parkinson's, osteoporosis, varicose veins, migraines, arthritis, hearing, vision, and orthopedic problems.

> ... in old age we really don't want to get rid of the diseases that kill us before we've got rid of the diseases that slow us down, that rob us of our independence, that put us at the mercy of someone else. (Gladwell, 1996, p. 65)

Life extension as a means of sustaining youth is probably a fantasy. If there is any real lengthening of the life span, it will probably result in a prolonged late middle age. Gladwell cites Dr. Michael Rose, who has done the pioneer work on telomeres. Rose sees life extension as a trade-off. (*La vie en rose?*) The "high testosterone surge of insanity" will be lost, but the acquisition of knowledge and the development of a personal philosophy will be gained. Currently, people die just as they are at the top of their productive ability, particularly in the sciences and in philosophy. (It has been pointed out *ad nauseam* that this is strikingly untrue of mathematics.)

Will people live longer and better as a result of new surgical procedures? Will organ transplants enable us to become more like machines with replaceable parts? Certainly for the victim of a heart attack, a coronary bypass or balloon angioplasty can add a few years of life, and can often restore remarkably good functioning. Angioplasty has to be repeated in almost half the cases.

Endarterectomy (typically on a clogged carotid artery) can clear out plaque, and greatly diminish the chance of a stroke. In the past, men who were unable to get an erection (impotence) as they grew older needed penile implants. Alternatively, they could have used self-injections of a chemical that would allow them a rigid half-hour. The advent of Viagra has made it possible for a majority of impotent males to have erections without pain. Hearts, corneas, livers, and kidneys can be transplanted, if the patient is lucky enough to find a compatible organ donor. We have entered the age of preventive remedial surgery, the era of the "bionic man." It is clear, however, that while these procedures may make living less painful, and even more enjoyable, they do not significantly extend the average life span.

There is a saying, "Be careful what you wish for. Your wish may come true." The wish for longevity may be just such a nightmare, ending with a world full of ancient cripples. It reminds me of the short story, "The Monkey's Paw." A magical shriveled monkey's paw allows a family to have three wishes. They wish their son were alive again, and that he might return home. Their son, a bloody misshapen creature after being crushed by the machinery where he worked, comes scratching at the door. His parents see him, and terrified, make the third and last wish, to have him dead again. If we live into the hundreds, will we also be misshapen creatures? Will our children and grandchildren want us dead?

Are we living better as a result of our growing obsession with health? Are we a nation, or even a world, of hypochondriacs, or are we just exhibiting a healthy self-concern? Hypochondria is defined as "excessive preoccupation with one's health, usually focused on some particular symptom, such as cardiac or gastric problems" (Flexner, 1987, p. 943). As usual, the problem is to define what is excessive, and definitions of what is normal or excessive can be conditioned by culture, by the environment, or many other factors.

Expressions of concern about health have been described as more frequent among Italians and Jews in the United States. In contrast, there has been a stereotype of the Protestant, especially the New Englander, as being stoic, and denying health problems even when they are serious. Which of these is more pathological: the obsession with health problems or their denial? Certainly severe denial of illness can be fatal, and studies at Cornell Medical College (by Harold Wolff and Lawrence Hinckle) showed that men had fewer illness episodes than women, but a much larger proportion of the male episodes were fatal. This denial is clearly part of the "macho" complex, or what Talcott Parsons called the "sissy complex." It is a platitude that men have to break their identification with their mothers who are almost always the early primary caretakers, while women don't need to disidentify with their mothers. This complex, which is evidenced, for example, by a boy's refusal to comb his hair and a (very temporary) disgust with girls, also includes an avoidance of crying or concern over injuries. This is carried over into adult life, and if extreme, can result in death by illness or accident.

Concern with health is not new. There is an American tradition of selling and using nostrums, patent medicines, formulas, and various drugs to ensure health and cure disease. The term "snake oil" describes well the usually ineffective medicines that used to be sold by pitch men at county fairs and circuses. A large number of these mixtures contained alcohol, and if they didn't cure the disease, they at least produced a pleasant alcoholic glow in the self-medicating patient.

Times have not changed much, and the over-the-counter drug market today is a multibillion dollar industry. Most of the drugs sold only by prescription in the United States. are sold over the counter in developing countries. While great strides have been made in creating antibiotics to counteract infectious diseases, there are often severe side effects and drug interactions, particularly among the elderly and children.

The drug companies promote their products by giving physicians free samples, paying travel and expenses for seminars on their products at professional meetings, and by visits from trained salesmen who describe and recommend their latest products. The public hears about new drugs, and clamors for them, often when the drugs have not even been tested or approved by the FDA. This is like a *folie-a-trois*, involving the drug companies, the doctors, and the health-obsessed public.

I have always been concerned with my health. Upon turning 70, I subscribed to no less than three health newsletters. I found them useful in learning about advances in medicine, about drugs and their side effects and interactions, and about various types of prevention and intervention. Reading these newsletters helped me to ask more intelligent questions of my doctors. Am I a hypochondriac? Yes. Am I obsessive about my health? Yes. Do I feel that it is pathological or dysfunctional? No. I have been able to make better decisions and get more information from my physicians.

It is interesting that prostate cancer topped the list of the ten topics most frequently covered by 30 health newsletters in 1995 (the ranks are shown in parentheses) (Hamlin, 1995, p. C2). Clearly, the list is slanted toward older people, but some items, such as antioxidants (3), saturated fats (5), and Prozac (8) could apply equally to the whole age range. Topics such as heart disease (6) and Alzheimer's disease (10) seem to apply equally to men and women. Prostate cancer (1) and impotence (7) are balanced by breast cancer (4), estrogen therapy (2), and natural progesterone (9).

Not in the first ten, but close behind, were low-carbohydrate diet, gene therapy, diabetes, weight training versus aerobics, and chronic fatigue. These subjects, with the exception of diabetes, seem to apply to a wide age range.

The subscribership of the five newsletters with the largest circulation ranges between 425,000 and 750,000. Most health newsletters are published nationwide, range in price from $24 to $50 per year, and are aimed at nonprofessionals. They are more evidence of our nation's concern with health, as if more proof were needed.

Added to newsletters, television programs, and newspaper columns about health is the ever-increasing flood of books on every imaginable disease and condition known to man (and animal). There are health books for men and women; on child and infant disorders; for those over 50; for victims of heart attack, diabetes, prostate cancer, and so on. Then there are the autobiographies of people who have had these diseases, or are in the process of dying from them, such as AIDS, cancer, and so forth. There are even books on pet health, farm animal health, recovery from drug addiction, alcoholism (as far back as *The Lost Weekend*), sex addiction, spousal abuse, and childhood sexual abuse, among others. There is no dearth of information. There is probably an overload of it, but it may be difficult for some of us to obtain.

Not all of this concern with health is bad. The goal seems to be to make everyone an informed medical consumer, and with the revolutionary changes going on in the U.S. medical system today, it behooves us to be well informed. Many people cannot afford 20–40 dollars for a subscription to a newsletter or to buy a medical self-help book. Does this mean that concern with medical care is limited to the wealthy? I think not. The concern is there, but the information is not readily available to the poor. It has been repeatedly shown that the lower the socioeconomic status, the less information is obtainable about your health, and the less you can ask your doctor questions (assuming you even have a doctor). In the past, women were less apt than men to ask for and to get information from their doctors. This is slowly changing, as women demand more information and respect from their physicians, and as more women become doctors.

Despite all the improvements in medical technology, its distribution is spotty, just as medical information is unevenly distributed. While organ transplants and coronary bypass operations may be more available to the wealthy, heart attacks don't discriminate by social class. Sudden cardiac arrest kills 250,000 people in the United States each year. The only way to treat it and save lives is to apply electric shock to the heart. This is done with a defibrillator, but most ambulances don't carry them

> Every minute's delay in returning the heart to its normal pattern of beating decreases the patient's chance of survival by 10 percent, experts said at a meeting held by the American Heart Association. This means, they said, that a person's fate is essentially decided within 10 minutes of the attack. (Leary, 1994, p. C3)

Plans are under way to develop less expensive defibrillators that could be placed in all ambulances, and in police and rescue vehicles. In addition, they could be placed in office buildings, malls, bus and train terminals, and airports. The current heart attack survival rate is under 10%, and in New York City it is 2%! We may scoff at the idea of saving the heart attack victim and decry the expense involved, but for the survivor and his or her family (in most cases) no expense will have seemed too great.

It seems cruel and inhuman that cost–benefit analysis and the practice of triage (first helping those most likely to survive, a procedure initially developed on the battlefield) are being applied to needy patients.

In my own recent experience with "bottom line" triage, my cousin, who was slowly dying of bladder and kidney cancer, previously had both organs removed. He was on dialysis, when his Medicare funds were suddenly denied. The doctor in charge of all services came to the hospital room where he was being dialyzed, and shouted at him, "We want you out of here. There is nothing more we can do for you. We want to make room for someone we can help …" He had not looked at my cousin's chart, or he would have seen that the patient had not been told that he was terminal. This was a tremendous shock to a man in his mid 60s, already weakened by his disease. He died the next day.

Although there are knotty ethical dilemmas and insoluble economic problems arising in medicine, there is no excuse among medical staff or family members for harsh treatment or lack of compassion for the sick and the dying. The anger of caretakers at patients who "refuse" to get well, or the rage of family members whose money, time, and patience are being eaten up by the patient's illness, are well documented.

It is hardly necessary, in the light of these problems, to point out again that living longer, and getting "better" health care, may have negative effects on the patient, his or her survivors, and on the society as a whole.

Beauty, Health, and Sex: Living Better?

Most people believe that looking better will lead to living better. Some may feel that their self-esteem is enhanced by changing the way they look. Heightened self-esteem is a key weapon in the fight against death fear and anxiety. Looking better was formerly effected mostly by the use of stylish clothing and makeup. The beauty industry now permeates almost every aspects of our lives, but it has been, up until recently, more focused on women than on men. Don't forget that rich men's clothing was quite expressive and competitive during the Middle Ages and the Renaissance. Lace, satin breeches, and wigs were still common among the wealthier American colonists.

Although makeup, such as kohl, has been used to darken eyebrows and eyelids since early Egyptian times, the use of beauty aids has only recently grown to massive proportions. Naomi Wolf, in *The Beauty Myth*, claims that beauty work took over from housework over the last 35 years (Jefferson, 1996, p. 109). She documents an "alternative female world":

> … by recording just about every form of obsession and exploitation a $20 billion-a-year cosmetics industry, a $33 billion diet industry, a $300 million cosmetic surgery industry and a $7 billion pornography industry can nurture and supply.

Most importantly, Ms. Wolf claims that this alternative female world is just as repressive as the former world of women, which relegated them to the home, childbearing and childrearing, and the church. (The German motto for the female ghetto was *Kinder, Küche, und Kirche*, or children, kitchen, and church.) Wolf sees children and young men and women "being imprinted with a sexuality that is mass-produced, deliberately dehumanizing and inhuman." I see no reason to limit this indictment of the beauty culture to any age group. Eleanor Dana O'Connell is an example of how the search for a positive self-image through good looks has spanned the age range She became a Ziegfeld Girl in 1921 when she was 17. She is now 92.

> A widow for 25 years, she is on the lookout for 'a light love affair,' though she doubts the, ahem, agility of gentlemen her age. Two months ago she spent $4000 to have her eyes touched up by a plastic surgeon. 'If I only live two years so what?' said Mrs. O'Connell, her blue eyes dancing mischievously. 'I've had two years of joy' (Martin, 1996, p. B17)

As usual, from the observer's viewpoint, Eleanor may have been "dehumanized" early on by being labeled a "girl" and valued only for her beauty. Her cosmetic surgery could be viewed as vain, wasteful, exploitative, and even risky at her age. From her own point of view, she received "joy" and hope from the operation. Her good looks made her good life possible, and she wants to preserve them, and the possibility of meeting a "gentleman." You can't help but admire her vitality.

Approximately 400,000 cosmetic surgeries were done in 1994, and fewer than half of the people involved could be considered at all wealthy. These operations are not covered by health insurance, so the motivation to undergo them must be very strong. One motive is certainly to avoid the effects of aging. A second (and not necessarily a secondary one) is the wish to be sexually attractive. Other factors have influenced the growth of this industry.

> This growing acceptance of plastic surgery may reflect more than America's peculiar (?) inability to let go of youth or the advances in surgical techniques. We are witnessing a fundamental change in our thinking about the body...(We) mark upon our increasingly disengaged, physically disappointed selves (by tattoos and body jewelry). Selves that, with the proliferation of Instamatic cameras and video camcorders and computer-imaging machines, we now routinely contemplate from afar. (Siebert, 1996, p. 22)

Siebert lists some of the reconstructive surgery now available: hair replacement, brow lifts, drooping eyelids and puffy bags, ears, noses, liposuction (removing fat deposits), chemical skin peeling, dermabrasion (acne removal), face lifts, facial implants (for receding chins or shallow cheekbones), tightening upper-arm skin, breast enlargements or lifts, male breast reduction, tummy tucks, pectoral and calf implants, buttock restructuring, and phalloplasty (lengthening and thickening of the penis). The risks of these procedures have been greatly reduced, but are still a factor to consider before opting for this type of surgery.

Men have increasing flocked to plastic surgeons. Hair transplants have been in vogue for some time. Rogaine (minoxidil) and Retin-A (retinoic acid) are applied in the hope of sprouting new growth. Male pattern baldness is evidence of a high level of testosterone. In spite of the macho implications, male baldness is viewed primarily as another sign of aging, and therefore undesirable. Even the popularity of the stage and screen star Yul Brynner's shining bald head could not turn the tide of public opinion. Baldness can be very beautiful. The Samburu women of Kenya have shaved heads, and I think they are among the most beautiful women in the world. Wigs have always been in style for women, and were signs of noble birth or of the judiciary for men. Now transplants and hair weaving have become more popular. Ads show a depressed looking man "before" and a smiling Adonis "after" the procedure.

Physical fitness has been both in and out of vogue several times in our history. Now, in addition to workouts by the lone runner or the home calisthenics or aerobics devotee, the health club has come of age. Health is ostensibly a primary goal of people joining such a club. Lowering low-density cholesterol, raising high-density cholesterol, obtaining cardiovascular fitness, losing weight, and obtaining muscle strength and joint flexibility are all health benefits these clubs can offer.

A second, but perhaps not secondary, benefit of the health club is the opportunity to meet like-minded members of the opposite sex. Membership is limited to people of moderate to high incomes, for the price is steep. Even more money can be spent by hiring a "personal trainer." Cosmetic makeovers combined with aerobics, saunas, and massage can be had for several thousand dollars, and include special diets. Such spas cater mostly to women.

For those who can afford them, home exercise machines are now widely available, and cost less than joining a club. They range from treadmills to rowing and skiing machines and many others to trim specific areas or build specific muscle sets. A variety of aerobic, yoga, and low-impact exercise videotapes are now sold for home use.

Team sports are often valued over education in many of our schools. Yet the physical fitness of the nation has declined over the years, and the proportion of overweight Americans has grown. Some 65 percent of our population are said to be sedentary. So the exercise canon is honored more in the breach than in the observance. Only a small portion of the population exercise for the recommended minimum half hour three times a week or better.

What of the effect of exercise on death fear? My impression is that some of the motivation for exercising is based on fear of dying. On the positive side, there are improvements in mood, and exercise has an anxiety-reducing effect. The endorphins are mood elevators, and are produced by the body during the "runner's high," and during most other types of aerobic exercise. Walking, gardening, and other mild forms of exercise can provide a pleasant routine and perhaps relieve some tension as well. Almost any repeated behavior, if enjoyable, can act as a life-quality enhancer and diminish obsession with death.

Exercise can have a peculiar masochistic quality when done to excess. It can diminish death fear by numbing, but it can also take much of the joy out of living. It is more often obsessive when used as an antidepressant. There is then such a strong need for exercise to control angry or sad feelings that it takes over many other functions. The time spent training for a marathon, for example, can take away from family, work, and friends. The ascetic aspect of excessive exercise is seen in the great number of musculoskeletal injuries sustained. Long-distance runners also frequently suffer from hematuria (blood in the urine), and women distance runners often stop menstruating.

Last but not least in the growing health craze is the food and diet fad. There is no need to elaborate on our national obsession with vitamins and low-fat or high-carbohydrate, all-protein, or thousands of other diets. There is great concern with food additives, with "natural" foods, with the cruciform vegetables and their anticancer benefits. There is a rage for fiber, a quest for bioflavins, and so on. Surely reasonable dieting is good for you, and life-enhancing, and losing weight through diet is cheaper and better than a tummy-tuck. But anorexia nervosa, which can be fatal, is widespread among our young women, and has been for years. Girls are taught through ads that they should look like match-stick thin models, like the famous "Twiggy." Again the downside is not health, but depression, obsession, and debility.

What can finally be concluded about the value of living to the hilt, living longer, or better? These are coping styles that color almost every aspect of our behavior. Each has advantages and disadvantages, and may be more adaptive for one individual in one historic period or one culture than another. Living to the hilt, the uninhibited pleasure-seeking mode, may sustain against death fear over the short term. It acts in part by keeping the person so busy that he or she doesn't have time for insight or rumination, which might result in depression. The drugs and alcohol and excessive food intake can all deaden feeling to an extent, thus reducing anxiety and depression. It is in between flings and binges that the unpleasant moods come to the surface. This coping mode may be better suited to young people, who are capable of sustaining such constant sexual and other orgiastic activity. It is almost doomed to failure in later life.

Living longer is certainly a rational goal, given the recent improvements in medicine. Taking reasonable steps to prolong life and to avoid pain and disability seems more than justifiable. The down side is that great risks are often involved in surgical procedures. They are almost all expensive, and the body seems to be programmed nonetheless to disintegrate according to its cellular clocks. There is an ascetic quality to much of the exercise, dieting, and health fads. In the extreme it borders on masochism, as in the case of polysurgery (seeking successive elective surgical interventions). There is a monotony to exercise that can induce trance-like or dissociative states. The crash dieters, the high-impact aerobic exercisers, and the long distance runners may be the monks, nuns, and anchorites of today. The "loneliness of the long distance runner" is a large price to pay for what may be just an anesthetic to relieve the pain of depression and death fear.

As in all behavior, the Golden Mean or happy medium is ideal. Living it up too much and its opposite, ascetic and obsessive preoccupation with health, diet, exercise, and one's looks, are both unlikely to control basic anxiety and fear of dying. In fact, such excessive activity is a symptom of death fear, not a solution for it.

10

GROUP MEMBERSHIP

Durkheim noted that there is something inside you but is also outside you and is larger than you. He said it was society that you had within you. This offered feelings of belongingness, and set limits and norms for behavior. Freud focused on the mechanism for the entry of society into one's own self, which he said was due to the introjection of the parental images. (Robert K. Merton pointed out this difference in emphasis in a lecture comparing Freud and Durkheim.) Group membership affords some of the emotional supports of human contact (along with its demands and deficits). It also gives one some hint of immortality, since one's family or nation will go on beyond one's own life. Georg Simmel noted, however, that some groups do not survive their members. He mentions the "Society of the Broken Plate." Each member had one piece broken from a plate. As each member died, his piece was glued back into place. The last member, of course, was not able to glue his shard, leaving a gap in the end product.

Perhaps the support of groups goes back to early man, who had to hunt larger animals, such as bison, mammoths, and saber-toothed tigers, in hunting packs. Some social animals still hunt in packs or groups: wolves, African hunting dogs, lionesses. This may have been the source of human male bonding. The pack, then, was a direct defense against death caused by the large or predatory animals. Today the armed forces of nations and the police stand between citizens and death. Being members of a nation offers, if not immortality, then some protection against death.

What evidence is there for the power of group membership, and how does it operate to diminish fear of dying? The feeling of support and strength that one gets from belonging to a group is often intangible, yet there are times in each person's life that these feelings become strong and conscious. These feelings have been eloquently described in an article on religion: "the rituals of the rock concert and the Catholic Church alike tap into this effect—the collective intoxicating rush" (a quotation from Elias Canetti's book, *Crowds and Power*, in *The New Yorker*, April 8, 1996, p. 68)

Assuming that we agree that such powerful feelings exist, we must ask, "Where do they come from?" We are all born into a group of two: mother and child. Soon the infant recognizes that there is a father (if present), and also brothers and sisters. We are by our biological nature forced into a dyadic relationship, and become a member of the family group. No one except a wolf-child is alone. Even Romulus and Remus had a wolf-mother. We "belong" first to our mother; then to our family; and later to our peer groups, our schools, our ethnic, religious, and national groups. There are also loyalties to corporations and groups larger than the family but smaller than the state. (Loyalty to corporations has decreased sharply in the United States due to massive downsizings. It has been pointed out that in Japan, corporate loyalty is still high, but waning.)

Francis Fukuyama has labeled private groups that are "larger than the family but smaller than the state" as "intermediate institutions." These charities, church study groups, choral societies, book clubs, and discussion groups enable people to work together without the legalistic rules of the larger society. He sees these informal groups as helping both democracy and capitalism, since they are based on trust (shades of *Gemeinschaft*!). A reviewer of his book, Fareed Zakaria, points out that it is not the existence of local groups, but rather their political philosophy, that promotes democracy.

> We like intermediate institutions when they have good effects, and dislike them when they have bad ones. What we want, it would seem, is not civil society, but civics—what the Romans called *civitas*; that is, public spiritedness, sacrifice for the community, citizenship, even nobility. But not all of civil society is civic minded. (Zakaria, 1996, p. 25)

Zakaria cites a glaring example of how an "intermediate institution" does not necessarily lead to liberal political institutions, which Mr. Fukuyama has claimed. Timothy McVeigh, who blew up the Federal Building in Oklahoma, belonged to a bowling group. Are we to believe that this automatically imbued him with a deep democratic philosophy, or instead, that this group brought together some friends and enabled them to plan the bombing?

The sense of power and security that derives from belonging to a group is psychologically supportive because it is originally (in infancy) and in later life physically supportive and protective. Society is made up of institutions that are meant to provide for the well-being of its citizens. There are the military and police for protection; schools for education; various government and private organizations for providing food, clothing, shelter, and health; and the institution of religion for spiritual and moral guidance, as well as the institution of the family. (Mae West, that great sociologist, said, "Marriage is a great institution, but who's ready for an institution?")

These institutions provide physical protection. In the case of the infant (whose helplessness is a developmental platitude), the protective function of the family is self-evident. For the older individual, these institutions stand between him and starvation;

dehydration (and other illnesses and conditions); natural disasters (involving exposure to heat, cold, water); and man-made disasters such as crime, enemy attacks in war, airplane, train, and car crashes, toxic pollution, and so forth. Belonging to a group, particularly to a nation that provides well for its citizens, serves to allay fears of death and dying. I believe that these feelings of protection and security are laid down in infancy and early childhood, assuming reasonable parental love and support. This is what is called "basic trust." If the various societal institutions continue to support that individual, then the feeling of basic trust is reinforced.

It is by this series of early and later supports that the fear of abandonment and its later form, the fear of death and dying, are held at bay. However, when the mother, family, school, or government fails to provide protection, fear of abandonment/dying and consequent rage follow.

A good example of this rage attributable to underprotection is described in *The American Soldier* (Stauffer, 1949–1950) as a failure of the "psychodynamic bargain" between the enlisted man and his officer. During World War II, as the percentage of casualties rose in a platoon or company, officers were sometimes shot or "fragged" (with hand grenades) by their own troops. The "bargain" was ostensibly made by the soldier giving over his superego to his officer. He would obey commands as long as the officer protected his life. When casualties rose sharply, the basic trust was broken, and murder or desertion followed.

Being a member of a group provides physical and psychological security, and it also supplies a good part of an essential psychological ingredient, identity. The loss of identity through divorce, death of a loved one, job loss, or illness is one of life's greatest stresses. People say things such as, "I lost my better half," or "This felt like an amputation" (or castration).

There have been many recent instances of murder in cases of divorce or where a person is summarily fired from a job after long and devoted service. A husband will ignore an order of restraint, and shoot his divorcing wife or unfaithful girlfriend dead in broad daylight. He will often commit suicide after that. If there are children, he may kill them too. Recently there have been several people who, after being fired, have gone into their former place of employment and killed many people with bursts of automatic gunfire.

If we look at marriage or holding a job as a "psychodynamic bargain," then divorce or firing constitutes a breach of that bargain. You could almost call the marriage and the job "contracts of commitment." If you marry me, I will support you and stick with you in sickness and in health "till death do us part." Or, "I will work hard for you if you will pay me and give me benefits." When the bargain is breached, or the contract broken, there is loss of protection, loss of identity, and a loss of some equivalent of love and/or respect. These breaches of contract are the ultimate "dissing." (Dissing is a ghetto slang term meaning major disrespect.)

So abandonment by a parent; by your peer group at school; and later by a spouse, boss, close friend, or your local or national government (whether real or imagined abandonment) is a breach of an unconscious contract (in the case of marriage often a written prenuptial contract). The intensity of the feeling engendered by this breach of contract is enormous. While depression is common, the underlying rage may also lead to assault and murder.

The belief that the government is guilty of a breach of contract with its citizens has given rise to an army of antigovernment militias. It has also spawned presidential and local political campaigns based on "running against the government." How can the governors run against themselves? Simply by saying they will cut down on government control and spending.

> America's increasingly look-alike parties present the country once again with the paradox of swarms of political bureaucrats who have spent most of their lives working for the government in Washington spending the better part of the campaign savaging the Washington governmental bureaucracy ... there is the irony of women and men who among them have notched centuries of service in the federal capital wanting us to believe that the very government they have been serving these many years is the enemy of our freedom. In democracies, representative institutions do not steal our liberties from us, they are the precious medium through which we secure those liberties. (Barber, 1996, p. 20)

There is a massive mistrust of politicians. Both Clinton and Dole were accused of obtaining presidential campaign funds illegally. The president and congressmen are seen as puppets "bought and paid for" by special interest groups. This mistrust is not a new phenomenon. Murray Levin wrote way back in 1962 that:

> Our analysis of this post-election survey has shown that a large proportion of the electorate feels politically powerless because it believes that the community is controlled by a small group of powerful and selfish individuals who use public office for personal gain. (Levin, 1962, p. 227)

This analysis was not based on the Clinton–Dole presidential campaigns of 1996 (as it might seem on first reading), but on the Boston mayoralty election of 1959, 41 years ago! Voters remarks were heavy with political alienation — "Collins is the lesser of two evils," "Voting wouldn't do any good," "I think, they're all the same." This sounds like "déja vu all over again." Levin notes that the powerful figures seen as controlling society are not necessarily capitalists, but are often politicians, labor leaders, the Mafia, or small-scale businessmen.

Political alienation is only one form of alienation from society. Levin lists powerlessness, meaninglessness, the lowering of norms (e.g., bribery is OK), and estrangement (the inability to find satisfaction in political or other societal activities as a responsible citizen).

How are political and other forms of alienation, such as work alienation and religious alienation, related to death fear? If you derive your identity and your feeling of being protected and loved from your country, your family, or other membership groups, and any or all of those groups fail to offer you security, then the usual good effects of membership are weakened or obliterated. It is the feeling of being wanted, loved, and part of something bigger than the self that is so crucial in protecting us against fear of dying. Alienation from the group recalls and reinforces any earlier feelings of abandonment, loss of parental love, or rejection by one's peers. Early loss sensitizes the individual, so that adult alienation becomes more devastating psychologically. This can be seen in the high rates of suicide in children of parents who committed suicide (for example, Ernest Hemingway and his father, and later his grand-daughter). The rates of divorce for children of divorce are much higher than for children of nondivorced parents.

Meaninglessness, estrangement, and powerlessness are found not only in alienation, but also in depression. The depressive individual is often described as feeling hopeless and helpless. I feel that alienation is really a term for depression, but on a societal rather than an individual level. We are more likely to say that "workers are alienated" or "teen-agers are alienated," and to say that a single worker is depressed after losing his job, or an individual teen is rebellious (angry and depressed).

One way of combating alienation, depression, and fear of dying is by identification with a charismatic leader, or by starting or joining some political, religious, or other (charitable, environmental, military, human rights) action group. As mentioned before, these groups can be constructive to the society as a whole, or destructive to everyone else except their members.

The rise of Nazism in Germany has often been attributed to the alienation of the "Kleinbeampter," the small official (the street car conductor, the primary school teacher) after World War I. These people had lost what little authority they had, and the Nazi party offered them power. (In this case, the intermediate institution of the beer hall gang again led away from democracy, not toward it.)

Alienation usually applies to some segment of a society, some subgroup, such as women, minorities, the Luddites, the working class, the rural populists. This may have harmful effects on the rest of society, or it may make for some positive changes in the social structure (women's right to vote, equal opportunity, minimum wages). In the case of the right-wing militias, or the Nazi movement in Germany, the net result has been very destructive, although briefly supportive for its members. Remember, the "Thousand Year Reich" lasted only for about 12 years. Sometimes there is no alienation *within* a society. Some societies integrate all their members and give them emotional, physical, and economic support. This sounds ideal, except that some of these cultures, tribes, or nations are extremely destructive to all outsiders. This is true to some extent of warlike nations led by such charismatic leaders as Alexander the Great and Genghis Khan.

As a graduate student in sociology at Columbia University I took part in a seminar on cultural psychodynamics taught by Dr. Abram Kardiner, a psychiatrist and psychoanalyst. He said that of all the tribes and cultures he had studied, the Apaches were the best adjusted (Kardiner, 1945).* Their society was well integrated, so that everyone had a function, a meaningful life, a feeling of being needed and important. For example, the berdache was an institution that created a protective niche for homosexuals. Gay youths and men were trained to be pages, to carry the shields and weapons of warriors, and to take care of their horses. One of the students in the seminar pointed out that while the Apache might be "well adjusted and integrated," they were known for killing many of the people in the surrounding tribes.

Alienation of a subgroup is not the only cause of conflict and killing. I discuss this at length in a later chapter on Projection, Killing, and the Problem of Evil. To this day the causes of war are not well understood, but warfare and killing have gone on since the dawn of mankind. On a percentage basis, killing has not escalated. In fact, in early times whole populations were more likely to be wiped out with no survivors.

Since the world's population has increased enormously (geometrically), the number (as opposed to the percentage) of people killed in war has exploded. In World War I there were 8.5 million military deaths, and in World War II there were 15.8 million, eclipsing the casualties of all other wars. From the earliest recorded history to the present, there have been 45 million battle deaths. This does not include civilian deaths due to war!

About 60 million more have been killed as a result of political or religious persecution (Long, 1985, pp. 145, 150, and 155–159). This presents a terrible paradox. Group membership is one of the greatest supports we have against the fear of dying, *yet it is one of the prime causes of the fear of death and dying because it is a rationale for and a cause of war.*

If group membership is to help in combating rather than promoting fear of dying (depression, alienation, and consequent anger and "acting out"), the institutions of a society should strike a balance between supporting (and controlling) the individual and a total lack of support and control (anarchy or anomie). When the institutions in a society are highly correlated (interwoven or connected) you have a traditional society, such as ancient China, Japan, or India.

Bali is still an example of a highly integrated and controlled society. Music, art, agriculture, marriage, child rearing, and almost all behavior is integrated through religion. Religious dances are held often, cementing communal bonds. Religious shrines are erected in rice paddies. Carvings and decorations of all kinds bear a religious message. The extreme control of life in Bali has been attributed to the need to distribute scarce water equally to all families. If one farmer removed part of a dam so that more water would flow into *his* terraced rice paddy, others below him on the steep hillside would suffer.

---

* Kardiner wrote about the Apache, basing his analysis on the field work of Ralph Linton.

This is in contrast with the United States, for example, where there is much greater freedom of choice, and established religion no longer holds sway over the community. Without controls, a condition that approaches anarchy may ensue. When the Soviet Union, which had been under very strict control as a Communist dictatorship, broke up, the people seemed to lose their sense of protection and direction. There has been a sharp increase in crime. An American businessman who ran a leading hotel in Moscow was recently shot down in broad daylight by rival businessmen. This is what Durkheim called a state of *anomie,* or normlessness. The usual constraints are lacking. In such times people again look to a charismatic leader who will bring order to the society. Often that means a return to dictatorship, an "escape from freedom." In most cases, people don't experience this normlessness as "freedom." They feel it as a life threatening chaos. The balance between freedom and control is hard to maintain. We see it as a constant struggle in developing children and in the ambivalence of their parents. It is also ever present in our political debates. So many want less government control (interference, regulation) but they also want the government to provide benefits, such as medical care and Social Security, when they get older.

The intensity of feelings of belonging inspired by group membership (outside of the family) is nowhere as clearly expressed as in national anthems. Many of these songs have martial or warlike themes. The French "Marseillaise" inspires its citizens to arms:

> Allons, enfants de la patrie, le jour de gloire est arrivé …
> Aux armes, citoyens! Formez vos batallions.
> Marchons, marchons! Qu'un sang impure abreuve nos sillons.
> (Arise, children of the fatherland. The day of glory has come.
> Against us the blood-stained banner of tyranny is raised.
> Hear, in the fields, the roar of her fierce soldiers.
> They come right into our arms to slaughter our sons and our consorts.
> Patriots, to arms! Form your battalions. Let's march, let's march!
> May the tyrant's foul blood water our furrows!)
> (Words and music by Claude-Joseph Rouget de L' Isle) (Reed, 1993)*

Slightly less warlike is the "Star Spangled Banner" of the United States:

> Oh say, can you see, by the dawn's early light,
> What so proudly we hailed, at the twilight's last gleaming.
> Whose broad stripes and bright stars, through the perilous fight,
> O'er the ramparts we watched, were so gallantly streaming?
> And the rockets' red glare, the bombs bursting in air,
> Gave proof through the night, that our flag was still there.
> O say, does that Star-Spangled Banner yet wave
> O'er the land of the free, and the home of the brave?

---

* Translations are given for all anthems in this remarkable volume.

(Third verse) ... Then conquer we must, for our cause it is just,
And this be our motto, 'In God is our trust.'
And the Star-Spangled Banner in triumph shall wave,
O'er the land of the free, and the home of the brave.
(Words by Francis Scott Key) (Reed, 1993)*

The German national anthem used to be more direct about it all — no holds barred:

Deutschland, Deutschland, über alles, über alles in der Welt. (Original version was first officially adopted in 1922)
(Germany, Germany, above everything, above everything in the world).

After the union of West and East Germany in 1990, new words were adopted, to be sung to the original melody of Franz Joseph Haydn. They are in sharp contrast with the older martial words:

Einigkeit und Recht und Freiheit, Für das Deutsche Vaterland! etc. (Unity and Right and Freedom, for the German Fatherland!)
After these let us all strive, Brotherly with heart and hand...) (Reed, 1993)

Many of the anthems are exhortations to fight the enemy, and to die for one's country, as in the "Marseillaise." The "Mameli Hymn" of Italy (adopted in 1946) says, "Italian Brothers, Italy has awakened. Let us band together. We are ready to die. Italy has called us" (Reed, 1993). The "March of the Volunteers" (China, written in 1935 and adopted in 1949) has similar commands:

Arise, ye who refuse to be slaves! With our flesh and blood, let us build our new Great Wall.
The Chinese nation faces its greatest dangers.
From each one the urgent call for action comes forth.
Arise! Arise! Arise! Millions with but one heart,
Braving the enemy's fire. March on! Braving the enemy's fire (3 times) On! (Reed, 1993)†

Upon browsing through about 200 anthems in this book, I was struck by the fact that there seemed to be no correlation between the warlike qualities of nations and their anthems. Among the anthems with the more "peaceful" words were those of Japan, Jordan, Denmark, Israel, Nepal, Sweden, India, Finland, Croatia, and Austria. The more warlike anthems were those of Portugal, the Irish Republic, Greece, El Salvador, Poland, Mexico, Iraq, and Iran.

All these anthems declare and are meant to inculcate love for and strong attachment to one's country. Anecdotes and mottoes serve the same function.

---

* The composer is unknown, but the melody is based on the tune, "To Anacreon in Heaven." Despite my pacifist leanings, tears come to my eyes as I type the words to the "Star-Spangled Banner." Such is the power of patriotism and group membership! I and many others would much prefer that "America the Beautiful" were our national anthem.
† The similarity to the Internationale, "Arise, ye prisoners of starvation," is striking.

As children, we were taught the story of Nathan Hale, who spied against the British in the Revolutionary War. As he was about to be hanged, his last words were, "I only regret that I have but one life to lose for my country" (Bartlett, 1995). We had a steady diet of patriotic tales and quotations. The ones that have stayed with me (although in slightly distorted form) are "Don't one of you fire until you see the whites of their eyes" (William Prescott at Bunker Hill, 1775); "Tell the men to fire faster and not to give up the ship; fight her till she sinks" (James Lawrence, on the U.S. frigate Chesapeake, 1813); "We shall not flag or fail. We shall go on to the end. We shall fight in France … we shall never surrender" (Winston Churchill, speech on Dunkirk, House of Commons, 1940); "Damn the torpedoes—full speed ahead!" (Admiral David Glasgow Farragut, Battle of Manila Bay, 1864); and "The summer soldier and the sunshine patriot will, in this crisis, shrink from the service of their country, but he that stands it now deserves the love and thanks of man and woman" (Thomas Paine, 1776) (Bartlett, 1995).

Perhaps today such sentiments sound almost kamikaze-like. In the United States (with some notable pacifist exceptions) wars generally used to be seen as "righteous." The enemy, were they British, German, or Japanese, were always 100% in the wrong. Then came Vietnam, and the killing of innocent villagers (women and children) at My Lai by American soldiers. War was no longer automatically justified. In the United States a majority finally sickened of war, if only briefly.

There has always been support for war and patriotism in our popular songs and poetry. In World War I, "Pack Up Your Troubles in Your Old Kit Bag" (and smile, smile, smile) was very popular. George M. Cohan's songs were often patriotic, even in peacetime ("The Yankee Doodle Boy" 1904*, and "You're a Grand Old Flag, 1906). His song, "Over There" (1917) ("The Yanks are coming over there") kept up spirits at home and in the trenches. Irving Berlin's "God Bless America" is almost a second national anthem. He also wrote "This Is the Army" (Mr. Jones). Frank Loesser added patriotic fuel to the fire with "Praise the Lord and Pass the Ammunition" (1942) and "What Do You Do in the Infantry?" These are notable among hundreds of patriotic songs, some of them martial, some humorous. Sometimes songs were not martial, but offered support or solace for soldiers. In World War II, "Lili Marlene," a German song with a wonderful melody and nostalgia for the girl who was left behind, became immensely popular on both sides of the conflict. Movies oozed with patriotism. Many starred John Wayne (World War II). Later on Sylvester Stallone as "Rambo" fought the Vietnam War almost single-handed, or rescued American soldiers who were missing in action after Vietnam. These martial sentiments were supplemented between major wars by movies about cowboys and pioneers versus Indians, or dirt farmers versus ranchers, who hated the barbed wire that kept their cattle from roaming freely over the tender crops of the farmers.

* "I'm a Yankee Doodle dandy, Yankee Doodle do or die … born on the 4th of July."

Against this tidal wave of martial patriotism there was always a trickle of pacifist sentiment. Among the most notable was Jonathan Swift's satire of war, *Gulliver's Travels*. His Lilliputians fought a major war over which end of the egg to crack open first—the large or small end. "All Quiet On The Western Front," by Erich Maria Remarque, both as a novel and film, was a scathing indictment of war. "The Thin Red Line," by James Jones, didn't have the success of "From Here to Eternity," but it had an even stronger antiwar message about killing and male bonding. After Vietnam, many books revealed a more realistic and negative picture of war. Movies such as "Platoon" are outright indictments of war, and would have dismayed John Wayne. They are a far cry from Gary Cooper shooting Germans like turkeys in "Sergeant York" (1941), or Audie Murphy reenacting his war exploits. Bertolt Brecht viciously satirized war and patriotism in "The Threepenny Opera" (1928, with music by Kurt Weill) One of Brecht's lyrics about young soldiers says "We chop 'em (the enemy) to bits because we like our hamburger raw." The chorus reads in part "Let's all go blarmy, let's join the Army, see the world we never saw." The last verse shows how, after recruitment, these young men die in battle, become amputees, or are disfigured.

Patriotic songs, poems, movies, and quotations promoting war or praising one nation or group over another far outnumber those that are pacifist or promote internationalism. This is because they are the artistic (or attempt to be the artistic) expression of group membership. Many musical compositions dedicated to national or group themes are true works of art: The Moldau (part of Má Vlast, or "My Fatherland" by Smetana) ; The German Requiem (Brahms); "Finlandia" (Sibelius); and Mozart's anthem for the Masons ("Brüder reicht die Hand zum Bunde") are among hundreds that were inspired by group membership. This does not include the music of the Baroque and Renaissance periods, which was heavily inspired by religious membership, a subject treated in the next chapter.

George Herbert Mead showed how children learn the rules of society by playing games (Mead, 1962). Boys are socialized into the macho role through contact sports in high school and college, such as football, soccer, boxing, and wrestling. There is also early socialization with cowboy and soldier outfits, toy guns, and military dolls. In the basic training films soldiers saw in World War II, the metaphor of a football team was used *ad nauseam* to illustrate how, in combat, your life would depend on the teamwork of your platoon. The loyalty to sports teams can literally lead to warfare, and hundreds of fans have been killed in riots. This sometimes happens when teams are from the same nation, but is more frequent during international matches. Race riots, tribal warfare, and gang warfare are a few more examples of the negative side of group membership. Political parties often stoop to open warfare, especially before elections (if the citizens are lucky enough to have more than one party). In many countries people are shot to prevent their voting. The "team spirit" is carried too far. The nastiness of U.S. political campaigns has always been with us, but seems to have reached new depths of muds linging. Allegations of sexual or business improprieties have been part of campaign battles since the birth of this nation, and apparently will continue into the future. It is this moralistic focus on indecency, rather than on appropriate political issues such as jobs, education, public safety, and health, that makes for much of the current political alienation and disgust with government.

In sum, what is the up side of group membership? It offers economic opportunity and often a "safety net" for those unable to work. It also provides physical protection in the form of police and the military, and services such as health and education. Family members usually protect and provide for each other. "Intermediate institutions" and the family provide psychological support and all groups offer the individual member some modicum of identity. *The feeling of belonging, of protection, of heightened identity, and of continuity provide a strong bulwark against the fear of death and dying.*

On the down side, loyalty to the in-group very often (but not necessarily) leads to aggression against the out-group, the stranger, the enemy. It is a paradox that groups that are originally homogenous tend to split up into new subgroups. This was pointed out by Michael Ignatieff in speaking about the Serbs, Croats, and Bosnian Muslims; they share language, folkways, and political culture and have a common history, yet they have been in conflict (with the urging of demagogic leaders).

The struggle is driven by what Freud called "the narcissism of minor difference," in which essentially similar peoples exaggerate what separates them in a desperate search for identity (Fukuyama, 1994). The search for identity, then, can become a divisive force in society, just as it can in a family, as children mature and want to separate. Some examples of these fine divisions are the "lace curtain" Irish and the poorer Irish immigrants; the German, Ashkenazi, and Sephardic Jews; the many sects of Protestantism; the North versus the South during the American Civil War; social class divisions; the war of the sexes; the war of the generations; and so on. The breakdown of support by the group, especially by the nation, can lead to the popularity of charismatic and demagogic leaders who often offer security in exchange for freedom (extremes of "law and order" and curtailment of civil liberties). New groups offer the possibility for constructive social action and change, but some of these groups may be more destructive than constructive. During transitional periods, the usual supports of the society are damaged or absent, leading to such states as anomie, alienation, or chaos. The breakdown of the family can lead to physical illness and to psychological and psychosocial disorders, especially depression and antisocial behavior, which are prevalent. Defenses against death fear are greatly diminished, especially in depression.

11

RELIGION

Two problems lower the rank of this adaptation for me. First, a focus on the afterlife may mean less devotion to this present life, creating a type of religious withdrawal, and possibly fatalism. Second, I have mentioned the eternal association of religion with war and persecution. (Other group memberships such as nations and races can be the rationale for just as much destructiveness, the list is endless). Perhaps the ideas of redemption, of forgiveness for sins, and the belief in life after death have encouraged much homicidal behavior. (Becker ranks religion as the highest level of four levels of coping, but he defines it in such a way as to avoid any of its worldly consequences. Higher order religious philosophies, such as Albert Schweitzer's, focus on the life-loving aspects, but not the destructive group-membership aspects. If defined this way, religion would be in the top ranks of my coping hierarchy.)

In the introductory section, the coping mode of religion was described as another form of denial, or illusion. While to some people such tricks may be anathema, a perpetual parade of great minds has seen religion as the one salvation for the sufferings of man while on this earth. Not only is life hard, but death always threatens. In view of this constant threat, it may be a good bargain to sacrifice rationality in one area in order to function without unremitting fear. Since religion is such a universal phenomenon, and seems to be more or less effective, I would place it among the better coping modes, but not among the very best, for reasons I shall discuss later.

The major functions of religion, in my view, are:

1. The reduction of the fear of death and dying through belief in an afterlife, metamorphosis (rebirth in different forms), and in the spirit world.
2. Providing individuals with a group identity (I am a Catholic, Muslim, Buddhist, Protestant, Jew, etc.).
3. Offering an interpretation of the invisible world, a cosmology, and an explanation of our origins.

4. Providing meaning and purpose in our lives. Clearly, religion is not the only institution that provides such guidance and information. Families, the schools, the police, governments, philosophers, and scientists also perform many of these functions. Increasingly in Western society, religion provides less, and society more guidance in these areas.
5. Setting rules for interpersonal conduct, and for ritual and prayer. Defining what it is to be a "good person."
6. In confessional religions, religion offers a diminution of guilt feelings.

Our primary concern is with the reduction of fear of death and dying, but religion overlaps many of the other "coping modes" dealing with death.

The unique contribution of religion is the belief in the afterlife. While religion provides us with a group identity, we can also get this benefit from belonging to the Knights of Columbus, the United Auto Workers, or the local Rat Pack. We can also gain some identity by rooting for our favorite football, baseball, or basketball team, being a Marine (or former Marine) or veteran, or by joining any of thousands of charitable and volunteer organizations. Being a fan of Elvis Presley or the Who, the Beatles, or the latest rock group gives some people a sense of identity. Yet none of these groups confer immortality, while religious belief and membership does. (Groups that outlast the lives of their members do offer a sort of immortality, but this is rather indirect when compared with the promise of eternal life in the hereafter offered by some religions.)

As religion has weakened as an institution in Western society, so has the belief in the afterlife. Geoffrey Gorer felt that people are less able to contemplate death today, because of this loss of religious faith (Feifel, 1959, p. 116). Suppose the afterlife is an illusion. Is this to deny that it has important functions? In psychotherapy at present, the importance of illusion is recognized more and more. One does not try to strip another person—friend or patient—of all his hopes and dreams, as impossible as they may be. For most people, doing so would leave only grim reality. This is the message of Eugene O'Neill's play, "The Iceman Cometh," mentioned previously.

Freud, in *The Future of an Illusion* (Freud, 1957), asked where the idea of religion originated. To simplify his thesis, one could say that the religious figures were simply projections of the human family. For example, Joseph, Mary, and the infant Jesus are projections of parent and child. However, Mary conceives immaculately, so Jesus is the son of God. Depending on the culture, Jesus, Mary, or an abstract God-the-Father may be emphasized. It has often been pointed out that Latin Catholic cultures tend to worship Mary, while most Protestant countries focus more on Jesus. Bruce Bartlett, a successful entrepreneur, once wrote about Jesus returning to earth as a businessman (an extreme example of the influence of the Protestant Ethic in a capitalist society). The Old Testament god, Jehovah, is fierce and punitive. Mark Twain satirized the Old Testament in his book *Letters from the Earth* (Twain, 1962). He asked why God smote all those innocent children in Sodom and Gomorrah, when it was the adults who were fornicating? Wouldn't he, being all powerful, have better aim with his thunderbolts? Why, Twain asked, did he put a male and female mosquito on board the Ark? To punish man forever? What about germs?

Christ, on the other hand, is a forgiving figure. He says, "Cast first the mote from thine own eye." He suffers and dies, and is reborn. There are angry gods and kind gods. The Greeks had some jealous gods, such as Juno, who changed the nymph Io into a cow, to be eternally plagued by cow flies. Io had the audacity to be attractive to Zeus, and so had to be punished. Such nerve was known as hubris.

A major theme in Christianity is the resurrection ("I am the resurrection and the life"). Jesus' return represents the victory over death that every one wishes for. Through the resurrection he vanquishes death. Identification with him (love and worship) serves to reduce fear and disappointment.

The Easter hymn "Jesus Christ Is Risen Today" recounts the resurrection, and clarifies its purpose.

> Jesus Christ is risen today, alleluia
> Our triumphant holy day, alleluia
> Born to die upon the cross, alleluia
> Suffered to redeem our loss, alleluia.

I assume that our "loss" is that of innocence. Christ is often referred to as "our Redeemer" (as in the beautiful aria in Händel's Messiah, "I know that my Redeemer liveth"). The verb "redeem" is defined (in its theological meaning) as "to deliver from sin and its consequences by means of a sacrifice offered for the sinner" (Flexner, 1987, p. 1202). The death by crucifixion, then, functions to relieve guilt (as in the fifth function listed) through sacrifice and forgiveness, as well as through the confessional. If you believe that someone has "died for you," you can feel better about some of the inevitable trespasses you will have committed during your life. The second part of the Christ story, the resurrection, takes care of death fears. If you believe, you can also come back.

The idea that body and soul are separate has been promoted by religion. Thus one's body can die, but one's soul lives on and is immortal. One needn't be Jesus, then, to have immortality—to be resurrected.

The death of Jesus, his suffering, and his sacrifice are believed to have redeemed our loss of innocence (and perhaps our current bad behavior). If you believe, you will be reborn. This idea of the scapegoat dying to relieve the community of its sins is a recurrent theme in mythology. Sir James Fraser wrote a whole volume of *The Golden Bough* (Fraser, 1923) on this subject.

The ideas of heaven, purgatory, and hell appear in some form in most religions. There has to be a place for souls to go after bodily death. Souls can migrate to different animal forms. In this case, the soul is still immortal, but the body changes. The ancient Jews believed that the bones were immortal, and carefully gathered the bodies of their dead, so that new flesh could be hung on those old bones. Hence the song lyrics, "Them bones shall rise again."

Strangely enough, the bones of "Lucy," the first proto-human, have lasted for more than three million years, which is as close to immortality as any one of us is likely to get.

As mentioned before, Freud in his treatment of religion focused on the mechanism of introjection, by means of which the parental images were taken into the child's unconscious mind. Durkheim (1915), in contrast, focused on the adult, and on the role of society in forming religious feelings in the individual. He asked, What could it be that is outside us and is larger than us, but which we feel within us?

His answer was that it is society, which, although larger than us, is still inside us. Robert K. Merton, in his lectures to us as graduate sociology students, said that Freud focused on the mechanism whereby society was internalized — that is, through introjection of the parental images. The parents were the representatives of society, the "socializers." Durkheim didn't discuss how society got inside us, but took it as a given. He focused instead on societal states, which could affect human behavior, such as religious activity or suicide.

If the gods are in fact projections of the family in the cultures in which those religions originated, then some of the extreme variation in the behavior of the gods can be accounted for. The kindly gods, the stern ones, the jealous, and the avenging gods may reflect the typical mothers and fathers of the families at the time those religions were conceived. (The character of the gods may have changed as the family structure and culture changed.) But if man has the freedom to create any god he wants, then why are the gods so often fearsome and punitive?

The answer to this question may lie in part in a discussion I had with my therapist during a session. Suffice it to say that I often wandered away from the issue at hand, to "intellectualize," and to derail the focus from some subject that was painful to me. I asked the question, "Why, if one internalizes the parental image, which contains both the good and bad qualities of the parent(s), does the object choice (read "loved one, mate, spouse, friend") so often exhibit mainly the negative aspects of the parents' character?" (In "repetition–compulsion," the object-choice is repeated, with seeming disregard for the fact that previous choices of the same type of person have been disastrous.) My therapist's answer was something like this: "It's very simple. You want to resolve some early problems with parental figures. You choose people who represent those problems, and will continue to make for those problems in your relationship. You don't care about the good characteristics of your parents. Those issues have been resolved, or never even became issues. It is the unresolved issues that remain to be explored. In choosing the unloving, the domineering, the punitive, or the distant and withdrawn love-object, you attempt to resolve these longstanding childhood issues."

Let's assume that this interpretation is correct (with all the injustice I have done it by oversimplifying). This suggests that the gods (who are projections of our parents) for the most part will also have the more negative features of our parents. They will tend to be more punitive and judgmental than loving. They will be more jealous than forgiving. A survey of religions worldwide would probably bear this out. For every god of light there is at least one of darkness. While all the great religions preach charity and love, some also ask their god to smite the enemy and the sinner. Of the religious person we can surely say that her god is a love-object. She chooses this love-object, just as she chooses any other, out of the need for resolving old psychological issues, and her god is then (felt to be) angry, cold, accusing, and so forth, according to her own needs.

You don't need someone to die so that your guilt can be relieved. This can be accomplished through the confessional. (In many religions beside Catholicism, the subject speaks his sins and is forgiven by the listening individual, group, or congregation.) Guilt can also be relieved through psychoanalysis or other forms of psychotherapy.

Since redemption or forgiveness is such an important function, it may be worthwhile to refer to one of my favorite films, "House of Games," written by David Mamet.

The plot, briefly, is as follows. A woman psychoanalyst has a teenage male patient, who tells her that he is about to be killed by loansharks because he owes them money. She, being soft-hearted, writes out a large check, so he can pay off the debt. He then introduces the analyst to a con man and his gang, who "teach" her about the tricks they use. They stage a false murder, and she thinks that the head con, with whom she has been having an affair, will be killed by the mob unless she antes up some escape money. He cons her out of thousands, all her savings. She then hears no more from him until, in a local bar, she overhears some of the gang laughing about how they cheated her. She finds her con-lover, and demands an apology. When he tells her he won't apologize, and that she is just a sucker, she shoots him dead. After this, she meets her mentor, an elderly woman analyst, whose heavy accent tells us she trained in Vienna. Over lunch, our heroine asks her, "What do you do when you've done something unforgivable?" The woman smiles, and says "You forgive yourself."

In this tale lies a clue to the main difference between the confessional and psychoanalysis. In the confessional, you must return to the priest for absolution. In the process of analysis, and in most psychotherapy, you must learn to forgive yourself. This means first going back to face your guilt (or "transgressions"), your anger, or your uncharitable behavior toward others.

A great deal has been written about the parallels between religion and psychoanalysis. Erich Fromm (1959) provided a thorough analysis, and several others have commented on the similarities. There is the Holy Book, the God (Freud), the disciples (Jung, Adler, Ferenczi, etc.), the membership ring that Freud gave to his inner circle, and the religious zeal with which the members proselytized.

Psychotherapy aims to release the patient eventually, while established religion seeks to keep the worshipper in the fold. Good therapy enables the patient to "stand on his own feet," while religion tends to breed dependency. Yet the new vocabulary, the myriad rules for conduct and living and loving, often seem similar.

In a way, religion and therapy are like the "total institutions" of Erving Goffman (1962). Your vocabulary, your dress, and your motives are all born anew. It is like entering the Army or a hospital, or any total institution. Your identity is changed. (Your wrist tag or dog tag testifies to that.) After psychoanalysis you might say, "I cathected" or "I have a new love-object" instead of "I have a new girlfriend." You might say to a friend, "You're fine, How am I?" (as in the old joke). In a religious culture you say "I'm reborn" or "God be with you" (good-bye) or "Vaya con Dios" (go with God) or "Inshallah" (praise Allah).

MEANING

One of the functions of religion is to provide meaning and purpose in life. I think this search for meaning comes down, again, to the inevitable separations that occur early in life. The parent figure, usually the mother, is seen as the all-powerful protector. Abandoning the infant, even for a few minutes, can result in anguished crying. If this happens enough times, the fear and rage subside, and the baby assumes an apparent indifference that masks a deep depression. Earlier it was thought that babies and young children didn't have the mental apparatus to become depressed. This view has changed radically. Rene Spitz (1965) early on described the withdrawn appearance of children in an orphanage, who were never touched or held. They also suffered from marasmus, or wasting syndrome. Everyone wants love and protection, at least at an early stage of life. The parent is supposed to provide this protection. Of course, in many families, both love and protection are missing. Later on in life, God (if we can assume that God is a projection of the parents) "looks after" you. Angels "watch over" you, in protective parental fashion. Totems and saints guard you against evil, sickness, and death. The fact that somebody cares about you gives "meaning" to your life. Meaning often comes down to the fact that you will go on living, that you are protected against death (mainly by illness, starvation, or physical attack). That, of course, is "meaning" at its most primitive level. It is primarily insurance that you will survive. Extended to the congregation, God is the shepherd, watching his flock. The worshippers are the lambs. How interesting that metaphors from a pastoral-nomadic society thousands of years old should still be so apposite! God protects even those who kill. During World War I, a German motto was "Gott mit uns" (God is on our side). Well, He is on both sides of every war, for He is always "mit uns." He is "mit everybody." He is the protector of the flock, and thus of society itself.

No infant, if he could speak, could have uttered a more plaintive cry for help to God-the-Parent-and-Shepherd than adult David, sick and set upon by bulls and dogs.

> My God, my God, why hast thou forsaken me? Why art thou so far from helping me, and from the words of my roaring? (Psalms XXII, 1, King James version of the Bible)

On a more sophisticated level, but probably deriving from the same early need for protection (and fear of abandonment), is the search for meaning as articulated by poets, philosophers, and prophets. These are usually individuals with sharpened sensibilities. Often they have become sensitized through personal loss. This search is evidenced by a series of subfears, all related to the fear of death. These are sometimes relevant to certain coping modes discussed in later chapters, but they are part and parcel of every religion:

1. Fear of the meaninglessness and purposelessness of life
2. Fear of the finitude of our species, and of the earth itself
3. Fear of annihilation of the individual, and of the groups (family, state, country, or humanity) to which he belongs

These fears are manifested in the apocalyptic predictions of both major and minor religions. As we approached the second millennium, there were more dire predictions of the end of the world, the "second coming of Christ," and Judgment Day. The fears of chaos due to the "Y2K" (year 2000) problem in computer dating programs was apparently very exaggerated. The millennium, with its two last digits of "00," came and went without widespread computer breakdowns, at a cost of billions in worldwide preparation.

These apocalyptic fears may be reinforced by the current evidence for the impact of a meteorite crater in the Gulf of Mexico, which scientists now believe wiped out many families of animals, including the dinosaurs. The belief in Darwinian gradualism (evolution in slow increments) is being replaced by theories of saltation (or great leaps) and catastrophism (Gould, 1994, p. 10).* Apocalyptic predictions are usually the work of the fundamentalist religious right. However, it has now become clear that we must pay attention to the influence of

---

* Gould points out that "the terms 'uniformitarian' and 'catastrophist' were coined by William Whewell, England's leading philosopher of science, in 1832." Lyell (who greatly influenced Darwin) rejected the idea of catastrophes, deluges, and glacial periods that could annihilate plants and animals. When the fragments of comet Shoemaker-Levy-9 bombarded Jupiter in July 1994, "the equivalent of about 40 million megatons of TNT—or some 500 times the power of all the earth's nuclear weapons combined" was released. Gould says that this event gave even greater credence to the theory of Luis Alvarez, who in 1979 said that a comet or asteroid 6 miles in diameter struck the earth at the end of the Cretaceous period 65 million years ago. This impact (which left a crater in the Gulf of Mexico 200 miles wide) is now widely believed to have led to the extinction of the dinosaurs and the rise of mammals.

chance. Chaos theory presently supports this view of nature as capricious (like a goat, from the Latin caper, leaping!). Both gradual and catastrophic change are at work to create our destiny. Catastrophes are both natural and man-made. Major wars, the slaughter of Armenians and the killings during the Nazi Holocaust, the Black Plague and the current plague of AIDS, and many other disasters have heightened the fear of death and the subfears of meaninglessness and finitude.

In the face of personal or social disaster, people ask, "Why hast thou forsaken me?" Often their faith in God is destroyed. The example of Lisa Foster, the wife of Vincent Foster (President Clinton's personal lawyer) who shot himself, was given in Chapter 8. Her cry to God is as bitter as that of David or Job. If she was "God's child," why wasn't she protected? This rage against God is like the rage of the abandoned or abused child against the parents. If turned against the self, it can lead to suicide (or suicidal thoughts, as in Lisa's case). If turned against parents or society, it can lead to murder (as in Gruen's case of the double ax murder, or the case of the Menendez brothers).

Becker paints a horrifying picture of the world as one big disaster. He uses terms such as "panic," "grotesque," and the "terror of creation" to describe reality. Organisms tear each other apart. It is the world view of Hieronymous Bosch, in his famous painting "Big Fish Eat Little Fish," or his description of hell. This is a "planet soaked in blood." "Whatever is achieved must be achieved without deadening, with the full exercise of passion, of vision, of pain, of fear, and of sorrow" (Becker, 1973, p. 284). He criticizes science when it tries to "smooth over" the terrible reality (as suggested by a famous psychologist who wanted to find a chemical to stop man's aggressiveness). We have started on this road, by using Ritalin to treat "antisocial behavior" in children, and massive doses of tranquilizers and antidepressants for adults. "If all the world were on Prozac, wouldn't it be a happy place?" one might ask. Becker says that science and religion sometimes encourage the deadening of the perception of "The Awful Truth" (to use an old movie title) and that:

> Science betrays us when it is willing to absorb lived truth all into itself. Here the criticism of behaviorist psychology, all manipulations of men, and all coercive utopianism comes to rest. These techniques try to make the world other than it is, legislate the grotesque out of it, inaugurate a 'proper' human condition. (Becker, 1973, p. 283)

He further indicts science as one more attempt to deny death. One might say that science was being employed as just another of many mechanisms for coping with this terrible reality.

> Science, after all, is a credo that has attempted to absorb into itself and to deny the fear of life and death; and it is only one more competitor in the spectrum of roles for cosmic heroics. (Becker, 1973, p. 283)

What does this brilliant social critic come up with as the solution for our survival in a terrifying, grotesque, and irrational world? He sees man's struggle for life, his vitality, and his expansiveness as "sacred" and "mysterious." He calls for "new heroisms that are basically matters of belief and will, dedication to a vision." He cites Norman Brown saying that:

> ... the only way to get beyond the natural contradictions of existence was the time-worn religious way; to project one's problems onto a god-figure, to be healed by an all-embracing and all-justifying beyond. (Becker, 1973, p. 285)

He also leans on Rank, saying that:

> ... he (Rank) saw that the orientation of men has to be always beyond their bodies, has to be grounded in healthy repressions, and toward explicit immortality-ideologies, myths of heroic transcendence. (Becker, 1973, p. 285)

(Note that Brown waged war against repressions, in contrast to Rank and Becker.)

It is striking that a man who sees so clearly the destructive forces in nature and within man does not also see science and psychology as a step toward alleviating some of this pain and fear (not a "deadening" of the perception of the awful reality). Freud, too, saw religion as the illusion that was needed for the masses to get through life, but he held out the hope that rationality would eventually prevail. The fervor of Becker's argument for religion as a coping mode (my term) is shown in this excerpt:

> Best of all, of course, *religion solves the problem of death* (my italics) which no living individuals can solve, no matter how they would support us. Religion, then, gives the possibility of heroic victory in freedom and solves the problem of human dignity at the highest level. The two ontological motives of the human condition are both met: the need to surrender oneself in full to the rest of nature, to become a part of it by laying down one's whole existence to some higher meaning; and the need to expand oneself as an individual heroic personality. Finally, religion alone gives hope, because it holds open the dimension of the unknown and the unknowable, the fantastic mystery of creation that the human mind cannot even begin to approach. (Becker, 1973, pp. 203–204)

In a previous section, "Probable Causes of the Fear of Dying," I emphasized the role of parental behavior in producing fear of abandonment, and suggested that this was later translated into fear of death and dying, since early abandonment of a helpless infant or child is tantamount to death. These conclusions were based on overwhelming impressions gathered during a longitudinal study of 2000 families. Some years ago I stumbled on a copy of a 1974 review of Becker's "Denial of Death" in a second-hand bookstore. This review, by Lloyd Demause, was what might be called a sharp attack on a book that had just won the Pulitzer Prize for nonfiction! At this point I refer to it, because it reflects on Becker's apparent assault on science and psychology, and his exaltation of religion or faith. Demause sees good parenting as the ray of hope, and this is echoed by others, such as Gruen (1992). If my intuition about poor parenting and the genesis of the fear of death is correct, then psychology, to the extent that it can help parents to give love to their children, can be, or become, as important or more important than religion as a buffer against the fear of dying (and the fear of the "awfulness" of life). Demause, speaking in his role as a therapist and psychohistorian, criticizes Becker's philosophical roots (Brown and Kierkegaard) and his clinical mentors (Rank, Adler, and Jung) as people who know nothing about children.

> Given helping parents, children do not need heroics, and given love and under-standing they even manage to come to terms with death without repression. That few children today have parents who can provide this level of care is a psychohistorical fact, not an existential ultimate. Becker calls for a union of psychoanalysis with reli-gion, because 'only religion solves the problem of death;' he also calls for new illu-sions, new faiths, for man is 'stuck with his character' and 'can't evolve beyond it.' Little does he suspect that children all around him are evolving beyond our character even now. (Demause, 1974, p. 283)

Although I agree with Demause that Becker slights the potential of parent-ing for our salvation, I am also sure that no amount of parental love can protect us from the "awful truth" of sickness, catastrophe, war, and of the inevitability of our own death. It might help us to meet these assaults more bravely, but we will not avoid them through parental love. How often have we heard a parent say, "If only I could protect my children from the world and the sorrows that are sure to come to them in time!"

When Becker says, "Only religion solves the problem of death" we part company, because religion (with its belief in the afterlife) is only one of many solutions to the problem of (the fear of) death. This book was inspired by the fact that Becker, despite the brilliance of his ideas, put so much emphasis on killing as a coping mode. He and others mention various coping modes from time to time, but do not focus on them.

The point that Freud made, in his *Future of an Illusion* (Freud, 1957), is that if you take away religion, people will substitute something else. He pes-simistically said that these substitutes would probably be just as rigid and illusory as religion. The truth is that there are many other "solutions" to the problem of death, other than religion. It all amounts to how one "chooses" to live one's life. (This is not altogether a free choice, of course.)

Clairvoyantly, Freud was looking at political belief systems that might replace religion, and he became the victim of just such an illusory system in the form of Nazism. That system had its Thousand Year Reich, the myth of Aryan racial purity, its scapegoats and its Satans (the Jews and Gypsies), its god (Hitler), and its bible ("Mein Kampf").

Science, philosophy, and the arts may all be illusory, but they, in addition to religion, offer ways in which we can cope with death, and keep the "wolf from the door."

Incidentally, the wolf, like other large predators, is often a symbol of death. In fairy tales such as "The Three Little Pigs" or "Little Red Riding Hood", the death-figure of the wolf is defeated.

So many folk tales deal with the fight against death. Hansel and Gretel kill the witch, by shoving her into the oven in which they were to be baked. The Billy Goats Gruff conquer a troll hiding under a bridge. Jack the Giant Killer escapes with his life, and climbs down the beanstalk to safety. Many more fairy tales deal with abandonment or loss of status (a "mini-death"). Cinderella wins the Prince, although she has been disinherited by her wicked stepmother and two stepsisters, and made into a char-girl.

In "The Goose Girl" a princess's maid, noticing that her mistress' magical necklace has fallen off, makes her become a goose-girl in the palace of the Prince to whom her mistress was originally engaged. The false princess marries the Prince. Falada, the favorite horse of the true princess, can talk, so the false princess has him beheaded. The horse-head, though nailed to a gate, talks to the true princess every day: "Oh, Princess, if your mother could see you now!" When the Prince hears this, the true princess is restored to her rightful place beside the Prince. These tales all tell the child that there is death and misfortune in the world, but that it can be overcome. Again, art (in this case folkart) provides a bulwark against fear. If the lost status is a "mini-death," the restoration of the heroes and heroines to their rightful place is in effect a resurrection. For example, Sleeping Beauty is poisoned (again by a wicked stepmother), and is under a sleeping spell of 100 years. Awakening is resurrection.* Sleep and death are equivalents. Snow White is also poisoned. Both Snow White and Sleeping Beauty regain their position and marry into wealth. In fiction, the novels of Charles Dickens and the Horatio Alger stories are examples of the familiar "rags to riches" theme. Often upward mobility is due more to chance than to any effort on the part of the hero or heroine. The novels of Judith Krantz and other recent bestsellers repeat this familiar theme of rags to riches, but chance plays less of a part in success than hard work, social skills, and sex.

BENEFITS OF RELIGIOSITY

There have been numerous studies of the effects of religion on a range of outcome variables. Only a few can be mentioned here. One of the most famous is *Le Suicide*, by Emile Durkheim (1897). Durkheim found that Catholics had much lower rates of suicide than Protestants, regardless of the countries in which they lived. For example, French Catholics had lower rates than French Protestants, and Italian Catholics had lower rates than Italian Protestants. He attributed this effect to the strictures against suicide emphasized in Catholicism,

---

* It has been said that the awakening of Sleeping Beauty by the Prince's kiss represents the end of the sexual "latency" period. Thus she is no longer "asleep," and is sexually awakened by a kiss. The Prince is the only one who can wake her (arouse her)? These tales can be interpreted on many levels. On their face, they seem to say that you can escape death, or 100 years of sleep, or even being disinherited and degraded into a char-girl or a goose-girl.

making for lower rates, and conversely, to the sense of personal responsibility involved in Protestantism, which could make for higher rates.

In the Midtown Manhattan study (Srole, 1962, pp. 300–324; Langner, 1963) the differences in mental disorder between Protestants, Catholics, and Jews were confounded by the social class differences between these groups. Catholics in New York City happened to be of lower socioeconomic status than Protestants and Jews, on the average. If only the treated portion of the general population (public and private inpatients and clinic outpatients) was considered, Catholics had a rate of 659/100,000, Protestants 385/100,000, and Jews 250/100,000. When a home survey was conducted (which of course included both treated and untreated individuals), respondents reported their behavior and symptomatology in interviews, and were then rated by psychiatrists on this basis. The proportion rated as showing some impairment in functioning due to mental or emotional disorder was 17.2% of Jews, 23.5% of Protestants, and 24.7% of Catholics. (There were no black respondents in the sampled area.) The difference between Jews and Catholics was statistically significant. If we controlled for socioeconomic status, so that only the lowest stratum was examined, the three religious groups had almost equal proportions of "Well" ratings, but the percentage of Impaired was 30.5% of Catholics, 32.0% of Protestants, and 19.4% of Jews. Protestant–Catholic differences in impairment disappeared when age and socioeconomic status were controlled. However, Jews (contrary to earlier studies based on treated illness alone) remained significantly less impaired. Jews, nevertheless, did seek out psychotherapy in clinics in much greater numbers. By and large, those of all religions who sought clinic or private therapy tended to be less impaired, and of higher socioeconomic status than the average for their own groups!

Parental religiosity was not related to impairment in upper socioeconomic status individuals, or in Jews. However, such a correlation did exist among Protestants of low and middle socioeconomic status who showed greater impairment if they reported that religion was "very important" or "not at all important" to their parents. Those who said "somewhat important" had the lowest rates. A similar result was found among Catholics (with no socioeconomic status controls). Like low and middle socioeconomic status Protestants, Catholics at the extremes had higher rates. The explanation for this may be that in New York City, and on its upper east side in the early 1900s, it was probably normative for poorer Catholics and Protestants to be very religious, as shown by the proportions of parents so reported. The higher rates for the now-adult offspring of the parents who were the exceptions to this turn-of-the-century religiosity may be due to their parents' nonconformity. This is not true for Jews, but the evidence in their case is based on smaller numbers, and therefore not reliable.

In brief, Jews and Catholics have had lower rates of suicide than Protestants, owing to stronger injunctions against it. Mental disorder involving greater degrees of impairment is found more in Catholics and Protestants, because at least in the New York City area they comprise more of the lower socioeconomic levels. As of this writing, there is less and less adherence to religious precepts in the United States, but worldwide, religion is still one of the major influences on behavior.

There has been some question as to whether religiosity or social participation was behind the fact that religious individuals (not just those who attended church regularly) have been found to have lower death rates after surgery, and have also shown lower levels of stress-inducing chemicals in their blood. Several studies reviewed by Daniel Goleman (1995, p. 10) have found that getting comfort from religious belief was a key factor in the recovery of heart surgery patients.

> While those patients who said before heart surgery that they found no comfort in religious beliefs had a death rate almost three times higher than those who said they found some strength in their faith, other measures of religiosity were not nearly so strongly related to survival.

Churchgoing and a feeling of being "deeply religious" were not associated with a lower death rate. The study director, Dr. Thomas Oxman, said

> It seems that being able to give meaning to a precarious life-threatening situation—having faith there is some greater meaning or force at work—is medically helpful. If you can't make sense of what's going on, it's much harder to bear. (Goleman, 1995, p. 10)

The same study found that absence of participation in various social groups (church or other groups) was associated with a three-times-higher death risk in the six months after the surgery.

Dr. Oxman said, "It appears there is something life protective in belonging to a group and having a regular social activity of some kind." This finding may hold up in further research. Unfortunately, very large samples are needed to confirm hypotheses of this nature. There is a need to control all the important test variables in the analysis, and these variables are not always known before the study is conducted. For example, the degree of physical impairment due to circulatory and heart problems before the surgery may have prevented some of the sicker patients from participating in social groups. Depression associated with more severe cardiovascular conditions may have kept some patients away from groups they formerly attended. This would produce a spurious correlation between social participation and death rate. Of the 231 patients in the study, 21 died. A much larger sample, divided into patients with severe, moderate, and mild impairment prior to the heart attack, or one month after the attack, might have solved just this one problem of "pre-selection bias."

The levels of the chemicals produced by the body under stress have been found to be lower among individuals aged 70 to 79 who had "people in their lives who offered emotional support" (Goleman, 1995, p. 10 quoting Dr. Daniel Berkman, as epidemiologist at Yale University.) This seems in keeping with the general findings about norepinephrine and cortisol. Catecholamines were also elevated in people who had recently been told that they would lose their jobs.

On the other hand, levels of neurotransmitters, such as serotonin, have been found to increase after people have been exposed to humor. Serotonin is also involved in the "runner's high," a surge of good feeling reached after a fair amount of aerobic exercise.

Killer T cells, crucial in the immune system's function of fighting invading organisms, are found to be at low levels after an illness of a family member, or during bereavement. Perhaps this is why "Bad things come in threes." One illness is followed by another illness in the same family, owing to the lowering of the immune defenses in the family members who become depressed. All this evidence is not negated by preselection bias and circular reasoning.

However, one has to be very careful in identifying the exact independent variable (usually called a causal variable) responsible for differential rates of death and survival. (Of course, this is true of any research.) The upshot of Goleman's review is that religious faith and social participation are both independent factors influencing the outcome of heart surgery, other types of surgery, and survival rates in general.

RISKS OF RELIGIOSITY

Since "risk–benefit" analysis is applied to medical care, environmental laws, and almost every aspect of our lives, why not apply it to religion? The emotional support derived from being a church, mosque, or synagogue member, and the apparent psychophysiological support provided by religious faith, are counterbalanced by several negative correlates of religion, particularly established religion.

First, there is the problem of taking part in a magical and illusory system of beliefs. One faces reality "at one's own risk," as the road signs say when there is repair work going on. Yet this realism, this rationality, is one of the great creations of man, the thinking animal. Religiosity may be a step backward, in my opinion, although so many great minds, including Freud, have said it is a necessary prop for most people.

Second are the consequences of fatalism. This is often associated with deep religious belief, whether in Eastern religions or in Western Protestantism. The latter formerly stood for individual responsibility, but it has become almost a non-religion in the United States, unless one is talking about some of the more revivalist sects, or the activist religious right.

Fatalism may be helpful in cases of terminal illness or threats of unavoidable death (as mentioned previously). During the life span, however, this blind acceptance may be a powerful deterrent to action in one's own self-interest. Fatalism is a politically inactive position. The "sweet lemon" of the Biblical

"Beatitudes" suggests the "cooling out of the mark" described by Goffman (1952). The marks (persons to be cheated) are all of mankind, but especially the poor, sick, and various minorities, such as women, children, and nonwhites. The "cooler" is the person who works with the con (confidence man) to steal from the "mark." When the mark finds out that she has been cheated, she gets angry (see the "House of Games" plot earlier). The cooler is a confederate of the con, and has made friends with the mark prior to the actual stealing. The mark, enraged, says, "I'll go to the police." The cooler says, "But think of the publicity. Also, you were greedy; you wanted to get this money too!" The mark is then dissuaded from action against the con. Goffman's coolers are the priests, rabbis, clergymen, psychiatrists, psychologists, social workers, judges, and some lawyers—any authority figure who may at times stop an individual from taking social, political, or legal action to better his lot. Good therapists and good clergymen (by my definition) encourage their clients to take some action to improve their situation. Very often, however, the focus of therapy is on the individual's inner problems, and how he or she handles his or her environment, not on the often noxious environment itself. Some churches, particularly black churches in the United States and Catholic churches in Latin America, have led the struggle for the underdog. This has not been true of most established religions.

The Beatitudes sum up the traditional role of the church:

> Blessed are the poor in spirit: for theirs is the kingdom of heaven.
> Blessed are the meek: for they shall inherit the earth. (Matthew V, 3–9)

Others who are blessed are the mourners, the righteous, the merciful, the pure in heart, and the peacemakers. There is nothing wrong with being any of these, but they are all on the more passive side of the fence. The Old Testament said, "Smite thine enemies" while the New Testament preached loving your enemies, forgiveness, and turning the other check. The poor and the meek have looked to the fatalism and passivity of the New Testament (the "sweet lemon") while the rich and powerful seem to have thrived on the philosophy of the Old Testament, the "eye for an eye" maxim (also called lex talionis in the discussions of Oedipal and castration-complexes).

Third, confession and absolution (in those religions in which it is central), while easing guilt feelings for the individual, may also lead to a society whose sins can be indulged for a price. This was one of the things Martin Luther raged against, in his attack on the Catholicism of his time. "Indulgences" were actually sold, with prices varying according to the degree of the sin, a practice supported by John Tetzel, which prompted Luther to post his theses on the church door, and led to the Reformation.

In our own society, no sin is so great that an "indulgence" can't be bought through the legal system. With enough money to pay top lawyers, one can buy absolution. For example, it is quite probable that O. J. Simpson killed his wife and her friend Ron Goldman, yet no prosecutor could have won a conviction against Simpson's top team of the leading defense lawyers and forensic experts in the country. What was new in this case was that a black man was able to be acquitted of killing a white woman with a great deal of evidence against him. In the past, only a wealthy white man could do so. Money and celebrity made the difference.

What was once a severe (Protestant) conscience has been externalized, and left to depend on the legal system. With a lack of consensus about what is right or justifiable, people look not to themselves, but to outer authority for rules. These rules operate by an elaborate, often arcane, system called "the law," which often fails in its attempt to reach its goal of justice.

Fourth, as previously mentioned, religion has been one of the primary sources of war and persecution There have been "holy wars" since time began, in large part because of the group-membership aspect of religion. It provides an identity, and when that identity is attacked, ideologically, economically, or physically, conflict results.

These four risks (among the many risks of religion, despite its great comforting powers) tell me that it belongs only in the second rank of defenses against the fear of death. Creativity, Love, Humor, Intellectualization, Procreation, Obsessive–Compulsive Behavior, Living to the Hilt, Better, or Longer, and Group Membership precede Religion in my somewhat arbitrary ranking.

Coping Modes in a Moral Framework

More important than the exact rank order of any particular adaptive or coping mode is the fact that I have thought it appropriate to place them in a moral framework. Their relative position is arguable. However, to say that the murderer and the artist are equal in ethical standing is, to my mind, nonsense. This may be the viewpoint of the therapist, whose job it is to help and protect the patient. If he sees the patient as immoral, he is accused of counter-transference, or hostility, or being judgmental. Nevertheless, the therapist also has a duty to protect society. Judgments must constantly be made as to the severity of the patient's behavior, and this involves weighing possible damage by, or benefit of, the behavior to the self or society. After the initial interview, the individual is usually referred for in-patient or out-patient treatment, or sent home as a nonpatient. This is called a disposition.

Since everyone makes these judgments of damage potential (the policeman must decide whether to bring his suspect to the local mental hospital or to prison, and family members must make a choice in bringing their oddly behaving relative to a psychiatrist, social worker, or mental hospital, or to call the police), I think it more than justifiable to arrange behaviors in some sort of continuum of severity and potential damage.

Is putting coping strategies into a moral hierarchy in terms of damage to self and others perhaps a reversion to the philosopher's eternal search for the "good," for proper behavior among human beings? Yes, this echoes the absolute values of Plato. However, the coping hierarchy is a continuum. The top of the list contains the ideal behaviors, such as creativity and love, which are seldom fully achieved, but worth striving for. At the bottom is homicide or killing. The privileged relationship of doctor–patient or priest–penitent must be breached when a rape, torture, or murder is confessed. This has become part of our framework of laws, and unreported crimes may leave therapists open to major lawsuits.

Good behavior and the ideal life are of course not absolutes. Their definitions vary over time, and between cultures. For example, in a few hundred years, homosexuality has gone from behavior punishable by death, to a mental disorder as defined by the Diagnostic and Statistical Manual (DSM) of the American Psychiatric Association, to recently being dropped as a diagnosable entity in DSM IV. The psychiatric profession and the general public have changed their minds about what constitutes pathology. Values are not engraved in stone for eternity.

Still, taking the life of another person other than in self-defense is hard for most of us to accept as excusable behavior. Perhaps there is at least a bottom line to be drawn, beyond which we will call an act evil, heinous, and unforgivable. The hobgoblin of moral relativism is less frightening when we realize that we can draw a (bottom) line in the sand. But the line in the sand is constantly shifting, and we must (and we do) fit our ethics to the times. This makes for a greater effort, a constant balancing act. It is much more difficult than clinging to absolute values.

RISKS OF THE BETTER COPING MODES: THE DOWN SIDE

The risks of many of these "better" coping modes are still considerable. For example, creativity produced the atomic and the hydrogen bomb which have threatened to destroy life on this planet. (We assume that the preservation of life is a universal and positive value, although after Auschwitz, Armenia, Bosnia, Rwanda, Kosovo, and so on, one sometimes wonders.)

Humor, so effective in the fight against death, is often used as a weapon to cut down various human targets, such as minorities, religious groups, women, the young and the elderly, rural folks, and racial and tribal groups.

Procreation in excess may eventually make the earth uninhabitable, if the "population bomb" scientists are correct. The earth's population appears to be doubling every 20 years. A good defense against individual death fear may at the same time contribute to the death of our species by overcrowding. Workaholism blinds one to life's enjoyment and to creativity, even though it keeps death fears at bay. Conspicuous consumption and national hypochondriasis are the result of wanting to live better and longer.

Belonging to groups feeds war and other deadly competition, as well as providing emotional support for the individual.

There is a down side to each coping mode. Some, like suicide and killing, are primarily on the down side. Religion seems to me to lie somewhere just above the middle on the risk–benefit scale.

From time to time there are voices that offer the hope that religion and science together can promise a new way of believing, give us guidance, and add meaning to our lives. Essayists such as Lewis Thomas and Stephen Jay Gould, coming from medicine and biology, certainly have helped in this fusion of apparently disparate disciplines. Hundreds of others from philosophy and theology have contributed. Artists (especially great poets, novelists, and playwrights) have shown us models for behavior. The social sciences have made many contributions. An interesting new voice, Loyal Rue, has been heard, attempting to be realistic about illusion:

> ... society is caught up in a Kulturkampf with nihilists promoting intellectual and moral relativism and realists defending objective and universal truths. The noble lie would introduce a third voice, one which first agrees with the nihilists that universal myths are pretentious lies, but then insists, against the nihilists, that without such lies humanity cannot survive...it remains for the artists, poets, musicians, filmmakers, and other masters of illusion to seduce us into an embrace with a noble lie. We need a new myth that tells us how we should live together, to say how things really are and what really matters. (Rue, 1994)*

Rue echoes Freud's conviction that man currently cannot live without illusion ("lies"). He seems to ask that the artist make those lies more "noble," more aesthetic, more palatable, or in Becker's words, more "heroic." Freud, in contrast, hoped that man's intellect would eventually overcome the need to harbor illusion. The illusion he referred to was religion.

---

* This quote is from Rue's jacket copy, which describes succinctly what composes his "third voice." Of special interest is his knock on "moral relativism." This seems to be a modern devil. It is one of the central modern evils in *The Death of Satan* by Andrew Delbanco, and appears as a whipping boy in writings of the right and the left.

12

Mementos and Monuments

Since the time of the Neanderthals and the Cro-Magnons, man has left his mark by drawing on cave walls, scratching figures on rocks, and building statues of gods in his own image. The Greeks had a word for it *hubris* excessive pride or arrogance. Shelley captured this incredible vanity in his poem "Ozymandias".

> ...Two vast and trunkless legs of stone
> Stand in the desert. Near them, on the sand,
> Half sunk, a shattered visage lies, whose frown,
> And wrinkled lip, and sneer of cold command
> Tell that its sculptor well those passions read
> ...And on the pedestal these words appear;
> 'My name is Ozymandias, king of kings;
> Look on my works, ye Mighty, and despair!'
> Nothing beside remains. Round the decay
> Of that colossal wreck, boundless and bare
> The lone and level sands stretch far away.
> (Marshall, 1966, p. 461) (Shelley, 1817)

Ramses II is the Ozymandias of Shelley's poem, "the god-king who boasted of his martial prowess in inscriptions and statues found from Abu Simbel near Aswan to the Nile Delta." He fathered 100 children, 52 of them sons, who were buried in 67 chambers of a large mausoleum.*

In our own small way we can mimic Ozymandias. Collecting mementos and building monuments are ways of achieving a sense of immortality. This can be done during one's lifetime, by building a small mausoleum, donating personal letters and furniture to a library, or buying a new laboratory for one's college. You stipulate, of course, that your name must appear prominently on the tomb, laboratory, or library entrance.

---

* A new find, a huge mausoleum, was discovered in 1995. The discovery and the identification of Ramses II as Ozymandias was described in an editorial in *The New York Times*, "In the Valley of the Kings."

Tax deductions encourage these charitable gifts. Wills and trusts can be made during one's lifetime. Most of them become active after one's death. Many are meant to control the survivors with a "dead hand from the grave."

There have always been attempts to preserve the image of oneself or one's family for posterity. Statues of the wealthy and powerful abound from the Ur and Nile valleys. Naturalistic oil portraits were made on some Egyptian coffins. Nobles and later the wealthy bourgeoisie commissioned portraits. These have in a sense prolonged the lives of the subjects. The walls of art museums the world over are adorned with portraits of monarchs, merchant princes, and in some cases more humble husbands and wives, youths, and workers (as in the paintings of Rembrandt or Murillo). Still photos, movies, and now videotapes capture the faces, movements, and even the voices of the past. These are the modern methods of embalming, of stopping time, of preserving the self and loved ones.

The nobility have always shown a great interest in genealogy, but lately this has been extended to people from all walks of life. An industry has sprung up that researches your family tree, and offers computer printouts of all possible family members. Diaries, memoirs, and autobiographies preserve the self in deeper ways. Inner thoughts and feelings are expressed that cannot be captured on film.

Many collections are undertaken with an eye to immortality. Museums house paintings, furniture, stuffed animals, and memorabilia of the rich and famous. These collections are often displayed in rooms or wings dedicated to the donor or his family. For example, the Rockefeller Wing of the Metropolitan Museum was donated in memory of Michael Rockefeller, who died collecting sculpture in the Asmat area of New Guinea.* Many of the carvings he collected are on exhibit there.

Most of the ceremonies and procedures associated with death suggest the striving to maintain life. Tombs, tombstones, epitaphs, elaborate funerals, and obituaries often eulogize the dead, and make pretensions to immortality.

The body-preserving customs and funeral rites are only a small part of the attempt to control fear of dying and proclaim the power of life and living.

> From the times of the earliest cave men, who kept their dead alive by dyeing the bones red and burying them near the family hearth, down to the Hollywood funeral cult, the flight from death has been, as Unamuno said, the heart of all religion. Pyramids and skyscrapers—monuments more lasting than bronze—suggest how much of the world's 'economic' activity also is really a flight from death. (Brown, 1959).

The writing of history is clearly a way of embalming and embroidering the past, just as a corpse is beautified for viewing at a funeral. The litany of wars, biographies of "great" men (both good and evil), famine, migration, art, science,

---

* The newpapers at the time of his death reported that he had drowned after falling overboard from a canoe about 2 miles off the Western shore of Irian Jaya. A Jesuit missionary to whom I spoke when visiting the area during a tour of the Indonesian Archipelago told me that story was untrue. He said that the head of any member of a powerful family was much prized, and that young Rockefeller had probably been killed for his head. He also stated that the victim was a very strong swimmer, and could easily have made it to shore, where he probably met his fate.

and all human experience is a testament to the continuity of man. Writing, reading, and teaching history has as one of its main functions the preservation of confidence that there is meaning, direction, and order in our lives (no matter how delusional this may be).

> Now what is history? It is the centuries of systematic explorations of the riddle of death, with a view of overcoming death. (Seldes, 1967, p. 478, quoting Boris Pasternak in *Doctor Zhivago*.)

Let's take a look at some of these mementos and monuments.

TOMBS, TOMBSTONES AND EPITAPHS, AND CEMETERIES

There is a vast literature on cemeteries, funerals, and ceremonies connected with death. Our focus is on how our customs and folkways help to control the fear of dying. Just how secure are our tombstones and graves? Are we justified in thinking that we are permanently protected in our graves?

> One clown asks another in Shakespeare's Hamlet, 'What is he that builds stronger than either the mason, the shipwright, or the carpenter?' 'Gravedigger' is the riddle's answer, because the 'houses he makes last till doomsday.' (Iserson, 1994, p. 525)

Iserson points out that, on the contrary, graves are far from permanent. He gives details of how skeletons and buried ceremonial objects have been pilfered from Native American graves. In medieval Europe, bones were dug up within a few years and placed in a charnel house. Many modern cemeteries rent graves for a few years and up to 30 years.

In the United States, cemeteries are not immune to the laws of eminent domain, and can be plowed under, or moved. In New York City, buildings went up over old cemeteries, and "the remains were rarely moved." Iserson quotes General Lew Wallace, the author of Ben Hur: "The monuments of the nations are all protests against nothingness after death; so are statues and inscriptions; so is history." Iserson remarks, "These 'protests' from most ancient grave markers have dissolved with time, since they were made of wood or soft stone. Those of hard stone, such as the millenia-old obelisks of Egypt, still exist" (Iserson, 1994, p. 533). In the United States, gravestones were once made of marble, slate, or sandstone. These stones eroded so quickly that they were eventually replaced with granite and bronze. Granite in Egyptian statues has lasted at least 5000 years. While this may seem "permanent," man has been on earth at least three million years, since "Lucy" was born. Even the beautiful temples of Greece (and Asia Minor) have been eaten away by the acids formed from automobile exhausts, and are in danger of being destroyed. They are only about 2000 years old.

Mausoleums, especially large ones, attest to the power of the deceased, or, as in the case of the Taj Mahal, the love of the living for the dead. Ambrose Bierce, in his usual acerbic style, called mausoleums "worm's meat," and said, "Probably the silliest work in which a human being can engage is construction of a tomb for himself" (Iserson, 1994, p. 540). Iserson feels that mausoleums are a product of conspicuous consumption. Some cost hundreds of thousands of dollars. He cites Hartsdale Cemetery's "Cathedral of Memories," which contains 8800 crypts, 250 private family rooms, and an 80-seat chapel.

In the past, many memorial plaques in churches and tombstones in cemeteries (dating from the 1700s) bore epitaphs. Some were reminders of man's grandiosity or vanity, and predicted the viewer's death.

> Such as thou art, so once was I,
> As I am now, so shalt thou be.
> (Tuchman, 1978, p. 295)[*]

There are many paintings entitled "Vanity," which usually depict a young woman in the pink of health gazing at herself in a mirror. In the mirror you see her reflection as a skull. The message is the same as on many tombstones. Some gravestones have humorous epitaphs:

> "Thorp's Corpse" Poor Martha Snell, hers gone away. Her would, if her could, but her couldn't stay. Her'd two bad legs, and a badish cough. But her legs it was as carried her off. (Iserson, 1994, p. 537)

The cemetery is usually a collection of individual graves, and it has a symbolic function as well as the practical one of disposing of dead bodies.

> The fundamental *sacred* problem of the graveyard is to provide suitable symbols to refer to and express man's hope of immortality through the sacred belief and ritual of Christianity and to reduce his anxiety and fear about death as marking the obliteration of his personality—the end of life for himself and for those he loves. (Fulton, 1970, p. 367)[†]

Obviously, the graveyard is almost universal, and is meaningful for people of many religions (not just Christians). As cremation becomes more popular in Western societies, the graveyard will probably become obsolete. The Balinese cremate their dead, and then send the ashes out on small boats into the ocean. Given the fact that populations increase geometrically rather than arithmetically, in a few centuries cremation may become a necessity rather than an option.

MONUMENTS

There is some overlap between tombs and monuments. The word "monument" comes from the Latin *monere*, to remind or warn. The primary meaning of "tomb" is "an excavation in the earth or rock for the burial of a corpse; a

---

[*] Inscribed on the monument of the Prince of Wales at Canterbury. He died in 1376. Verses were inscribed in French telling of the evanescence of earthly power, the Ozymandias message of vanity and hubris.

[†] The chapter is by W. Lloyd Warner, "The City of the Dead," reprinted from *The Living and the Dead*, Yale University Press, 1959, Chapter 9.

grave." Secondary meanings are "a mausoleum" or "monument for housing or commemorating a dead person." There is the "Tomb of the Unknown Soldier," which is really a monument, since it is not an excavation. Many gravesites could be called monuments, since they have statues on them rather than simple headstones. One example is a statue of Al Jolson, arms outstretched, obviously singing his signature song, "Mammy" ("Destinations", *The New York Times Magazine*, May 14, 1995, p. 92, photograph). Sir Richard Burton's monument is a carved Bedouin tent, appropriate for this Victorian explorer ("Destinations", op. cit.).

There are probably more monuments to wars and warriors than all the other types—presidents, martyrs (Joan of Arc), famous heroines (Alice in Wonderland), heroic animals (Balto), and so on. James Reston Jr. complains that the Washington D.C. mall is becoming cluttered with war monuments. He says that the Civil War, Korean War, and Vietnam War monuments are so close to one another that their impact is "diluted." In addition, a World War II Memorial and a Black Revolutionary War Patriots memorial are planned. Reston quotes Lewis Mumford:

> In their vanity the eminent and powerful seek a petrified immortality; they write their boasts upon tombstones, they incorporate their deeds in obelisks; they place their hopes of remembrance in solid stones joined to other solid stones...forgetful of the fact that stones that are deserted by the living are even more helpless than life that remains unprotected and unpreserved by stones. (Reston, 1995, p. 49)

While war monuments are initially memorials to the soldiers and sometimes the civilians killed in a particular war, they often turn into quasi-religious shrines. Gustav Niebuhr quotes various experts who say that the monument becomes an "altar," "a place where pilgrims come and devotions are paid." People come "to be transformed intellectually and spiritually at a place of power." The power, I think, is the power of continuity, of the affirmation of life of survivors and a nation that continues living even after the death of some of its members. The primary function for the bereaved is to communicate with the dead and commemorate them (they leave flowers, photos, and flags; touch the engraved names; or make tracings on paper). The majority of visitors who have not lost family or friends in the war derive some sense of personal and national immortality.

IMAGES OF THE SELF AND FAMILY: FREEZE FRAMES AND FROZEN BODIES

If there is any doubt that images, such as sculptures and portraits, can confer some sense of immortality on individuals, one need look no further than the limestone busts of Nefertiti (1372–1350 B.C.) and her husband Ikhnaton (1372–1354 B.C.). The Nefertiti statue has been widely reproduced. I doubt that she would have been so well remembered without her statue, even though she was the wife of a king who was probably the first monotheist.

While these two works of art, particularly the head of Ikhnaton, are unusually naturalistic for that period, most Egyptian and Babylonian statues were highly stylized. It was only through inscriptions that the subject could be identified.

The ages when statues or oil portraits of kings, nobles, and wealthy merchants were the primary means of immortalizing them have passed. In modern times the camera, film, movies, and camcorders are able to freeze images of the living and preserve them after death. They can also reproduce not only a physical likeness, but motion and speech as well. This has made it possible to feed back images of living family members to each other and to "preserve" the previous generations in living color. Now the family albums with fading snapshots of great grandpa and great-aunt Tillie will become videotapes with earlier generations speaking to their great grandchildren. This will require a large number of copies, since families tend to reproduce exponentially. What will happen to the tape of Uncle Albert, the child molester, who was videotaped before his arrest, is anyone's guess. Perhaps he will be deleted from the family tape archives, or he may make a tape from prison, excusing his behavior because he experienced an abusive childhood.

As long as these images are reasonably positive, and don't depict violent family quarrels or scenes of severe illness, the children of the video era will probably get an enhanced sense of their importance and some reassurance of the family continuity. Watching videos of one's own development is usually a positive experience, since parents automatically edit the filming. Scenes of children crying, parents scolding or spanking, and parental quarrels are typically not recorded. One unforeseen consequence of this archiving of experience is that some adults, in middle or old age, may look back on their childhood tapes with nostalgia mixed with regret at lost youth. More on that subject later.

Susan Sontag's book *On Photography* gives us brilliant insights primarily into the meaning and uses of still photography. What she has to say applies equally to film and videotape.

> Memorializing the achievements of individuals considered as members of families … is the earliest popular use of photography.
> … photography came along to memorialize, to restate symbolically, the imperiled continuity and vanishing extendedness of family life. (Sontag, 1977, pp. 7 and 8).

Sontag is right on target as she describes how photos help to maintain the "imperiled continuity" of families, and she cites the popular rite of the wedding picture. Baby snapshots and graduation photos are other favorites. However, she focuses on the preservation of the event, or talks of the mortality of other people than the self.

> After the event has ended, the picture will still exist, conferring on the event a kind of immortality (and importance) it would never otherwise have enjoyed. (Sontag, 1977, p. 10)

To take a picture is to have an interest in things as they are, in the status quo remaining unchanged... (Sontag, 1977, p. 11)

All photographs are *memento mori*. To take a photograph is to participate in another person's (or thing's) mortality, vulnerability, mutability. Precisely by slicing out this moment and freezing it, all photographs testify to time's relentless melt. (Sontag, 1977, p. 14)

In her discussion of photography as a "defense against anxiety," she first sees it (tourist photography) as a way of "soothing feelings of disorientation during travel" and of appeasing the anxiety of the work-driven ethic of the tourist on vacation, especially the Germans, Japanese, and Americans (Sontag, 1977, pp. 8–9). Later on she talks about photos of war and accidents, and again mentions anxiety reduction:

The feeling of being exempt from calamity stimulates interest in looking at painful pictures, and looking at them suggests and strengthens the feeling that one is exempt. (Sontag, 1977, pp. 147–148)

Her statements about the reductions of anxiety and *memento mori* (an object, such as a skull, serving as a reminder of death or mortality) (Flexner, 1987)* are relevant to the broad subject of photography, but seem to skirt around the obvious point that photos, film, and videos now have a major role in reducing the fear of death and dying. The continuity of *one's own life* is supported by the procession of pictures and tapes starting with birth. The immortality of one's family is proclaimed in the snapshots of past generations, and in the tapes of one's children and grandchildren. While photographs may be a reminder of one's mortality, they also have the opposite effect of reducing death anxiety. The feeling of group membership, as discussed previously, is one of the best remedies for fear in general, and especially for death fear. The family is the most intimate of all groups, and has the potential for giving more continuous love and support than other groups. So snapshots, enlarged portraits, home movies, and videotapes of loved ones are a great source of comfort. If anyone doubts this, just look at the sales of cameras and camcorders and the proliferation of "one-hour" photo shops. The humorist George Carlin, in his usual acerbic manner, has asked (and I paraphrase), "What's wrong with these people? They just *took* the pictures, and now they want them back in an hour? What's the rush?" The rush is, I think, that they are anxious to preserve their children, to preserve every fleeting moment of their hurried lives, to keep their family and themselves "alive" through photography.

There are two additional processes which a person can use to keep his image "alive." These are embalming and cryonics. The latter involves the deep-freezing of bodies at death for future defrosting at a time when the particular

* The first definition of *memento mori* is translated directly from the Latin, "Remember that you must die" ... The first definiton is as an "object ... "

disease that caused the death is conquered. Embalming is certainly a denial of death, because it preserves the visage of the deceased, and in fact usually enhances it. By injecting formalin and other preservative fluids, the corpse is made to look lifelike, so that viewers are not shocked by the ravages of a final illness. I remember viewing my father in the hospital emergency room after he had died of a heart attack, following cancer of the bladder and liver. He had been defibrillated, pounded on the chest, given oxygen, and all this with only two months to live because of the liver cancer! His mouth was wide open and his face was gaunt. He looked like the faces I had seen in Hieronymus Bosch's painting of hell. That face would haunt me for years. I can still see it clearly, although the image no longer comes up spontaneously. A final mental picture of him embalmed and lifelike would have been much easier to bear. Both Geoffrey Gorer and Robert Lifton thought that embalming interfered with the grief process and caused confusion in the minds of the survivors. Stephenson seems to disagree with them, although it remains (sic!) a heated controversy (Stephenson, 1985).*

In a South Pacific island tribe a party similar to the Irish wake is given. The deceased has been baked until the skin is leathery. He or she is in a sitting position, and "greets" the visitors as they enter. Each person shakes the hand of the corpse or touches the body in a greeting. I am sure that neither the wake nor the bake interfere with the grieving process of the survivors.

Woody Allen is not only the source of some of the best anxious jokes about death, but is also one of the first to arrange for a cryogenic future. He has made a movie called *Sleeper* about a Rip van Winkle type. I hope that he can be defrosted in 200 years, so that he can entertain another generation with his wonderful wit.

Cryogenics is certainly a more permanent solution to the problem of preserving one's image than embalming. While Lenin may last in an embalmed state for at most a few hundred years, the frozen dead may rise again, like Lazarus. Mummies, of course, have been with us for millenia, but they are neither very attractive nor recognizable as the people they were in life.

The cryogenic movement is probably the most extreme expression of our present-day denial of death. The members of this association believe that biological death is not necessary at all. Testimony to that belief lies in the fact that in 1996 several dozen corpses were immersed in canisters of liquid nitrogen in various repositories across the country, waiting for the day when medical science discovers the cure for what killed them. It is believed that by that time science will also have solved the problems associated with restoring a frozen body to life.

---

* See his discussion of embalming on pp. 230–231. "There are no studies to indicate that this confusion is a frequent occurrence, nor am I aware of any studies that imply that seeing the body in a beautified condition is unhealthy."

The motto of this movement, appropriately, is "Freeze, wait, reanimate." While the adherents of this movement believe themselves to be the ultimate secularists, it would appear that they are contemporary practitioners of what might be termed "refrigerated Christianity" (Stephenson, 1985, p. 7).

Images, whether frozen in marble, paintings, photographs, or in liquid nitrogen, give us the illusion of immortality. For the price of a roll of film, a blank videotape, or the many thousands of dollars it takes to get and stay frozen, we can order our imperishable and timeless counterparts. When our survivors look at one of these reproductions of ourselves, they can say, "That photo (film, tape) is a dead-ringer for Grandma," or whoever may be depicted.

GENEALOGY: THE FAMILY TREE INDUSTRY

I recently received a letter from a company that provides a list of people who share your last name. I had hoped that I would find some interesting relatives and perhaps some description of my origins. On receiving my "World Book of Langners," I was shocked to see how many Langners there were—5047 world-wide! Aside from a first cousin or two, I knew none of them. More of a shock was the discovery that there were hundreds of men named Thomas Langner living in Germany! My illusions of individuality were destroyed forever. The world was teeming with my Doppelgängers. Instead of feeling immortal because of my great family heritage, I felt totally replaceable by an army of the same name.

My daughter Lisa, during training as a family therapist, had to draw a chart of our family tree. Unfortunately, she also had to make estimates of the mental health of all the family members. The chart was yards long, and filled with persons of doubtful stability. Luckily, I had not given her the name of a second cousin, who is a convicted murderer. My first cousin's daughter had also made a chart, tracing the family back to the court of Queen Isabella. I knew that one distant relative had been Isabella's court doctor. I don't know if he failed to convert from Judaism during the Inquisition, or was forced out of Spain because he joined a managed care organization (HMO), but his descendants ended up in Germany and England.

As for mythology, there was Uncle Ike Bachmann, on my mother's side, who sold food and equipment to the miners during the gold rush of 1849, made his fortune, and returned East to start a huge woolen business. He became a multimillionaire. There was my Aunt Phyllis, thrice married, who divorced an East Indian Prince, then married a stockbroker, and later married her hairdresser when she was in her 60s. This, of course, scandalized the family. There was Harper, seen as a "failure" by my hard-driving relatives, because he went to New England and started a chicken farm. There was my maternal grandmother, Heddie, who carried on a rivalry with her sister Martha, taught "normal school" (the equivalent of junior college today), and worshipped her grandchildren. There was my paternal grandfather, who caught my grandmother having an affair with her music teacher. (Some said the stable boy.) She got pregnant. Grandpa kicked her out, and died shortly thereafter, temporarily orphaning his five children. She bore the illegitimate child, remarried, and had a seventh child. She collected her abandoned children and brought them back to semi-luxury in London, in the home of her solicitor husband. She once complained to her adult sons that the hand-crafted whalebone corset they had ordered for her (probably the last of its kind in the world) was the wrong size.

There was my Uncle Lawrence, who founded the Theater Guild, his wife Armina Marshall, and their son, my cousin Philip. My visits to their house or the theater often involved bumping into stars of stage and screen. Uncle Julian was known for owning most of Cape Canaveral, which he was forced to sell dirt cheap during the Depression. He would have been one of the richest men in America, he told my father, every time he came to borrow some money.

This extended family unit, with its living and dead, was surely a boon to me as I grew. It was at some level a bulwark against fear of dying, for there were always many loving relatives who cherished me. Those feelings of being part of a group are brought back by mental as well as photographic images. I can still see the huge Thanksgiving and Christmas dinners we had at my maternal great-grandma's house on 92nd Street and Riverside Drive. There would be upwards of 50 people, and the board groaned with turkey, roast beef, ham, and all kinds of pastries. Being German Jews primarily, they served Lebkuchen, Sachertort, and Baumkuchen. After a tremendous meal, which virtually immobilized everyone, the men would light up cigars and talk about business, golf, and such matters. The women would gather in another room and talk women talk. A strong male would be designated to lift the plaster bust of Alfred Lord Tennyson off the free-standing Victrola. I noticed that Tennyson's beard was always full of Carnauba wax, which stood out yellow against the white plaster. It was my job to wind up the machine with a large crank that fitted into a socket on the side of the beauti-ful wooden paneling. The records were mostly of the old Victor "His Master's Voice" type, with the red label, and the little dog listening attentively to the Victor logo. They ranged from magnificent recordings of Caruso to horrendous vaude-ville routines by the "Two Black Crows." There was an astonishing mixture of good and bad taste, which was easily recognized even by a youngster. I would retreat to the kitchen and help Bridie, the Irish maid, wash the dishes. I was madly in love with her, and it was a temporary haven from the talk and cigar smoke.

At age 70, I began to draw up a family tree of my own. I talked to my cousin Richard Danziger, who helped fill in some of the current details of marriages and births on my mother's side. There were no members of the "older generation" left on my father's side, except for his half-sister Estelle in England. My first cousin, Charles Robertson ("Carlo"), had talked at length with Estelle in 1999 while visiting her in Richmond, Surrey. He was armed with pages of questions I had written. He recorded the details of our family history as dictated by the last living source. On reading this, it suddenly struck me that I was the oldest survivor of that line, except for her. I think my chart of the family tree, instead of giving me a sense of pride and continuity, simply aroused more death anxiety in me. I was obviously "next."

There is a new twist to genealogy. Members of the Cohen (Cahan, Kahn, Cohn) tribe, which means "priest" in Hebrew, are now flocking to see if their DNA matches that of some ancient bones. It seems that many present-day Cohens are related to these ancient rabbis. This should give them a good feeling of continuity, and diminish death fear by boosting self-esteem. After all, they have a very elite gene pool, which in these times has a lot of cachet.

It seems as if the ability to trace your ancestors puts you one up on your neighbors. My Aunt Armina was very proud that her family way back had included a Blackfoot Indian. The Marshalls, of course, figured in the Gold Rush of '49. Armina's father was actually a marshal who killed an outlaw who was hiding behind a pot-bellied stove by shooting him through the stovepipe. In the Southwest, if you have "Indian blood," it proves your family was among the earliest settlers. When I was doing field work for my doctoral dissertation in southern Colorado, I found that "Anglos" with some American Indian ancestry took great pride in it. They were very prejudiced, however, against contemporary fullblooded Ute and Navajo Indians who lived in the area.

WILLS, TRUSTS, RULES FOR INHERITANCE: CONTROL FROM THE GRAVE

Wills and trusts are of course a way of conveying wealth to the following generations. They also serve a not-so-subtle purpose of maintaining the power of the deceased over the lives of the living. This has been known as the "dead hand from the grave." There are many examples of wills that locked the next generation into a straightjacket. One father left a will stipulating that his son receive a healthy stipend "as long as he was a student at Columbia University." This "student" managed to take course after course at Columbia, well into his later years.

Tommy Manville, the heir to the Johns–Manville fortune, was to be given money upon his marriage. He married 11 times, and each time received a large chunk of money. There was nothing unstable about his marital relationships. It was just that he occasionally ran out of money, and needed a new wife. (He was fortunate to die before the company was sued for causing asbestosis.)

Dr. Stephen T. Emlen has developed a theory of the evolution of the family. Natalie Angier describes how Emlen found families unstable because "restless non-breeding adults disperse ... as soon as better opportunities open up elsewhere." Some animals establish "property," such as granaries or hunting grounds, which lend stability to their families.

> In a similar vein, the privileged gentry among humans, with their coats-of-arms, their grand chateaux, and their ability to trace their ancestry back to William the Conqueror, survive as recognizable genetic units through the ages, while poorer families tend to disintegrate over time, becoming genealogically diluted. (Angier, 1995, p. C5)

Barbara Tuchman says that for northern France, in the mid-1300s, it is estimated that only 10% of the population were devout observers.

> At the moment of death, however, people took no chances: they confessed, made restitutions, endowed perpetual prayers for their souls, and often deprived their families by bequests to shrines, chapels, convents, hermits, and payments for pilgrimages by proxy. (Tuchman, 1978, p. 237)

Tuchman chose one medieval figure to tell her story of the Middle Ages; a member of the nobility, an Earl, Enguerrand de Coucy VII (1340–1397). He made a bequest to pay for two masses to be said every day for himself and his descendants. "Coucy counted on a perpetuity without change" (Tuchman, 1978, p. 272).

Belief in hellfire and damnation has eased since the Middle Ages. Large bequests are made to churches and other charities, but they seldom pauperize the next generations, as in medieval France. That function is now filled by the Internal Revenue Service of the United States. Without careful preparation, more than half of an estate can go to the federal and state government in inheritance taxes. Generally, money or property left to a wife is not taxed, but if left to children without special types of trusts to protect it, a wealthy family nest egg can soon be gutted (or at least scrambled). Gifts up to $10,000 can be given without inheritance taxes each year, and a married couple can gift $20,000 tax-free. There is currently a "Federal Unified Credit" of $600,000 (increasing annually for a few years to more than a million dollars) which can be given estate-tax-free during a lifetime. Beyond that, the federal and local taxes take a big bite unless elaborate trusts are drawn up by lawyers specializing in estates and wills. The George W. Bush administration has succeded in getting a bill passed that will exempt progressively larger amounts from estate (death) taxes ending with complete tax repeal in 2010. In 2011, estate taxes may be reinstated.

Inheritance patterns have varied over time and between nations and tribes. In England, the first-born son typically inherited the family fortune (primogeniture) and the others, in former times, were left to "seek their fortune" away from the family estate. Stories abound about the youngest son who must leave home after his father dies. ("Puss in Boots," "The Three Princes of Serendip.") In Ireland a century ago, there was no law of primogeniture. The favorite son was chosen to inherit the family farm. This produced a virtual slavery of the sons under a tyrannical father.

Family and Community in Ireland (Arensberg, 1940) describes how the sons, now age 50, were still being hired out by the father to neighboring farms, under a system called "cooring." In a strict Catholic country, it was very dangerous to get a girl pregnant, especially if you didn't know who would get the farm. Few solutions were open under this system. The sons took factory work, emigrated in droves to America, or drank heavily with their peers as a method of controlling their sexual desires. Marriage was late, if ever. This desolate picture was all laid at the door of an ambiguous inheritance pattern by the authors. Corroborating this father–son conflict is the brilliant play by Synge, *Playboy of the Western World*, in which a son claims to have killed his father with a blow to the head. All the girls go crazy for him, and he is a great hero, until they discover that his father was only bloodied, but not killed!

Much has been made of the classical inheritance of the Chinese peasant. This was essentially a "per stirpes" arrangement. The land was divided equally among the heirs. Soon "farms" became only narrow strips of land a few feet wide. This caused a great deal of migration and loss of family integrity.

Disinheritance plays a great role in folktales. Cinderella, of course, was begrudged clothing and food by her mean stepmother and two stepsisters. Only a fairy godmother and a glass slipper saved her from a permanent life as a chargirl. In "The Goose Girl" [Lang, 1966 (reprinted), see pp. 266–273],[*] a princess is given a handkerchief or a magic necklace with three drops of her queen mother's blood on it, which will protect her. As described in the previous chapter (11) she accidentally loses it, and her servant girl makes her mistress into a servant, taking her rightful place. She is in effect, disinherited. Once the Prince learns the truth, he has the impostor "put stark naked into a barrel lined with sharp nails ... dragged by two white horses up and down the street till she is dead." He then marries his true betrothed. Again, loss of inheritance, status, and power is the tragedy, and regaining it is the eventual triumph over evil and misfortune.

Snow White is also the daughter of a queen who dies. Her father remarries a jealous woman, who is enraged when her mirror tells her "Thou, Queen, may fair and lovely be, But Snow White is fairer still than thee." This stepmother gets a hit man (huntsman) to kill Snow White, but he spares her. She runs to the seven dwarfs. The queen, disguised as a peddler, laces her up with apron ties so she can't breathe. Failing to kill her, she runs a poison comb through Snow White's hair. Failing again, she tricks her victim into eating a poison apple. Of course, a prince rescues her. At the wedding the queen stepmother is forced to wear red-hot iron slippers and "dances" until she falls down dead. Stepmothers rather than stepfathers seem to be the villains. To this day, fathers are more likely than mothers to remarry after a divorce or after becoming widowers. These tales continue to resonate in our times, for children are still subject to disinheritance, to the loss or remarriage of parents, and to the possible predations of step parents. We hear of President Bill Clinton's having to stand up physically to his stepfather, who was abusive to his beloved mother.

---

[*] The imposter's death is described on p. 273. Lang adapted this tale from the German of the Grimm Brothers.

In any event, wills, trusts, and inheritance patterns wield a great deal of power over subsequent generations. They are a way of "living on" past death. In a sense, they are a legal form of immortality. If there is life after death, many ghosts are either praising or cursing their attorneys for the way they set up their endowments and bequests.

There is a close relationship between wills and monuments. Very often, a rich person's will leaves some of his or her money earmarked for a structure that is large, easily seen, and can bear the individual's name in perpetuity. Monuments nowadays are less likely to be tombs, and more likely to be donated hospitals, libraries, or, in the following case, gigantic telescopes!

> Typical of those who have sponsored big-time astronomy was James Lick, an immensely successful 19th-century real estate speculator. Lick wanted to build a monument to himself, *and he planned to erect a full-size replica of Egypt's Great Pyramid of Giza.* (italics ours). But astronomers talked him out of it, convincing him that the money could be better spent on an observatory.
>
> The result was the Lick Observatory near Santa Cruz. It inspired another philanthropist, Charles T. Yerkes, who had made a fortune developing Chicago's mass transportation system, to endow a competing observatory at Williams Bay, Wis. (Browne, 1997, p. C7)

The association in Lick's mind between a pyramid and a massive telescope is a wonderful demonstration of how modern moguls mimic the pharaohs, kings, and emperors of the past. Not to be outdone, William M. Keck, founder of the Superior Oil Company (now part of the Mobil Corporation), set up a foundation in 1954 that built twin telescopes larger than any predecessors. They were completed in 1996. The competition to be this year's Ozymandias is always keen.

DIARIES AND AUTOBIOGRAPHIES: THE SEARCH FOR THE SELF AND ITS PRESERVATION

Since long before the days of Samuel Pepys (1633–1703) men and women have kept diaries. Pepys' diary was in cipher, but most of it was deciphered in 1825. Did he mean to keep his life a secret? Perhaps, because of fear of political reprisal. Yet here was a detailed record of almost 10 years of his life in Restoration England. Diaries are one more way of time-stopping, of preserving one's life. Only a few diaries have actually brought some immortality to their authors. Pepys' descriptions of the plague (1665) and the great fire of London (1666) are memorable. Mary Chesnut's description of life in the Confederacy during the American Civil War, and Anne Frank's diary written while hiding from the Nazis in a house in Amsterdam, are also famous. Andre Gide, Franz Kafka, and Virginia Woolf also wrote well-known diaries.

The memoir, unlike the diary, is retrospective. It records the past, and is not written on a daily basis. For some, it is an attempt to freeze the past, and perhaps to convey one's early life to others. Autobiography is surely a monument to the self. One essayist said:

> ... literature was being taken over by a bunch of narcissists. Look Ma, I'm breathing. See me take my initial toddle, use the potty, scratch my sister, win spin the bottle. Gee whiz, my first adultery—what a guy! (Atlas, 1996, p. 26, quoting William Gass' essay in Harper's "The Art of Self-Autobiography in an Age of Narcissism.")

There is also a confessional aspect of the memoir and the autobiography. If one writes of one's own sexual escapades, violence, and chicanery, perhaps the new priest-confessors, the American Public, will forgive the sinner. Not the least of the motivation for such revelations is that they sell like hotcakes. The common man is titillated by the peccadilloes and indiscretions of the rich and famous. John Kennedy and now William Clinton have probably set all-time records for presidential sexual flings. Richard Nixon and Newt Gingrich probably set records for underhanded dealings. They are all admired, overtly or covertly. Loren Bacall, in her autobiography, tells how she slept with Frank Sinatra while "Bogey" (her husband, Humphrey Bogart) was dying of cancer. Liz Taylor's affairs and marriages are part of our national heritage. Even demure Grace Kelly, it seems, slept with almost every leading man she worked with. The confessional has turned into another performance.

Mental illness, alcoholism, drug addiction, and the attempts to overcome them seem to dominate our fiction and autobiography. How can we reconcile this with the wish to be immortal? Perhaps in a culture in which there is little or no shame, the sex, criminality, and psychopathology constitute a new claim to immortality. It is no longer a tale of sin and redemption, but a tale of sin and glory, much like the adolescent excesses of On the Road. Atlas says that Lasch's "culture of narcissism" has been replaced by a culture of confession, with a nation of voyeurs ready to lap it all up (Atlas, 1996, p. 26).

Biography and autobiography (much of which is disguised in the form of novels) is still a model for our behavior. In my own youth, there were collections of short biographies, such as Bolitho's Twelve Against the Gods. These lives of independent thinkers were an inspiration to me. Presidents, such as Lincoln and Washington, sports stars, generals such as Eisenhower and Stilwell, and endless movie stars were guiding lights for me to follow. Scientists such as Darwin, Wallace, Freud, and Einstein seemed like gods. Darwin's Voyage of the Beagle and Wallace's parallel discoveries filled me with wonder. Arcane questions bothered me, such as "Did Darwin retreat early in life because he got Chagas' disease from a "kissing bug" in South America?," or "What if Wallace had had the Royal Society and someone like Thomas Henry Huxley to go to bat for him? Would he have been as famous as Darwin?"

While some biographies are bought and paid for by wealthy folk who just want a public relations job done, most biographies and autobiographies deal with the innermost problems, joys, and sorrows of the subject. I tend to think of autobiography and memoir as a summing up of a life. But what if a life ends in the teens, like Anne Frank's? And what can we make of a memoir by Joyce Maynard, written at age 17, who has seen all and done all? Is having an affair with J. D. Salinger a sufficient excuse for such an early outpouring?

Many memoirs and autobiographies are a search for the lost self of childhood. This is in fact a mourning for the death of the past self, and by implication, an anticipatory grieving for the death to come. Robert Merton has written of "ancitipatory socialization" among the arrivistes and social climbers. Grieving, as this book has emphasized, is not just about others. It is as much or even more about the self. Any bookstore will have a hundred books on bereavement of widows, widowers, "creative divorce," the death of a child, or how to help children with the death of a parent or sibling. Few books deal with grief for a self—grief that can last a lifetime, as each period—infancy, childhood, adolescence, young adulthood, and middle age—slips away.

A poignant story of an author's academic search for Mignon, also known as the Little Watercress Girl (and maybe the Little Match Girl and so many starving heroes and heroines of folklore and novels) is found in "The Child Who Wasn't There" (Kendrick, 1995, p. 34). The review of Carolyn Steedman's book, *Childhood and the Idea of Human Interiority: 1780–1930,* tells of her search for Mignon, the "strange, deformed and piercingly beautiful child-acrobat." In Goethe's 1796 novel, *Wilhelm Meister's Apprenticeship,* Mignon appeared in many guises, and her figure fascinated the Victorians. Miss Steedman confesses to a "compulsive search for a child who did once actually exist." She searched through every household in Farringdon, enumerated in 1851, and found a possible candidate, 10-year-old Hannah Hardwick. After all the effort, she still cannot be sure. She finally admits that "Of course it is not her; she is not to be found ... The search is for the self, and the past that is lost and gone" (Kendrick, 1995, p. 34).

And so it is with social history, as well as the history of the self. The writing of history, as this case so clearly illustrates, is often motivated by a search for some message from the past—some historical figure who will speak to the historian's present life and its problems. This does not minimize the political aspects of history writing, which are often an exercise in jingoism.

The search for the childhood self has dominated psychoanalysis, yet this search was surely in vogue before the Victorian period. My own search for an explanation of my troubled early family life determined my career in psychiatric epidemiology, and wakened my interest in psychology and anthropology. My parents had a violent marriage, with verbal fights verging on physical violence. My father had affairs, and my mother retaliated in kind, in a sorrowful rage. I was the favored child, while my sister got little love from her father, and was often the object of my mother's jealousy. At age 30 my sister committed suicide by jumping out a tenth story window while my mother tried to save her. She was having a paranoid episode. She said that her then boyfriend, who was in jail on charges of statutory rape (he had seduced his 13-year-old stepdaughter) was blackmailing her. He may well have been. She also thought the FBI was after her. I didn't fare all that well in such a family atmosphere, even though I was favored. I suffered from mild depression, which was exacerbated by my sister's suicide. I had tried to help her, but still felt guilty that I hadn't done enough.

My research, at first as a junior member of a team, and later as head of a longitudinal project, looked at mental disorder and its origins in 2000 families in New York City. The great mass of research data, involving questionnaires dealing with parental behavior; children's psychiatric and physical illness symptoms, and social background variables such as socioeconomic status, race, religion, sex, and age, seemed atomistic at first. Regression analysis and cluster analysis reduced the variables to manageable proportions. Equations gave weights for early life events, parental practises, and various losses and illnesses. Since there were 16 behavioral (child symptom) variables, the impact of one set of predictors (let's say for delinquency) was soon displaced by the importance of another set of factors predicting depression or repetitive motor behavior or anxiety, and so on. The disparity between an individual case history, seemingly so clear, and the abstract equations and regression weights of the mass data was unbridgeable.

A friend who knew me well pointed out that I was motivated to undertake this massive research program in an attempt to understand the sources of my own depression and my sister's suicide. I later sought psychotherapy when my first marriage and my career came crashing down. *The "search for my childhood self" has dominated my whole working life and my choice of research subjects.* That search was as compulsive as the search for Mignon, and just as fruitless. That younger self is "lost and gone," and is in fact dead. The grieving for that self, and the struggle to reconstruct it, took place primarily in psychotherapy. That experience has not brought me back my distorted "golden" picture of my youth, but it has allowed me a more realistic appraisal of my early life, and reconciled me to those early losses. It was also the first trigger for a realistic appraisal of my life span, and along with my 70th birthday was probably the springboard for this book.

The search for understanding my childhood has not been without some secondary gain, since it has prompted me to follow a career in research that in turn has yielded several books and articles. These have had some impact on the field of social psychiatry

At age 58 I met my second wife, Susan. This dramatically changed my life for the better. After some time we married, and I recovered my early good feelings about myself and the world. We had a child named Laura (Sue's first, my sixth). My second wife and daughter, and my five older children, have given me a new grip on immortality, through Love and Procreation. This book has allowed me to cope with fear of death through Creativity and Intellectualization, and the Obsessional Behavior involved in this kind of writing and library research. (See Chapters 4 and 7, and 3, 6, and 8.) Being a member of a family has also helped. (See Chapter 10, Group Membership.)

Is this book an autobiography? No more than most novels, essays, histories, and even biographies of other people (chosen for their consonance with the biographer).

FUNERALS AND OBITUARIES

There is a voluminous literature on funerals. Since I am focusing on ways of coping with fear of death, the most relevant fact is that elaborate funerals prepare the departed for immortality or rebirth. In Bali, as in many other cultures, the size of funerals is directly related to the power or wealth of the deceased. A king is given a huge funeral with a seven-story structure that allows him to get to heaven. In the Celebes (north of Macassar, which is now named Sulawesi or Ujung Pandang) people are buried in cliffs. I will never forget looking up 100 feet, and seeing a whole "village" of 4 foot-high dressed wooden figures carved in the likeness of the dead, their palms outstretched as if in supplication, beseeching the living to remember them. Wealthier individuals are taken out of their tombs every 5 years or so, and given an additional funeral, with a feast of sacrificial water buffalo and pigs. Many buildings, which are really flimsy stage sets made of palm and bamboo, are burned in their honor.

While repeated funerals are rare, there are repeated memorial ceremonies for leaders and heroes. We celebrate Lincoln's and Washington's birthdays now under the heading of "President's Day." Martin Luther King Day has been added to our holidays. By amassing wealth and power, or by their sheer charisma, some people are able to be remembered longer than others. This yields a little bit of immortality.

The yearning for being remembered is satirized in a joke told among some New York City Jews. A man is talking to a funeral director. He asks that he be buried in Bloomingdale's Department Store. The funeral director is shocked, and wants to know why. The man says "At least, I know my wife will visit my grave several times a week, while she is shopping."

Some sources on funerals are Van Gennep (1960, pp. 145–165), Fulton (1970, No. 16, pp. 344–381), Rank (1932, reprinted 1989; see "Burial Customs"), and Iserson (1994, an excellent and detailed reference).

COLLECTIONS

The packrat instinct of hoarding seems just as powerful as the ratpack drive for group membership. We accuse rodents of being acquisitive. We even say that someone has "squirreled away" a lot of junk, or money. The Scots and the Jews are labeled as "thrifty" or "penny-pinching." Thrift, once seen as a virtue, has become a dirty word. In a culture dominated by "conspicuous consumption," frugality and parsimony are devalued. You have to show what you've got up front, by means of your clothing, your car, your yacht, or private plane. Packratting is deeply rooted, and probably stems, even in humans, from a simple desire to go on living—to acquire enough food. During floods, power outages, and snow-storms, there is always a rush on food stores to stock up. Flashlights, candles, matches, and bottled water are also high on the list. This is evidence of a healthy instinct for self-preservation. (Self-preservation is the positive side of the coin, while fear of dying may be the negative side of the same coin.)

Collecting combines packratting and conspicuous consumption in an ingenious way. It allows you to hoard something, but at the same time avoid the disapproval of your friends and neighbors, since that something is rare, beautiful, or valuable. Now it is true that some people will collect almost anything—book matches, coasters, baseball cards, toys, glass animal figures, hubcaps, and theater or concert programs. Nobody is struck by the beauty or value of their collec-tion—that is, until one baseball card fetches several thousand dollars at auction. Who would have thought that a Mickey Mouse wrist watch would sell for thou-sands? Years ago I clipped a cereal box top, added a quarter, and sent away for a Dick Tracy two-way wrist radio. I never received it, and at age 10 it was a major tragedy. Perhaps it still is a loss, since it may be worth big bucks as a "collectible."

The U.S. Internal Revenue Service has encouraged collecting on a grander scale, since gifts of expensive collections can be used as a tax deduction during one's life, or as a way of reducing estate taxes upon one's death. Such gifts are usually in the form of paintings, sculpture, and furniture. Pamela Harriman died in February of 1997. She left the Van Gogh painting, "White Roses," estimated to be worth 50 million dollars, to the National Gallery in Washington, D.C. No doubt, taxes were involved. She was a staunch Democrat, and also a collector of men, among them her husbands: Winston Churchill's son, Leyland Heyward; the theatrical producer, and Averell Harriman, the politician, diplomat, and heir to a railroad fortune.

Collections of paintings and sculpture often trigger the formation of a museum, or a new wing for an established museum. These art museums bear the names of the donors; the Hirshhorn Museum in Washington D.C. (industry), The J. Paul Getty Museum (oil), the Rockefeller Wing of the Metropolitan Museum of Art in New York City (Standard Oil), and the Barnes Collection of Impressionist art (bought with money made from inventing "Argyrol," a medicine using mild suspension of silver nitrate, which was widely used as nosedrops and to prevent eye infections in infants). Very often there are stipulations that the paintings and furniture be exhibited in their entirety, and in the same way as they were in the donor's home during his or her lifetime.

When I was an Assistant Professor of Sociology in the Division of Social Psychiatry at Cornell University-New York Hospital, located at Payne Whitney Psychiatric Clinic (long since bulldozed), I made friends with a wonderfully wise and kindly Swiss-born psychiatrist, Hans Syz. He was one of the first psychiatrists involved in the development of group psychotherapy in the United States, working with Dr. Trigant Burrow. Hans invited me to his home in Westport, Connecticut, where he and his wife housed a huge collection of Meissenware. It filled an entire room. He left it to a museum. I later found out that each piece was rare and worth a great deal of money. The "color of green" at that time impressed me more than the heavy blue color of the German porcelain. Meissen was the city near Dresden that actually produced the famous "Dresden china" after 1710.

Collecting may originally be a security blanket, and a way of fending off fear of dying. Through a process of "functional autonomy" (Gordon Allport) the coping mechanism (of collecting) becomes a way of life. An illustration of this process is a heart attack patient, who was told to take up golf in order to get back in shape. He became an expert player, and devoted the rest of his life to golf. The means became the end or goal. Similarly collecting, although it may originally be a defense against insecurity and death fear, offers great satisfaction to the collector. The hunt for a painting, a rare animal, or a fine old book can be an exciting adventure. In the past, African safaris yielded collections of stuffed animals that the rich gave to museums. The game-hunting safaris have changed to photographic safaris in this age of environmental awareness. A shot from a rifle is exchanged for a "shot" of a lion or elephant taken with a camera. The use of the word "shot" or "snapshot" suggests the violence underlying photography, and its invasion of privacy. In some countries, the snapshot of a person without permission is considered to be stealing an image, and can result in arrest and confiscation of film and camera. The paparazzi are often attacked by their victims, whom they stalk for a scandalous news shot.

Collecting, then, can be a one-way ticket to immortality. It can also be fun, and it can save taxes for the rich, and enrich some of the poor, who by luck and persistence find some valuable "collectible."

HISTORY

As I said before, history is a way of embalming and embroidering the past. The embalming function, the preservation of the body of the nation and the freeze-framing of an era (a written time- stopping) has the function of preserving confidence in the continuity of a culture and a way of life. It serves the individual who belongs to that culture or nation, and acts to overcome his fear of dying. The heroes of the past are trotted out—the great statesmen and the brilliant scholars and artists—while the list of wars won is trumpeted. Surely one can bask in the reflected glory of such a heritage, and feel special and protected against the grim reaper. Doctored history adds power to group membership, thus enhancing its role as an antidote to fear of dying. Only a confirmed outsider and social critic such as Groucho Marx would say that he wouldn't want to join any club that would have him as a member.

The embroidering of the past is like the injections of formaldehyde, wax, resins, and the Biblical frankincense and myrrh that have been used by embalmers to beautify and deodorize the bodies of the dead. If open caskets are requested, the deceased are made to look much better than they did at the time of death. This parallels the censorship and beautification that goes on in written history. The past is glorified, and the sins of the nation and its leaders are often buried with what may be viewed as a long eulogy rather than the unvarnished truth. Here's what some great skeptics have said:

> All great events have been distorted, most of the important causes concealed, some of the principal characters never appear, and all who figure are so misunderstood and misrepresented that the result is complete mystification. (Benjamin Disraeli)

> History is a fraud, agreed upon. (Napoleon Bonaparte)

> That huge Mississippi of falsehood called history. (Matthew Arnold)

> Reason creates science; sentiments and creeds shape history. (Gustave LeBon)

> Ancient histories…are but fables that have been agreed upon. (Voltaire) (Seldes, 1967).*

The point is that there is nothing new in deconstruction. Great minds and lesser ones have been debunking history for ages. A major latent or covert (as opposed to manifest) function of history is to smooth out the contradictions of a particular country's behavior. Slavery and the genocide of Native Americans were not big subjects in U.S. high school textbooks until recently. Exploitation of the powerless and the control of government by vested interests is still played down in most texts. The Boston Tea Party is depicted as a group of colonists who wanted freedom, instead of a group of British expatriate businessmen who were fighting against taxation by the British government.

Has history lost this supportive function, the ability to stir the heart of the child with tales of patriotism and sacrifice? Has it lost its role in preparing young men and women to sacrifice their lives in battle? To some degree, but youngsters are still enlisting in the armed forces, seeking a better lifestyle and income.

---

* All the above quotations are taken from the section on "History." There are, of course, some quotations praising history, but they are in the minority. Many decry the ignoring of history by politicians.

Lichtenstein (1977, 1983) refers to the "Protean" style of the present generation (a term invented by Robert Jay Lifton to describe the interchange-ability of identities of the same individual) (Lifton, 1971). This is discussed in the chapter on Dissociation. The rapidly changing values and identities of current generations can make history into "bunk" for successive waves of teenagers. There has always been some generational conflict and teen rebellion, but rapid social change has widened the generation gap into a Grand Canyon (Lichtenstein, 1977, 1983; see pp. 336–337, a case history of "Ronnie").

Is history *all* "bunk" to today's youth? Not by a long shot. There are still inspiring acts of heroism, creativity, and sacrifice described in history books. If Audie Murphy and Sergeant York were war heroes of the past, we now have General Powell directing General Schwartzkopf during "Operation Desert Storm." This was a public relations coup, with people glued to their TV sets, while we bombed Iraq into submission. Unfortunately, Saddam Hussein saved the major part of his armed forces, while civilian casualties were high. They are still high, due to the blockade of Iraq, whose civilians lack food and medicine.

History, with all its distortions, is an antidote to feelings of alienation, mean-inglessness, and valuelessness. These are all elements that are related to fear of dying. The existential question, "Why am I living?" is crucial to the developing child and teenager. History of the usual kind (not the debunking kind) takes out the contradictions that bother our youth. It skips over the killing of innocent Vietnamese women and children at My Lai. It ignores the suffering of Iraqi women and children. It doesn't point up the innumerable delays on the road to U.S. and European intervention in Bosnia, resulting in hundreds of thousands of deaths, rapes, and acts of torture. It doesn't take account of the belated aid to Tutsi and Hutu sufferers in Rwanda. It tells our youth that "God's in his Heaven, all's right with the world," as Robert Browning put it. German history, as reported in Hitler's *Mein Kampf*, is an extreme example of historical distortion. Yet it brought new meaning to an alienated people for a short time, and a set of com-mon values that are to this day a bloody blot on that nation. Social cohesion is not necessarily democratic.

No wonder there is so much hatred directed at Derrida and his decon-structionist heirs. They look under the hood of the car for the "secret," and ignore the paint job. No wonder that the multiculturalists are seen as enemies of the Republic. They are indeed. With their search for their own truths, they breed unrest, anxiety, and anger at our government and the "establishment." These are mainly the radicals of the left. Those on the right hate government too, but they focus on the right to bear arms, hate gun control and environmentalists, and are against paying taxes, against abortion, against separation of Church and State, against all government regulation, and against animal rights. The progressives, the liberals, the centrists, are fast disappearing. It is hard to have a strong agenda when you are trying to keep an open mind and hear both sides. That's why the middle is weak, and the tails of the political distribution have a clearer and stronger policy. Bipartisanship is just a temporary public relations smoke screen after the recent U.S. presidential elections; a pause, while the right and left (or is it the right and the center?) gird their loins for the next round.

And the next round is here! In the presidential election of the year 2000, all pretense of bipartisanship has disappeared, as Republicans and Democrats fought over the electoral votes of Florida. Even as I write, there are sharp divisions in the Senate and the House of Representative. The Supreme Court is also split along ideological lines.

National holidays, birthdays, and religious holidays "keep alive" past events. (Keeping something "alive" is obviously part of the fight against the death of events and our own death.) Lincoln's and Washington's birthdays recall the Civil War and the Revolutionary War. Martin Luther King's birthday, now a national holiday, recalls the struggle for Black civil rights. Repeated behavior such as eating, working, walking, and making love are functions to which we cling as buttresses against the ravages of time and aging. They are our "signs of life." When we stop all of these activities, we are indeed dead. Written and oral history also "keep alive" past events. Families keep themselves alive with their own versions of family history and special celebrations, such as birthdays, family gatherings, and religious worship.

The daily, weekly, monthly, and annual repetitions of our lives are reflected in history books. Wars, elections, holidays, the march of the generations of our forebears, speak to the rhythm and ongoing stream of life. "Repetition is an attempt or a tendency to transcend the irreversibility of the flow of time" (Lichtenstein, 1977, 1983, p. 28). In a sense, then, repeated behavior is the most basic sign of continuing life, like breathing and a steady heartbeat. The protective function of repetition in the battle against fear of dying has been discussed in the chapter on Obsessive–Compulsive Behavior, but not in the general sense of pure biological survival. It focused instead on being enculturated in a blind and busy manner, so that death anxiety and time were stopped through a numbing process.

I can see a parallel between national history and the recall of the history of an individual's childhood during some types of psychotherapy. It is now widely accepted that the patient and therapist eventually develop a scenario about the early childhood and youthful experiences of the patient. This is partly a true rendition of what actually happened, and partly a new agreed-upon creation. Once the villains have been named, the heroes identified, and the complexes excavated, the scenario becomes a reservoir of meaning and hope for the patient. That scenario—that personal "history"—is a shield against anxiety, depression, and fear of dying. In a parallel way, written national history is also a scenario, a collaboration of the writer, his values, the times he is writing in, the politics of the day, and the reader. The historian (and her history book) is the therapist, and the reader is the patient. Once the reader accepts the scenario, he has a guide to current behavior and values, and gets a boost to his self-esteem at the same time. How fine to be a citizen of a country with such a great history! What a great source of borrowed power!

The history of the issue of childhood sexual abuse illustrates how difficult it is to determine what happened in the past. Freud's denial of actual abuse and his positing of sexual fantasies and wish fulfillment has now been tempered by reports of widespread physical and sexual abuse of children. However, recall of sexual abuse by patients in psychotherapy became a cottage industry in the United States until some of the fathers who were victims of abuse lawsuits countersued the therapists. Some teachers who were accused of sexual abuse of children, both men and women, were later found to be innocent. Some children had been coached by police "psychologists."

So also with abuses in history. Some historians even denied the existence of the Nazi Holocaust. The character of some of our heroes has been impugned or distorted. Jefferson, for example, has lately been described as a slaveholder who may have had children with his black mistress, Sally Hemmings. Although he was a polymath—statesman, scientist, inventor, and musician—according to the revisionists he had major faults and value conflicts.

Janet Malcolm has accused biographers of actually writing autobiography. By projecting their own thoughts and values onto their subject's lives, they lose their presumed objectivity. Indeed, who would dig into another's life for years with such dedication if that life did not have some resonance or deeper meaning for their own?

Barbara Tuchman, in a lucid discussion of the hazards of writing history, reviews the sources of error:

1. Contradictory data; but "contradictory data are part of life," part of the different viewpoints and values of the people who kept records of their lives and the lives of others.
2. The "overload of the negative"; war, famine, and death (three of the Four Horsemen of the Apocalypse) are more newsworthy, and thus more often recorded than pleasant events, a fact I discussed elsewhere.
3. The difficulty of empathizing with a Weltanschauung or world view that is dead or distant; for example, Christianity so dominated the Middle Ages that it is hard for us to put ourselves in that place and time.
4. There are large gaps of information—times when no record was made, or records were destroyed (Tuchman, 1978; see pp. xvii, xviii, xix).

I would add to this the bias of the historian and the previous historians upon whom she bases her impressions.

The writing of history is a creative act of the highest order when it is done well. Tuchman's *A Distant Mirror* and *The Guns of August* are outstanding, and contain a great deal of interpretation and "inner dialogue" which helped me in understanding the motives and values of the main characters. These are not historical "facts;" they are conjectures, but they flesh out the narrative, which would be dull without them.

Another favorite of mine is *Truman*, by David McCullough (McCullough, 1992). The description of Truman's difficult decision to drop the atomic bombs on Hiroshima and Nagasaki gave me a mixed feeling of horror and thankfulness, since that decision kept me from being part of the planned invasion of the Japanese mainland. My chances of getting through that invasion unscathed, as an officer in a Chemical Corps mortar battalion temporarily based in the Philippines, would have been very slim. Reading about history that took place when I was 18 to 21 years of age and in the U.S. Army and World War II gave me a feeling that my President protected me from death. It diminished my fear of dying. That surge of gratitude and renewed confidence in my survival came to me in 1993 (a full 48 years after the dropping of the bomb in 1945)!

That feeling of protection by one's government and leaders is the selfsame psychological support against fear of dying that history, despite (and often because of) all its distortions, can offer the individual.

13

Counterphobic Behavior

What is it like to be a counterphobe, someone who seeks danger? The best way to find out would be to interview one. The choice was simple. I interviewed myself. I have been a mild counterphobe as long as I can remember. I traveled to East Africa twice, driving my own family through Uganda, Kenya, and Tanzania. A short journey to Rwanda ended in 12 hours when our host, a retired British colonial, warned our family that the Tutsis and the Hutus were about to start fighting a few miles away.

In Kenya my son Josh and I were chased by an angry rhino, who tried to overturn our Landrover. At a lodge in Tanzania we watched in horror as a cape buffalo gored a woman to death right outside our cabin.

A trip with a group of 12 tourists to 10 West African countries was bound to be dangerous and exciting. This time I went without my family. Ten of the twelve members dropped out after a few weeks, owing to the rigors of the trip, and the various diseases to which we were exposed. An 8-hour hike to see mountain gorillas in Eastern Zaire brought me face to face with "Musha Muka," an alpha male gorilla twice the size of any I had seen in the zoo. He was beating his chest in the approved manner and screaming at me. I averted my gaze, as I had been told to, so as not to challenge him. We were only a few feet apart. The three pygmy guides later told our French-speaking guide that Musha had killed another male a few days ago, but had received a large shoulder wound which made him very irritable. I got more than my money's worth of fear, but of course survived, which is the joy of being a counterphobe.

Years ago I took my family to Tobago. I had not learned to scuba dive, so I bought a floating compressor that had two 50-foot hoses to which face masks were attached. I put one on, and my guide, a very friendly, large, and athletic Tobagan named Courtney, put on the other. We dove down. Buccoo Reef was a paradise then. It had not been destroyed by too many divers such as myself. Suddenly I was gasping for air. I looked over at Courtney, and saw that he had thrown off his mask and was kicking his fins to get to the surface. I did the same.

159

A large wave had overturned the compressor, and it conked out. When I got to the surface, I took a huge breath of air, and suddenly began to sink to the bottom. I had panicked, and was confused by lack of oxygen. I kicked to the surface again, breathed, and sank. I was desperate. I swam to a coral head, and crawled on it into fresh air. Then I looked down. In my panic I had forgotten to throw off my weight belt. I had come very near to drowning.

This search for adventure and danger has never stopped. Around 1975 I took a trip up the Mahakam River in what used to be called Borneo (now Kalimantan) to visit a tribe of headhunters. My only companions were a retired guide and a young Swiss steeplejack/travel agent, who was reading *Future Shock* while we dodged huge logs coming down the river as we went upstream. The steeplejack was reconnoitering a swamp where the only black orchids in the world grew, in preparation for a trip by the Swiss Orchid Society. He got off about half-way, and I never saw him again. He was a wonderful companion for that short time. Later on, in one village, a sword dancer made his local audience laugh by pretending to behead me while I photographed him with flashgun and camera. Then a wild boar hunt proved to be rather tame, but I must admit being scared of the poison darts in the blowguns.

With my present wife, Susan, I went to Iquitos on the Upper Amazon. From there we took trips to a few headhunting tribes, and got stuck sideways in a light canoe in the middle of the Amazon with waves breaking over us. Our guide Moises, always cheerful, gave us his usual reassurance, "No problema!"

Some of the natives unfortunately had traded in their shrunken heads for Adidas T-shirts, which reduced the danger considerably. A spider the size of a small plate seemed drawn to Susan's hammock, but she bravely brushed it off. We fished for piranhas. Sue caught a large one, and another guide, "Secundo," pointing to the large teeth, got too close and lost the tip of his finger. What bothered me terribly, in addition to his lost fingertip, was that he wouldn't let me fix his wound with my antibiotics and first aid kit. (Half the fun for a counterphobe is being "prepared" for danger.) Instead he used a greasy rag, with which he wiped the motor, to stop the bleeding!

Our guide to various tribes, "Moises," wanted us to try "ayawaska," a hallucinogenic root that he claimed could make you see clearly in the jungle at night. He gave us a copy of an article from *High Times* magazine, which was apparently a Bible for U.S. druggies. We turned down his "drug trip." The other alternatives were living on roots for 2 weeks, or visits to tribes. We chose the latter.

It is clear to me that I have had a lifelong fear of death and dying. Counterphobic behavior was only one of many mechanisms I used to cope with my fears. I had to prove that I could take risks and still live. I review my own "choice" of coping mechanisms at the end of this book.

Everyone has taken a dare at some time—to leap from an overhanging rock into a lake or river, to ride a bike with no hands, or to snatch some object in a store and pocket it without getting caught. These relatively innocent episodes can't compare with skydiving, scuba diving, or bungee jumping, but they seem to be part of the process of growing up for all but the most timid souls. Some of us (such as myself) never grow out of it.

Probably one of the earliest and best discussions of counterphobic behavior was by Otto Fenichel (1939). He refers to:

> ... a definite type of these fear-defences, which is usually referred to under the inexact name of 'overcompensation against fear', but which could much more precisely be called the 'counter-phobic attitude' (Fenichel, 1939, p. 263)

> It often happens that a person shows a preference for the very situations of which he is apparently afraid. And even more frequently he will later on develop a preference for the situations which he formerly feared. (Fenichel, 1939, p. 264)

Fenichel explored the conditions under which counterphobia might turn out well—that is, succeed as a defense mechanism. The first condition occurs when a passive position is made into an active one. "We frequently see that in adults too, the search for situations which were formerly feared become pleasurable precisely because they are actively sought..."

The second condition has to do with a feeling of trust or protection.

> Children overcome their anxiety not only by playing actively at what has threatened them, but also by letting a loved person, whom they trust, do to (with) them what they fear to do themselves... pleasure may be enjoyed so long as one believes in the protection of an outsider. (Fenichel, 1939, p. 264) (parentheses added)

The third condition involves pleasure or excitation from the counterphobic activity:

> Fear, like any other excitation, may be a source of sexual excitation. But this is true—just as in the case of pain—only so long as the unpleasure remains within certain limits, for example, in feeling sympathy for the hero of a tragedy. (Fenichel, 1939, p. 271)

The fourth condition is a little obscure. The counterphobe is testing out the reality of his fears, to convince himself that they were imaginary, and that he is safe.

> Search for the anxiety situation has the character of a 'flight to reality.' This means that the reality of the situation with which imaginary expectations of punishment were connected is sought, presumably to convince the subject that this connection was purely imaginary and that actually only the situation itself occurs. (Fenichel, 1939, pp. 271–272)

This continual testing of the reality of the fearful situation is due to the fact that "there is no proof that the punishment will not occur eventually." In addition, the pleasure of the release of the tension that is created by seeking the danger is sought over and over again, in a sort of addictive process.

Fenichel was one of the first to point out that part of the joy in sports is that "one actively brings about in play certain tensions which were formerly feared" (or one is actively trying to overcome a fear of sports, and gain of sense of accomplishment and the kudos that goes with it). He also calls mountaineers the "true counterphobic subjects." He suggests that artists often paint what they fear "to achieve a belated mastery." "The same holds true for scientists, who want to have an object (onto which they have projected their anxiety) under control" (Fenichel, 1939, p. 274). (The sharp insights of Fenichel's mind are a pleasure to read, though he sometimes drags in what might now be considered some far-fetched theory such as the "sadistic component of infantile sexual excitement" as interfering with successful counterphobia.)

Karl Menninger's definition of counterphobic behavior is similar to Fenichel's. However, he raises the subject of cowardice, which to my mind detracts from his definition:

> The *counterphobic mechanism* is similar (to reaction formation); instead of being avoided and run away from, danger is eagerly sought and even produced. One sees it in childish form in the defiance of feared danger, 'whistling in the graveyard.' This symptom is of particular social importance in adolescents when the temptation to over-come fear by bravado is uncontrolled by mature judgment, with the result that the laws of reality and of the community are apt to be flouted, not so much in contempt of law as in fear of cowardice. (Menninger, 1963, p. 144, quoted in Farberow, 1980, p. 401)

To my way of thinking, Menninger (and Delk) have missed the more basic point by bringing cowardice into their description of counterphobic behavior. Delk says that the skydiver is compelled to jump "because of an unconscious fear of cow-ardice." "His fear of being labeled a coward by others or *himself* is stronger than his fear of death." In actual fact, it is because they fear death, rather than cow-ardice, that they jump. Delk even says later that "they must engage in counter-phobic *defiance of death*" (italics mine). Cowardice is just the social reinforcement of the individual fear of death of skydivers, racing car drivers, and scuba divers who have been individually recruited and self-selected to join those sporting groups.

In the face of death, which is part and parcel of life, almost every one of us is a coward. Considering that women and men both face eventual death, there is a striking difference in favor of male counterphobic behavior. For example, males constituted about 94% of the total fatalities for skin diving and scuba div-ing between 1970 and 1975 (Blau, 1980, p. 413, see Table 2). Rates are not given, but the participation in racing, motorcycling, and skydiving is known to be predominantly male. There are obviously great differences in the way men and women handle fear of death and dying. Given the "macho" male culture of most of Western civilization, we could expect men to take a more blustering and defiant path to deny death. Women, in contrast, give birth, and this is closer to immortality than most males ever get. In the past, at least, women were trained for passivity and acceptance of their lot. As this changes, we can expect to see more women divers, racers, and climbers.

Recently the first U.S. woman jet-fighter pilot, Lt. Kelly Flinn, was forced out of the service for having an affair. The charge was that she lied about her adultery. In contrast, an Air Force general, Joseph Ralston, accused of an extramarital affair, was allowed to stay in the service. He did, however, withdraw as (the favored) candidate for chairman of the Joint Chiefs of Staff, the highest military post in the United States. Times haven't changed all that much. Hillary Clinton, and Eleanor Roosevelt before her, have been resented because of their lack of passivity.

Counterphobic behavior has some close relatives, which are worth discussing briefly. It must be distinguished from "stress." Klausner (Klausner, 1980, p. 377) sees stress seeking as a cognate of "struggle," "arousal-seeking," "risk-taking," and "counterphobic attitude." However, he makes it clear that in stress seeking the individual does not seek danger, while in counterphobic behavior this is the central feature.

Synonyms for stress seeking might be "striving" or "effort." The concept is related to the coping modes of Creativity and Obsessive–Compulsive Behavior, discussed in an earlier chapter. These modes do not necessarily involve the seeking of danger, although they may at times.

"Risk taking" may seem identical with counterphobic behavior, but when closely examined, it appears somewhat different. There are all sorts of risks in life. These range from the everyday risks of walking across the street to driving in traffic, taking transportation, and eating. These are calculated risks, and the activities are necessary for most of us. There are environmental risks from chemicals in the air we breathe, the water we drink, and in or on the foods we eat. We continue to breathe, drink, and eat, because these are necessary activities. Some anxious people severely curtail even these activities.

It is only when the risks are really great, and the chances of death considerable, that we talk about "high-risk" activities, such as sports or occupations. Miners, steeplejacks, lumberjacks, and X-ray technicians are in high-risk occupations. Whether they are counterphobic has not been determined, but the conquering of fears may well be involved in these occupational choices. This motivation may also be predominant in choosing to become a policeman or fireman, both of which are hazardous jobs.

Tension reduction and tension seeking are related concepts. In the counterphobic behaviors, the tension of a feared situation is sought time and again, and the relief of this tension is extremely pleasurable, helping to make it addictive. In my view, these fears come out of early fears of abandonment, and later on out of direct fears of death and dying. The tension and its reduction are like having a brief immunization against fear, because you've survived, tested whether you were fated to die or be injured, and you get the satisfaction and relief of the tension reduction (a tension that you yourself created by choice). The popularity of horror films and violence on TV has often been linked to this tension creation/tension reduction process.

"Arousal seeking" is a central concept for Michael Apter 1992. I cannot do justice here to his well-worked-out theoretical framework. In brief, he believes that people have a basic need for physiological arousal. When they are too aroused, they avoid stimulation. When they are bored, they seek arousal. He does not believe, as do some theorists in this field, that each person has a particular fixed level of arousal that satisfies them. Our society, he feels, is now too protective, so that many of us seek arousal through thrills and danger. He thinks we should encourage high-risk sports, and structured risks such as the running of the bulls at Pamplona (an annual event in Spain). He also notes that arousal is interactive, so that sexual arousal and fear of heights (for example) are synergistic. A famous experiment showed that men who walked a risky bridge were more likely to ask an attractive woman guide for a date afterwards than those who hadn't been exposed to any risk.

Apter doesn't deal with the concept of counterphobia at all. His index doesn't mention the word death. He emphasizes the importance of the "protective frame," much as Fenichel did:

> ... the seeming paradoxes of human nature make sense *if* we understand that emotions are 'turned upside down' when experienced within a protective frame. (Apter, 1992, p. 196)

Apter's general theoretical framework is called "reversal theory" in which pairs of mental states, such as arousal–avoidance, pervade all our emotions. Interestingly, the behaviors that he deals with so expertly, "surfing" (riding on the outside of cars, trains, and elevator roofs), scarfing (autoerotic asphyxiation), bungee jumping, eating fugu (a poisonous puffer fish popular in Japan), among others, all have a high rate of fatalities. These behaviors are clearly counterphobic, but Apter's focus is on arousal, and he seems to carefully avoid the idea that subconscious fears of abandonment and death motivate so many of us. Obviously, arousal and seeking excitement are an important part of dangerous behavior. To me, the much greater part is the defiance of death, the conquering of fear of death by constant testing and risk taking.

What are the counterphobic activities? Do they differ to any extent in their effects and risks? Are the people who are attracted to these activities different from the general population, and do they differ between sports?

SKYDIVING

Delk (1980) offers us some of the details of skydiving and a picture of the skydiver's character. Most of those who are engaged in high-risk sports are males between 15 and 40 years of age. Out of some 40,000 people who skydive each year, there are about 12 fatal jumps. That might not seem like a high figure, but among those who have jumped for 3 years or more, 715 suffered injuries. It is of interest that former President George Bush, after his term ended, completed his lifelong wish of making a parachute jump. He had been a fighter pilot in World War II. John Kennedy sought danger, even after his severe back injury, incurred when his torpedo boat was sunk in World War II. Do we select our presidents for special personality characteristics, including counterphobia? Teddy Roosevelt is almost a classic example. "The delicate son of a distinguished family, he made determined efforts to overcome the frail health that would markedly affect his character" (Levey, 1983, p. 730). He formed and led the "Rough Riders" regiment which fought in the Spanish–American War, and spent much of his spare time big-game hunting in Africa. He might almost be a character invented by Ernest Hemingway.

Delk studied 41 adult male skydivers. These men averaged 546 parachute jumps, most of which involved free fall. They averaged two jumps per week. Three fourths admitted to thoughts of death, mostly just before the jump. Their pleasure was greatest during free fall, and their anxiety high just before the jump and at the point of their chute opening. (At the latter point their anxiety was higher than their pleasure.)

On the MMPI (Minnesota Multiphasic Personality Inventory) the skydivers' profiles showed a clear pattern. They seemed to be free from anxiety, phobias, and depression, due to an underdeveloped superego (conscience). They were socially deviant and anticonventional. They were open and nondefensive. They rejected traditional religious beliefs. They showed high self-confidence, and were impulsive and action-oriented. They were hedonistic risk takers, which also involved unusual sex practices, thrill seeking, and excessive use of alcohol. They sought immediate gratification, were sociable and extroverted, and didn't worry about their health. Their profiles "show clear manifestation of psychopathic behavior" (Delk, 1980, p. 404).

That skydivers might also be sociopaths is of special theoretical interest. We would probably not think of mountain climbers as sociopathic, and they are clearly recruited from a different stratum of society. While skydivers don't injure others during their high-risk behavior, as serial killers do, they may engage in antisocial behavior when not diving, when their drinking or drug taking gets out of hand. One major contrast between counterphobic behavior and sociopathy is that the counterphobe usually doesn't intend to put anybody else except himself at risk. The sociopath also seeks thrills, but his thrills come mainly from inflicting damage or controlling and manipulating others, and his risks from getting injured by his victim or arrested by the police. An excellent discussion of thrill-seeking in psychopaths is given by Rieber (1997, pp. 43, 45–46, 56–57). The counterphobes share only the first of the four "salient characteristics" of psychopaths which Rieber calls the Mephisto Syndrome:

"thrill-seeking, pathological glibness, antisocial pursuit of power, and absence of guilt" (Rieber, 1997, pp. 44–45). He distinguishes normal "pursuit of excitement" from psychopathic thrill-seeking, which "seeks to break the rules."

A joke about skydiving illustrates both the fear involved and the importance of the protective frame, in this case provided by Buddha. A novice skydiver about to take his first jump asks the instructor what to do if his parachute doesn't open. "Well, you pull on the D ring." "And what if that doesn't work?" "Well, just pray to Buddha." The novice jumps, and his chute doesn't open. He pulls the D ring, with no results. He lands in the palm of a huge hand that comes out of the clouds. Relieved, he shouts "Thank God!" The huge hand turns upside down, and dumps him out into space.

MOUNTAIN CLIMBING

There is clearly some overlap between sociopathy and counterphobic behavior, possibly owing to the differential recruitment for various sports activities. While skydiving may attract many who have some of the features of psychopaths, mountain climbing seems to be a case in which psychopathy is at a minimum. This may be due in part to the great expense of this activity. Recent expeditions to the Himalayas have charged $75,000 per person. Many of these are inexperienced climbers, who have achieved high professional status in their fields. If they come to conquer and subdue, it is not other people, but their own fears, and the mountain and the forces of nature that they wish to defeat.

On May 13th, 1996, a report from New Delhi brought the bad news that 11 people had died in a severe storm on Mt. Everest. They were members of several expeditions. Some of them were very experienced climbers and expedition leaders. One of them was Robert Hall, a "charismatic guide."

> ... a 35-year-old New Zealander made a satellite telephone call to his pregnant wife from a snow hole just below the summit of the world's highest peak. His voice weak from frostbite, the climber, Rob Hall, murmured what may have been his last words before he died. 'Hey look, don't worry about me.' he said. ... Mr. Hall told his wife that he was trapped, unable to move because of the frostbite in his legs, with no tent, sleeping bag, oxygen, fluids or food, but was confident that rescuers would reach him when the weather cleared. (Burns, 1996, pp. A1 and A3)

It is clear that when a storm hits, mountaineering skills may not be enough to save your life. The 11 who died, along with the survivors, were suddenly enveloped in the fatal blizzard.

> ... a storm blew up in minutes on Friday afternoon, turning what had been a good climbing day into a nightmare of temperatures that plunged to 40 degrees below zero, of swirling snowstorms that climbers call whiteouts, and fateful choices that determined which of the climbers died and which survived. (Burns, 1996, p. A3)

Elizabeth Hawley, an American who lives in Nepal, has kept records on climbers who died on Everest. Since 1921 there have been 142 deaths "Since the first successful ascent of Everest (in 1953) more than 4000 climbers have tried to reach the summit. Of these, 615 ... had made it to the top" (Burns, 1996, p. A1). Assuming that climbing Everest became popular after 1953, the death rate would be somewhat smaller than 142/4000, or 3.5% (0.035). That is a high rate for any high-risk activity. It exceeds the death rates for other sports listed later. Clearly, the risk is a central part of the appeal to the counterphobe. The protective frame was apparently maintained by Rob Hall until the moments before his death. He still believed he would be rescued.

Edith Wyschogrod is a philosopher. She approaches high-risk activities from an existentialist standpoint.

> ... enjoyment in the elemental is pleasure in the face of death, that in fact the surrender of the individual to the elemental includes death as an element of the pleasure experienced.
>
> Contemporary man retains a yearning for identification with the being of the elemental despite its concomitant with the risk of death It is the elemental itself which is the antagonist and which may exact the penalty of life. (Wyschogrod, 1973, pp. 168–169, "Sport, Death, and the Elemental.")

There is a bit of mysticism about this explanation of counterphobic behavior. The "yearning for the elemental" may be the same phenomenon Apter stresses—a search for danger or arousal because of the boredom of our overprotected modern life (which Whyschogrod calls the "utilitarian character of contemporary existence").

In describing an ascent on Everest in 1924, Wyschogrod hits on a phrase that captures the essence of counterphobic behavior.

> One of the great mysteries of existence is that what is most awful and most terrible does not deter man but draws him to it—to his temporary disaster, perhaps, but in the end to an intensity of joy which without the risk he could never have experienced (italics mine) (Wyschogrod, 1973, op. cit., p. 191. She refers to Younghusband, Epic of Mt. Everest, p. 292)

There is always the sportsman's hope that the disaster he is courting is merely temporary, yet in so many cases it is permanent and ends in death.

SKIING AND SNOW SPORTS

Everyone knows that skiing has kept our orthopedists, neurologists, physiatrists, osteopaths, and chiropractors busy with injuries to legs, arms, backs, muscles, tendons, bones, and nerves. Although the *death and injury* rates are probably not as high on a percentage basis as in hang gliding (7%), many more people are involved, so the problem is greater.

Various high-risk sports have different rates of fatality. I calculated these crudely, based on numbers given by Delk (1980, p. 395).*

Sport	Death rate
Balloon flying	0.02
Glider plane flying	0.005
Hang gliding (delta kites)	0.003
Motorcycle racing	0.0006
Auto drag racing	0.0005
Sport parachuting	0.0003
Scuba and Sky diving	0.00007†

The risks of snow sports involve deaths not only from downhill and cross-country skiing, but also from snowboarding and snowmobiling. Avalanches are a frequent cause of death. In 1996, between January 1 and February 7, five people were killed by avalanches outside defined ski areas in Colorado alone: two snowboarders, a snowmobiler, a downhill skier, and a cross-country skier.

> Buried under four feet of snow, Michael Merick clung to life for three hours until a search dog found him, just as daylight faded from a Rocky Mountain slope west of here (Evergreen, Colorado). Pulled from his icy tomb with a faint pulse, the 23 year old snowboarder died on the way to a hospital on Sunday afternoon…. (Brooke, 1996, p. A13)

The age of the victims, and the grandiosity apparent in their belief in their protective frame, despite strong evidence to the contrary, help to fill out our picture of the counterphobe. The director of the Colorado Avalanche Information Center says:

> 'The average victim is 26 years old,' Mr. Knox said referring to his center's study of people caught in Colorado avalanches. "He's a young athletic guy, who thinks 'I'm immortal, I'm a great athlete, I'll just ride it out.'" (Brooke, 1996, op. cit.)

It is grandiose to think that you will not be injured while climbing Annapurna or Everest, or that you will not die from skydiving or bungee jumping. You must have an exaggerated idea of your own importance, and fantasies about protection by God, a saint, a lucky coin, or a rabbit's foot. This is juvenile thinking. It fits in with Freud's idea of the grandiose "oceanic feeling" of the infant. The young males seem to have almost exclusive rights to these grandiose feelings, as evidenced by their participation in high-risk activities, and their high accidental death rates compared with other age–sex categories.

---

* Delk's figures are based on *Accident Facts*, National Safety Council, 1976. Since many more people engage in high-risk sports now, the figures given by Delk are probably on the low side.
† Figures were taken from Blau (1980, p. 413). He estimates that there were 2 million Scuba divers in the United States around the year 1977. (He gives no numbers for skin divers.) The average skin and scuba diving fatalities between 1970 and 1975 were 147 per year. That yields a very rough estimate of the fatality rate, of 0.00007, or seven per 10,000 divers. It is also, to me, a very low figure compared with some of the other sports.

Racing Car Driving

Cornering provides much greater exhilaration for the racing car driver than driving on a straightaway.

> To handle a corner properly at the limit (*of speed*) is one of the finest human sensations, one of the ultimate experiences we can have. It brings us right to the edge of life. (Wyschogrod, 1973, p. 176, quoted from Jackie Stewart with Gwilym S. Brown, "Racing's Most Frightening Corners." *Sports Illustrated*, Oct. 12, 1970)

The edge of life is, of course, also the edge of death; it is where life and death intersect. The slogan of the counterphobe might be "I like living on the edge." On a trip to Alaska, which involved a stay on an island off the coast which was inhabited by large grizzly bears, the two young male guides told me repeatedly how they liked "living on the edge," and that Alaskan wildlife, rough waters, and severe winters offered them the risks they sought.

Wyschogrod describes the importance of the uniform and helmet of the driver as a symbol of his skill and "his victory over death."

> Castellotti, Italy's champion driver, looked like a movie idol in his white helmet and blue uniform, and was known as "Il Bello." (He) came in first leading a parade of Ferraris in a race in which five people had died and sixteen were injured. (Wyschogrod, 1973, p. 178)

There are risks to the spectators as well as the drivers in auto racing, and there have been accidents when cars hurtled into spectators standing 5 feet deep, decapitating and killing many.

Motorcycle Racing

Balance and contact with the earth are elements that distinguish the motorcyclist from the car racer. Wyschogrod points out that the biker is on his vehicle, not in it, and thus not as protected as the motorist, the seaman, or the pilot.

Legitimate bikers complain of the cultists, such as Hell's Angels.

> You dress the part—tooled boots, tight leather jacket (with studs), metal flake helmets with leopard skin lining … Easy Rider! (Wyschogrod, 1973, p. 184, quoting Melvin Maddocks, *Sports Illustrated*, Nov. 16, 1970, "Just Another Face in the Rearview Mirror", p. 47, who is writing of Colin Newell, a "legitimate biker")

Miscellaneous High-Risk Activities

People are always finding new ways to risk their lives. The sheer variety of these activities is mind boggling, but only a few need be mentioned, to give a sense of their range and perhaps their futility or horror.

Fugu

Fugu is a poisonous puffer fish, widely eaten in Japan for centuries. Between 50 and 200 people are estimated to die from eating fugu each year, but these deaths occur in the general population, and not in restaurants, where a properly prepared fugu dinner can cost $400. There are 1500 licensed fugu restaurants in Japan, which carefully detoxify the fish. Since 1949, only one person, a famous kabuki actor, Mitsugoro Bando, has died in a licensed restaurant, because he demanded to eat the fish's liver, where much of the poison is concentrated. The poison, "a neurotoxin known as tetrodotoxin (TTX) (is) 1250 times more powerful than sodium cyanide" (Sietsma, 1997, p. 46).

Fugu was not always relatively safe. In 1958, 176 people died of fugu poisoning in Japan. The liver is especially prized by men, because of the belief that it increases virility.

> A tiny amount of liver also sometimes gives a numbing sensation, a very mild form of paralysis that can also kill. Some diners find this thrilling, a kind of fishy high. (Kristof, 1996, p. A4)

The testicles are also believed to impart potency. This is another example of contagious magic. If you eat lion meat, you'll be brave; oysters will increase your virility (because they look like semen?). In the case of fugu, the counterphobia is combined with a display of affluence and a quest for virility. These are all intimately connected with immortality—worldly success and reproduction.

Car Surfing

Jessica Quire, an 18-year-old, sat on the hood of a car, leaning back against the windshield with a friend while the driver raced down the road. She fell off the hood, hit her head on the curb, and died (McQuiston, 1995, p. B5). Drag racers used this road in Hauppage, Long Island, for car surfing, a new fad in the United States. Rollerbladers also hang on the bumpers of cars. Elevator surfing consists of jumping from the roof of one elevator to another, an often deadly sport. Trains also provide a means of "surfing."

Volcanology

> In 1993, six volcanologists studying the Galeras volcano, a smoky colossus in the Colombian Andes, died when it exploded in a riot of lava, ash and incandescent boulders, some flung miles high. A seventh member of the team gathering data in the crater at the time of the eruption lived to tell about it, though with a fractured skull, crushed ear, broken nose, broken jaw, broken legs, and extensive burns. (Broad, 1996, p. C1)

You would think that after this experience, the motto of Dr. Stanley Williams, the sole survivor, would be "Don't gather data in the crater!" But no! He is:

> now healed and armed with a new instrument (and) headed for Popocatépetl, a 3.4 mile high volcano 45 miles from Mexico City ... El Popo, as it is called, shows signs of getting ready to explode. (Broad, 1996, ibid.)

His new instrument measures volcanic gases from a distance of 25 miles, and may be able to help predict eruptions. This activity, while bearing a great resemblance to counterphobic behavior, has the positive goal of helping to save the lives of thousands living near the volcano. Dr. Williams also plans to fly over the smoke plume of the volcano in a plane, to measure the gases. Dr. Rose, another volcanologist, says, "None of us in this business are trying to get blown up" (Broad, 1996, p. C6). As they say in England, "I believe you; thousands wouldn't."

Dangerous Animals

Most people are fascinated by lions, tigers, elephants, bulls, boa constrictors, rattlesnakes, Gila monsters, and tarantulas, to name a few of the more dangerous or poisonous creatures of this earth. The recent interest in dinosaurs, propelled by Stephen Spielberg's two movies about Jurassic Park, is just a continuation of a trend. Dinosaurs are the most popular exhibits in museums of natural history. Whether or not they represent scary father figures, as one book of cartoons would have it, they may eventually replace the "Big Bad Wolf" of the "Three Little Pigs" and "Little Red Riding Hood" in children's imagination.

The tensions created by stories or movies about dangerous animals are minor "temporary disasters." (Younghusband's term). Not many of us would actually like face to face contact with a lion, a rattler, or an elephant. Yet every year, thousands of tourists go on safari in Africa to see and be (safely) near dangerous wild animals. Except for hunters, these travelers are protected by their vehicles from attacks by all except elephants and rhinos.

Another 1000 to 3000 people annually seek direct contact with the dangerous fighting bulls of Pamplona, Spain. Six bulls are released in the town's narrow streets for a half-mile run to the bull ring. This is repeated each day of the festival. Precautions of all kinds are taken. Marshals, first aid crews, and ambulances are placed along the course of the run. Loudspeakers broadcast advice in five languages. A printed brochure features a 16-item safety checklist.

> The incident that added urgency to publishing the brochure, city officials said, was the fatal goring of a 22-year-old man from suburban Chicago last year (1995). He was the first person killed in 15 years and only the 13th since 1924, when record keeping began ... Some Pamplona officials believe the young American made a fatal mistake when, after falling to the ground as the bulls approached, he got up and started to run again, instead of remaining motionless on the ground and covering his head with his hands until the herd thundered past. (Anon, 1996, p. A3)

Ernest Hemingway celebrated the running of the bulls at Pamplona in his novel, *The Sun Also Rises* (1926). Hemingway was no doubt a counterphobe. He sought danger (and found pleasure) in big game hunting, in boxing, and in the bull run. His search for danger, and the fact that he committed suicide by gunshot in the mouth, exactly as his physician father had done before him, suggests that he was struggling with fear of death most of his life. Suicide is one way of resolving that fear, and by definition it is fatal.

Further insight into the counterphobic experience as quasi-religious, as an epiphany, comes from an account of snake handling by a complete novice. Dennis Covington went to Scottsboro, Alabama, to cover the trial of pastor Glendel Buford Summerford, "a small time hoodlum who had repented and been called to preach, routinely handled poisonous snakes, drank strychnine and stuck his fingers into live electrical sockets" (Abbott, 1996, p. 14. A review of *Salvation on Sand Mountain*, by Dennis Covington, pp. 240, Addison-Wesley, Reading, MA). The pastor was sentenced to 99 years in prison for attempting to murder his wife using rattlesnakes. Not content with his search for meaning and excitement, Covington looked for his roots in the Old Rock House Holiness Church, where he handled:

> ... the big rattler, the one with my name on it, acrid-smelling, carnal, alive ... I felt no fear...The snake seemed to be an extension of myself...There seemed to be nothing in the room but me and the snake ... The air was silent and still and filled with that strong even light. And I realized that I, too, was fading into the white. I was losing myself by degrees, like the incredible shrinking man. It is a feeling ... of victory in the loss of self, close to our conception of paradise, what it's like before you're born or after you die. (Abbott, 1996, op. cit.)

The "feeling of victory in the loss of self" seems to me to add a new dimension to counterphobia. It is the familiar mechanism of dissociation. The white light, the shrinking of the self, seem identical to the descriptions of "near-death" experiences so widely recounted in recent best-selling books. To die and then return to life is to prove your immortality. It also lifts the curtain on the great unknown—what happens to us after death. To face the rattler or the bulls is to almost die, and to find you are still alive is to gain a bit of immortality. In the dissociated state, the intense fear fades, the (frightened) self shrinks, and one is reborn. Covington, a recovered alcoholic, really found his "salvation on Sand Mountain."

War

So much has been written about war and the quest for danger that I hesitate to bring it up. It is the best opportunity for the counterphobe to prove himself, yet it is much riskier than all the sports combined. Eight million military men were killed in World War I and 20 million in World War II. Whole platoons, companies, regiments, and armies have been wiped out. Replacements have sometimes mounted to 300% or 400% in a short period. How is it possible that young men don't run for their lives at the first rumblings of a military draft? Why do so many volunteer for duty, when the odds are not good at all?

In earlier days there was a military tradition. The officer corps of France, England, and Germany were men trained to be part of an elite group, with an elaborate code of honor. This was also true of the Japanese samurai. Knighthood had been restricted to the nobility. The "right to bear arms" was not for the common man. Chivalry was for the chevalier, the man on horseback. As wars grew more mechanized and impersonal, the spirit of chivalry faded.

> As late as 1912 … a military textbook set forth the ideal qualities of a prospective young cavalry officer thus. 'We particularly want the hunting breed of man, because he goes into danger for the love of it … We draw upon a class who have not been used to much brain work' (Botsford, 1997, p. 6. A review of *The Soldier's Tale: Bearing Witness to Modern War* by Samuel Hynes, 318 pp. Allen Lane/Penguin, New York)

The elite hunters are not the only young males attracted to danger. In the United States and other countries there is a tradition of training boys in contact sports. In the training films to which I was exposed in World War II, war was presented as a game, and football was constantly used as a metaphor. There had to be teamwork, individual responsibility for a particular task (the line, halfbacks, and quarterback), memorization of plays, and a code of honor about "fair play," which was clearly to be breached when the going got rough. Winning was everything. Games, and then sports, provide the child with the ability to learn rules and work with others, as George Herbert Mead (1962) taught us. They are one of the principal means of socialization. They also prepare youth for warfare.

Apter tells of the actual use of footballs in combat, as if a real game of football was being played.

> The best known example (of sporting metaphors in war) is that of a certain Captain Nevill—who, as company commander, presented a football to each of his four platoons before an offensive on the Somme, (World War I) offering a prize to the platoon that first kicked its ball up to the enemy's front line. Unfortunately, Nevill wasn't able to award the prize; he was killed during the subsequent attack. (Apter, 1992, p. 166)*

While the presentation of war to recruits (as just another game, or "a chance to learn a trade" or a chance to get away from home, get a uniform, and be attractive to girls) may be part of a not-so-subtle propaganda campaign, what really sells war to the young male is the chance to test himself in real danger.

> Every new generation will respond anew to war's great seduction … Not to the uniforms and the parades but to the chance to be where danger is … In matters of war, cautionary literature and the evidence of experience do not change many minds or alter many romantic expectations. (Botsford, 1997, quoting Samuel Hynes)

---

* Apter is citing P. Fussell, *The Great War and Modern Memory*, Oxford University Press, New York, 1977, p. 27. Fussell and Apter both discuss the use of game and sports metaphors in war at length.

It remains to be seen whether the Vietnam War, with its political divisiveness, will make it very difficult to recruit or draft young men into the armed services. The "good wars," World Wars I and II, were seen as legitimate by most of the U.S. and European population. After that, thousands of men dodged the Vietnam draft, fleeing to Canada rather than serve in a war they deemed unethical. President Bill Clinton has been both praised and criticized for obtaining an exemption from service during that period. In a previous century he would never have been elected, owing to the pro-military sentiment of that time.

Even after volunteering or being inducted, and in the midst of combat, the viewing of war as a game acts to protect the soldier from panic. The leaders promote the metaphor, and the soldier seizes on it, for it gives him a false sense of security. "... the soldier has the illusion of being in the safety zone when in fact he is in the danger zone" (Apter, 1992, p. 167). The soldier sees himself as a "spectator," as being an actor on a stage or "starring in our very own war movie" (Apter, 1992, pp. 166–170). Dissociation, often working in conjunction with counterphobia, in this case protects the combatant from fear of death. However, it is society that gains and the soldier who loses, for this dissociation is dysfunctional for the individual. He or she often dies, or is severely wounded and crippled for life. How many war amputees, such as former Senator Bob Dole, make it to the top of our society despite their wounds, their rage, and constant pain?

Without a doubt, war has been, and will probably continue to be, a haven for the counterphobes of the world. They will often perform deeds of great daring, for their motivation is so strong that their protective frame is damaged and illusory.

More Fun for the Counterphobe: A Listing of Other High-Risk-Behaviors*

Most of these activities are obviously connected with counterphobic behavior. Not all people who engage in them are counterphobes. Motivations for these activities can vary widely.

Antisocial behavior: This is risky because one can get caught by the police, or injured by the victim. An example is "wilding," a term used by a teen gang that raped and battered a woman jogging in Central Park, New York City. The term suggests "looking for trouble" or running wild. It may include rape, vandalism, and various other crimes, including shoplifting (especially when not done for monetary gain), assault, battery, and murder.

Autoerotic asphyxiation: Hanging by the neck while masturbating, which heightens the orgasm. It is often fatal.

---

* The majority of these activities were taken from Apter's index; see Apter (1992).

Bullfighting: Especially in the case of a novice getting in the ring.

Bear wrestling (no comment, very grisly).

Bungee jumping: Jumping and then bouncing from a rubber cord attached to a bridge, building, cliff or balloon, etc. An estimated 1000 jumps are made a week in the United States. Banned in France owing to fatalities.

Driving dangerously: For example, passing on a hill, a curve, or on the right, speeding, tailgating—that is, the way most people drive presently. Consider the risk of 40,000 to 50,000 deaths a year in the United States from automobile accidents. Perhaps "road rage" is also related to fear of dying?

Dueling: By pistol, saber or sword. Now generally out of style, it was relatively safe, but not safe enough to save Alexander Hamilton.

Exhibitionism: The risk is in getting caught.

Fireworks: Firecrackers are sometimes thrown about randomly during the Chinese New Year festival. The Fourth of July fireworks in the United States are now much more supervised, as many children lost fingers and eyes in the past. Insurance costs have forced some towns to abandon the traditional spectacle.

Good samaritanism: Highly counterphobic. Altruism seems to be mostly absent, contrary to popular belief. "The interveners ... rarely expressed to us any sympathy for the persons they had assisted, or much satisfaction at having alleviated distress" (Farberow, 1980, p. 370).*

Kicking parties: British teens strip to their boots, dance, and kick each other, often resulting in broken arms and legs. A combination of voyeurism and sadism. Given the risks, also counterphobic.

Rappelling: Letting oneself down to the ground on a rope quickly from a height. This is often done down a rock face, by successive leaps outward from the rock wall.

Rock-climbing: In some ways the opposite of rappelling, since the general direction is up. Often the climber must use hand or finger holds, and climb upside-down to get over a ledge or overhang.

Russian roulette: Usually five of the six chambers of a revolver are emptied of bullets. Each player in turn spins the cylinder, points the muzzle at his head, and pulls the trigger. The high fatality rate has made "Russian roulette" a term that can be applied to any high-risk activity.

Speedy activities: Rollerskating, skateboarding, go karting, biking, hot rodding, motorcycling, skiing, water skiing, and power boating (Apter, 1992, p. 97), as well as roller-coasting and various carnival rides.

---

* "Altruism, Risk-Taking, and Self-Destructiveness: A Study of Interveners into Violent Criminal Events," by Gilbert Geis and Ted L. Huston. The authors found that "intervention into criminal situations represents neither untoward risk-taking nor self-destructive behavior." I would still insist that the intervener is probably a counterphobe, and also gets kudos from society for his heroism, as a secondary gain.

Surfing: Using a surfboard made of wood or plastic to ride the crest of large waves moving toward the shore, a sport originating in Hawaii. Car surfing consists of riding on the hood of speeding cars. Elevator surfing, an urban sport, involves leaping from the roof of one elevator to the roof of a passing elevator, with high fatalities. Train surfing consists of hanging onto fast moving trains.

Voyeurism: The risk is in being caught. The thrill is in seeing somebody in the nude who doesn't want to be seen in the nude.

What, finally, is the essence of counterphobic behavior? I think there are two main elements. The first of these is *control*. The counterphobe wants to control death itself, and his fear of death and dying. He wants to do this on his own terms. By his own choice, he exposes himself to death. He only wants to prove his immortality, to defy death. Wyshograd puts it in an existential framework:

> Death in these sports is the adversary ... In sport as in suicide, death does not choose its victim, but is rather chosen, in the former case as the conquered, in the latter as the conqueror ... sports ... are ... attempts to mitigate fate. The pleasure experienced is the pleasure of freedom (to choose, to control) (parentheses are my comments) (Wyschogrod, 1973, pp. 196)

Apter's view is that the counterphobe is seeking *arousal* and avoiding boredom. In his scheme, the pleasure is derived from creating the tension and then resolving it. Arousal seeking is surely part of counterphobic behavior. The pleasure of counterphobic behavior, the "addicting" part of it, can come from both tension resolution and the sense of control.

To me, in keeping with the theme of this book, *the fight against death fear is the primary explanation for counterphobic behavior*. In addition, it seems "self-destructive" only from the standpoint of the observer. From the point of view of the actor, it is a life-enhancing (even lifesaving) device in the face of overwhelming fear, anxiety, and depression. It becomes "self-destructive" only if the parachute fails to open, the scuba tank runs out of air, or the weather on Mt. Everest suddenly turns bad.

14

GAMBLING

Gambling is often called an addiction. Repetitive behaviors that are beyond the power of the individual to control may be addictions. Similarly, ideas beyond control are obsessions. There is an inability to get away from the slot machine or to get the horse race out of one's mind. The terms "drug addict," "sex addict," "food addict," and "workaholic" are used freely to describe people who can't stop their activity. Gambling, however, has a special quality. There is always the dim hope that one can "break the bank" and be rich beyond one's wildest dreams. Hope is one of the things we all need so badly.

In this aspect of preserving hope, gambling works like belief in the afterlife. Your lucky number may come up eventually, so keep trying. Poor people are more likely to gamble on the numbers, or Lotto and Bingo, or at the race track. Wealthy people gamble in stocks, bonds, commodities, and leveraged buyouts.

Rank saw a connection between human sacrifice and games (Rank, 1932, reprinted in 1989, pp. 294 and 303). At a later stage of sacrifice, a substitute (human or animal) could be found, and "an element of deceit crept in; a 'gambling with fate.'" This gambling with or tricking of fate was a game of life and death.

> The competitive character of games, too, seems to be primitive, though playing to win a prize is a very late development. The original victor in the competition ... did not content himself with honor alone: what he won was his life, which the defeated rival usually forfeit. (Rank, 1932, reprinted in 1989, p. 303)

We all remember (from the movies) the Roman gladiators and the crowd that turns thumbs down on the loser. The gamble with death has become transmuted into a gamble for money and power in most major sports. If one has any doubt, think of the infamous attack by Tonya Harding and her henchmen on her fellow figure skater and rival, Nancy Kerrigan. Harding's ex-husband and his co-conspirators arranged to hit Kerrigan in the knee with a baton, thus putting her temporarily out of commission. This enabled Harding to get on the Olympic team in 1994. There was worldwide shock, perhaps because a woman was involved, and because it happened in a sport usually considered to be nonviolent. Yet gambling is widespread in such sports as football, basketball, hockey, and boxing. Attacks during play, or even off the field, court, or out of the rink or ring, are common.

Gambling for money has been substituted for gambling for life or death, but the violent aspects of the Roman gladiator games linger on. Let's not forget that the Greek Olympic games were originally a preparation for war (running, wrestling, the javelin, the discus).

Rank (Rank, 1932, reprinted in 1989, p. 304) also describes how Tarot cards and other games foretold of death. Games and fortune telling are linked. We all would like to know what "hand" fate will deal us. So games, whether sports or card games, are in some derivative fashion a way of dealing with death.

While I have not researched the prevalence of gambling in other countries, an article in *The New York Times* magazine, by Gerri Hirshey (1994, p. 36ff.) gives some astounding statistics about its popularity in the United States.

> More Americans went to casinos than to major league ballparks in 1993. Ninety-two million visits! Legal gambling revenues reached $30 billion, which is more than the combined take for movies, books, recorded music and park and arcade attractions … The amount Americans spent on all forms of legal wagering last year, $330 billion—has set a historical precedent of its own. (Hirshey, 1994, p. 36)

Hirshey attributes this apparent sharp increase in gambling to several factors. The most important of these is the depressed national mood, triggered by the loss of jobs (especially good jobs), forced retirements, the "downsizing" of many corporations, and the loss of medical coverage and pension plans. This loss of security makes a gambling "fling" more attractive.

A second factor is the drive of politicians at the state and federal levels to raise money for governmental expenses without raising taxes, which are political poison. Hirshey says the government takes in $25 billion on lotteries each year.

A third factor is the selling of gambling via the mass media. Ads for racetracks and gaming and professional sports (where illegal gambling is rampant) are legion. There are billions to be made by corporations that finance the casinos and sports arenas.

> *Gambling and Wagering Business* magazine, in its most recent survey, figured the aggregate *illegal* take for horses and sports betting books, cards and numbers to be $43 billion. (Hirshey, 1994, p. 37)

The legal take of 30 billion and the illegal take of 43 billion makes an estimated total of $73 billion dollars. This is probably a gross underestimation, since there is a lot of informal betting, such as football pools and card games where money changes hands.

If gambling raises the hopes of many, how many people does it damage? If people who are down on their luck in general—the jobless, the divorced or separated, the crippled, the aged, the minorities—are more likely to gamble, then they are inevitably going to slide further down the slope. If you look outside an Off Track Betting (OTB) storefront, you will invariably see a collection of the outcasts of our society, trying for "one more chance." Of course, the government is taking their last dollar to finance schools, welfare, wars, prisons, and road building, and thus contributing to their downfall. You don't have to be a fundamentalist born-again Christian to be against the government's promotion of gambling.

And what of the great middle-class of gamblers? Are some of them at risk of self-destruction through gambling?

> At Harrah's (a casino), a special employee training program helps spot customers losing control. Estimates on the percentage of the American population at risk for the problem vary between 1 and 3 percent. (Hirshey, 1994, p. 53)

Again, this is probably a severe underestimate. When a customer is so reckless that the casino thinks he will be a troublemaker, or may not be able to pay his losses, the staff may intervene. They are not psychotherapists, however, and profit is their motive. They generally do not plead with clients to keep their money for the house or car mortgage, or to save it to pay their medical bills.

Even if we assume that the economic outlook in the United States is not always positive or stable across the socioeconomic range, can it account for the widespread gambling urge? If 10% of our households (perhaps 20% of our population) visit casinos each year, and some unknown but greater number bet on horses, sports, numbers, and cards, it is unlikely that there has been a sharp increase in gambling lately. If you look back at the riverboat gambling, and the gambling (and killing) over cards throughout our history, it is hard to believe that this was due to a contraction of hope. Betting was a booming business just as the westward expansion took place. The nation had never been so brimming with hope and opportunity. You could homestead and get 160 acres free if you farmed it. You could join the gold rush (an opportunity, but also a gamble). The government wasn't promoting gambling then. It just grew by itself. And of course, gambling is not limited to the United States. Gambling is a worldwide phenomenon, and as old as mankind.

More basic than economics is the fact that each of us is gambling every day. We gamble with our lives. We take chances crossing the street, working in an office or factory, and eating food. We might be hit by a car, or get injured by machinery in a factory or a mine. We might die of a heart attack brought on by stress in some corporate jungle. Even CEOs are vulnerable to sudden dismissal at the hands of stockholders (especially holders of mutual funds) and through hostile takeovers. Sex in this age of AIDS is a bet with death. Food poisoning reports are in the papers every day, as are stories about environmental contaminants that kill or disable us. Murder by guns and knives is part of the main course on nightly television news shows.

By betting, by gambling on sports, horses, dogs, or numbers, we take our attention away from our daily gamble with death. We defy death. We court "lady luck." We want this mother figure to be good to us. We keep up our hopes of a breakthrough, of "seeing our ship come in." In effect, we tempt fate, laugh in the face of our finitude, and hope for life eternal.

The strength of this "addiction," then, is in its power to conquer our fear of death—to give us an occasional victory over our basic bad luck, which is to be born human and fated to die. To return to Rank's idea, we would all like to see what hand Fate will deal us, but know we cannot predict the future. A game of cards (or any bet) is a small test case of the final hand of Fate. The repetition–compulsion of gambling finds its power in the repeated efforts to trick Fate, to force her to spare our lives and give us security. Each hand we win gives us hope, even though the odds are against us. Yet the odds in cards, numbers, and even in slot machines are much better than the odds of our living forever. The odds of dying versus living to age 200 are infinity versus zero. No one gets through life alive. The only odds that are minimally realistic are the odds of living long, living well, living creatively, and living happily, and they are almost impossible to predict for any one individual. The most we can get from the Dealer is a helping hand—the worst is the Ace of Spades.

15

DISSOCIATION*

Any mechanism, behavior, or personality style that can reduce or even temporarily eliminate the fear of dying may become a means of psychological and physical survival. A major mechanism, known as "dissociation," reduces or casts out fear from the conscious mind. It is a very generalized response to threat, and appears in many forms (at least when interpreted in a broad way).

Dissociation is defined in the dictionary (Flexner, 1987) as "The splitting off of a group of mental processes from the main body of consciousness, as in amnesia or certain forms of hysteria." The basic meaning of "dissociation," which applies to its use in other fields as well as psychiatry, is "separation." H. Spiegel described it as a fragmentation process. "The fragmentation can occur from central awareness to the unconscious, or it can surge from the unconscious toward central awareness" (Spiegel, 1963, p. 374). The separation, then, is between central awareness (conscious awareness) and the unconscious.

Dissociation is closely linked with the mechanism of repression, but is not synonymous with it. "Repression consists of withholding from conscious awareness an idea or a feeling" (Mardi Horowitz in Singer, 1990, p. 82). This is an involuntary unidirectional process. Dissociation is a two-way process. "Levels of awareness are in a constant state of flux" (Spiegel, 1963, N175, p. 374).

A further element in the definition of dissociation is the concept of identity. "In dissociation, one deals with emotional conflicts, or internal or external stress, by a temporary alteration in the integrative functions of consciousness or identity" (Mardi Horowitz in Singer, 1990, p. 80). This immediately brings to mind the multiple personality disorder (MPD) that has been such a favorite of novelists and movie makers. *The Three Faces of Eve* is about alterations of identity.

---

* I originally entitled this chapter "Withdrawal/Dissociation." Once I started to write it, I realized that dissociation is the more basic mechanism. Anyone who has dissociation as severe as multiple personality disorder or amnesia, or is an alcoholic or drug addict, is bound to be withdrawn. Withdrawal sounds more descriptive, while dissociation seems to get at the actual mechanics of what goes on in our minds. For this reason, I dropped the term "withdrawal."

Originally a case history (Thigpen, 1957), it was made into a movie. (See Movies section later.)

I would like to use the term "dissociation" in a much broader sense, to mean any altered state of consciousness. This state of separation or fragmentation is widespread in the general population. It is induced with drugs, alcohol, meditation, hypnosis, or trauma. There is group facilitation of dissociative states, such as during prolonged dancing and some emotional religious rites.

There is also a type of dissociation that is not induced by ingestion of drugs or brought on by any manipulation by oneself or others. This kind of dissociation is a human propensity that almost everyone employs from time to time. It could be called a Dissociative Personality Style. I shall discuss it later, after reviewing the more maladaptive modes of dissociation.

Multiple identity, fugue states, and amnesia can be seen as one end of a continuum of dissociative severity. (I owe this view to a suggestion by J. Jaffe. Previously I had viewed "pathological" dissociation as discontinuous with other types.) At the other end of this continuum I would place Dissociative Personality Style. There is also a rough correspondence between the dissociative severity continuum and the proportion of conscious versus unconscious control. The individual with MPD or the amnesiac has very little conscious control over the dissociation. The average American, especially the average businessman, lawyer, or politician, has a great deal of conscious control over his dissociation. He is living in a culture that has institutionalized lying, prevarication, "spin," and "public relations." This is discussed further at length later.

MULTIPLE IDENTITY, OR PROTEAN PERSONALITY STYLE?

Multiple personality disorder clearly involves an alteration of consciousness, but of a very special kind. Different elements of the conscious and unconscious are assigned to different characters, who usually have individual names and separate identities.

H. Spiegel points out that these cases have only one personality, but many identities. MPD, in his view, is a misnomer. The diagnosis has recently been changed to "Dissociative Identity Disorder," or DID, in DSM IV (*Diagnostic and Statistical Manual*).

The term "multiple personality" gained popularity after it appeared in Morton Prince's *The Dissociation of a Personality* (Prince, 1906). Prince's patient, a "Miss Christine Beauchamp" (pronounced "Beecham"), was a bright student in English Literature at Radcliffe, and later became the subject of plays and movies.* She had three "personalities" (alters). With the exception of Sally,

---

* For a brief description of the interest stirred up by "Miss Beauchamp," see Schwartz, 1996, p. 84.

they had amnesia for what had gone before, and for the other alters. Prince had put the term "multiple personality" in quotes, but clearly stated that only one personality was really involved. After Prince, the quotation marks disappeared!

Cases of this kind are commonly known as 'double' or 'multiple personality,' according to the number of persons represented, but a more correct term is disintegrated personality, for each secondary personality is a part only of a normal whole self. (Prince, 1906, p. 3)

The fact that so many "classical" cases of MPD involved women who had been sexually abused in childhood suggests that the fragmentation of identity is in itself a defense. Eve White and Eve Black (Thigpen, 1957) can play the good girl and the bad girl, but the conflict that would normally be felt by an associated (as opposed to a dissociated) individual is absent. There is little "cognitive dissonance," owing to the amnesia of one alter for the others. The conscience of the good girl doesn't punish her for what she imagines is her own bad behavior. It's that other girl, Eve Black, who is bad. When being abused, it is a dissociated part of the self that is suffering, not the whole self.

Cognitive dissonance is "anxiety that results from simultaneously holding contradictory or otherwise incompatible attitudes or beliefs"(Flexner, 1987, p. 399). It is of crucial importance in any discussion of dissociation. Dissonance in music is the opposite of consonance, and means inharmonious, unresolved, or discordant. The attitudes of a person suffering cognitive dissonance are in discord, and "want" to be resolved, just as dissonances (from dissonare, "to sound harsh") in classical music are usually resolved to a consonant interval, such as a dissonant second going to a third, fifth, or sixth. Dissociation is a primary mechanism utilized in the reduction and resolution of cognitive dissonance and other stresses.

In a discussion of MPD, Schwartz (1996)quotes a psychiatrist who sees a "play-acting quality" in some of these patients: a "monumental put on." Taking the opposite view, many therapists have argued that far from parading their many selves, these patients hide them, and have a high rate of attempted suicide.

What is so puzzling about the MPD individual is that she or he is either/or, a constantly shifting ambiguity that intrigues us. This is what fascinates us about cross-dressers and drag queens. Are they or aren't they? Some of our greatest movie stars, such as Marlene Dietrich and Judy Garland, specialized in song-and-dance routines dressed as men, often in top hat and tails. One element of their special appeal to the gay community has been the vague quality of their sexual identity. The operatic diva, who is female but appears to be cool, dominant, and unapproachable, is also very appealing to some in the gay community, which points to the complexity of the attraction. Prima donna is a synonym for diva. The use of the term prima donna to connote a willful, temperamental, petulant personality (not necessarily limited to the female leads in opera) completes the picture of this love "object."

There has been an increase in the appearance of sexual ambiguity in art, film, and literature, along with the very gradual acceptance of the lesbian, gay, and bisexual communities. There was

> ...an explosion after 1968 of photographic objects focusing on gender ambiguity...The radical social changes initiated in the 1960's—especially the rise of feminism, gay rights, and unconventional notions of masculinity—prompted modifications in accepted standards of gender presentation. (Quoted from explanatory notes at an exhibit at the Guggenheim Museum in New York City, entitled "Rose Is a Rose Is a Rose: Gender Performance in Photography," March, 1997)

Central features of the modern scene are ambiguity and irony. During times of rapid social change, people are forced to look at two sides of an issue. There is more criticism of the establishment. The old values are questioned. Authority figures are found to be hollow. "The Emperor has no clothes." The Wizard of Oz is a phony. (President Clinton might have qualified for the first condition if any more women accuse him of sexual abuse, and Nixon for the second.) Irony, cultural relativism, and deconstruction are necessary for social change. But, as Andrew Delbanco (1995) points out, these approaches are better at tearing down than at building up. This general ambiguity has its effect on identity as well. Lifton's concept of the "Protean personality style" may be a milder form of this ambiguous identity. Proteus, like Loki, could change his shape at will.

Lichtenstein, noting Lifton's concept of Protean style, saw it in some of his adolescent patients:

> Ronnie maintained a kind of traditional identity insofar as he aimed to become a professional person after finishing his studies. But he enjoyed as well the Hell's Angel image (a notorious motorcycle gang) into which he could slip with ease...He also liked the role of a kind of master craftsman. He mostly thought of himself as a kind of (sexual) guru...That his various ways of defining himself were often in conflict with one another was to be expected. (Lichtenstein, 1977, 1983, p. 337). (Parentheses are my comments.)

Today we see the phrase "reinventing the self" everywhere. Is it that easy to start over again, to build a new personality? How deep can the new self be? Is this a case of multiple "put-ons?" Are we dealing with charlatanism, with deliberate deceit? You may remember "The Great Impostor," a 1960 movie starring Tony Curtis, in which the antihero is able to pose even as a surgeon without ever having gone to medical school. He flits from one impersonation of a professional to another, until he is finally arrested. The film was based on the actual career of Ferdinand Demara, a master protean.

You might ask, "How could one person be so skillful?" On the other hand, how is it possible that professional roles in our society are so easily imitated? Are they hollow authorities too?

I think that the Loki-like personality style is a direct result of rapid social change and a shifting occupational structure. Today's youth may be better equipped for life as a broken field runner than as a staunch linebacker. Multiple careers are "in." Job-nomadism is a way of coping with rapid shifts in opportunity. Flexibility is more adaptive than solidity.

Clearly, the MPD/DID or the "near MPD" (Dissociative Disorder-Not Specified) individual is grappling with fears that are as close to death fears as a child can get. The painful sexual abuses to which Sybil* (Schreiber, 1973) was subjected by her mother are helpful in understanding the importance of dissociation as a mechanism for coping with the fear of dying.

I had chosen "Sybil" to illustrate MPD, since her case history was published and widely known. No sooner had I written several pages about her, than an article appeared in *The New York Review of Books*, consisting of an interview with Dr. Herbert Spiegel called "Sybil—The Making of a Disease." In effect, he was saying that Sybil didn't fit his criteria for an MPD.

> Back in those days, Multiple Personality Disorder was not yet in the DSM. To me, a multiple personality meant you had to have an 'alter'—that is, a distinct alternate personality—that was enduring, assuming control over the person for a considerable period of time, and that there was an amnesia barrier between one alter and another, as in the case, reported by William James, of Ansel Bourne, an American who forgot his identity and developed a second personality. I didn't see this at all in Sybil. I saw her 'personalities' rather as game-playing. (Borch-Jacobsen, 1997, p. 63)

I called Spiegel, rather upset over his criticism of Sybil, her therapist, and Flora Rheta Schreiber, the author of the book. We met to discuss the problem. If anyone knew about Sybil, he would, since he had regressed her under hypnosis several times at the request of Dr. Wilbur, her therapist. Both Wilbur and Schreiber had died. Spiegel told me that Sybil did not fit his criteria for an MPD (DID) for the following reasons:

1. No alter took charge for a fairly long period of time
2. There was collusion between the therapist and patient to "construct" her alters. (Note that some "scenario" is always created between therapist and patient.)
3. One of her alters knew the others. Sybil was aware of some of the different alters. In the pure case, they do not know one another. There is usually complete amnesia for events that happen to one alter as soon as another takes over.
4. Sybil didn't use the alter theme with Spiegel, although she did with Wilbur, her therapist.

On the other hand, there was strong evidence that Sybil was very close to being an MPD. She was highly hypnotizable. Spiegel regressed her easily. She

---

* From *Sybil* by Flora Rheta Schreiber, ©1973, H Regnery, reproduced with permission of McGraw-Hill Companies.

also dissociated quickly. He said "Wilbur reported that Sybil got distraught and smashed her fist through a window. When her analyst, Wilbur, became solicitous (because Sybil was bleeding), Sybil responded like a little girl, in a little girl's voice." (For Wilbur's own description of this event, see Kluft 1993, p. xxviii, "Cornelia B. Wilbur in her Own Words.")

Spiegel sketched out for me a continuum of dissociation, based upon his vast experience in hypnotizing hundreds of psychiatric patients.

LOW DISSOCIATION SCHIZOPHRENICS
SCHIZOIDS
MANIC DEPRESSIVES
HIGH DISSOCIATION DISSOCIATIVE DISORDER, NOT
SPECIFIED
DISSOCIATIVE IDENTITY
DISORDER (formerly MPD)

It is very difficult to hypnotize schizophrenics and others at the low end of the dissociative continuum.* In contrast, at the high end, patients go easily in and out of the hypnotic state. In fact, they often are able to hypnotize themselves spontaneously.

At the conclusion of our discussion, Spiegel said "Sybil is a good case for you, but she is a 'Dissociative Disorder, Not Specified' which is akin to MPD. She is as close as you can get to what MPD is in the current literature."

What were Sybil's symptoms, and what was her history?

> "Sybil had blackouts … During these periods … other … personalities would inhabit and control her mind: Vicky, stylish and sophisticated; the two Peggys, one tactful, one bull-headed; Marcia, assertive, speaking with a British accent; Mary, a maternal homemaker; and ten others. Sixteen selves existed within … Sybil Isabel Dorsett, 14 female and two male. (Schreiber, 1973, from flap copy)

Sybil's mother, Hattie, was severely depressed for 4 months after Sybil's birth (p. 94). Beginning when Sybil was 6 months old, her mother's "favorite ritual" was to separate Sybil's legs with a long wooden spoon, tie her feet to the spoon with dish towels, and then string her to the end of a light bulb cord, suspended from the ceiling … she would fill the adult-sized enema bag to capacity and return with it to her daughter. As the child swung in space, the mother would insert the enema tip into the child's urethra and fill the bladder with cold water. 'I did it!' Hattie would scream triumphantly, when her mission was accomplished. 'I did it!' The scream was followed by laughter, which went on and on (p. 160).

---

* Spiegel developed and tested an "eye-roll sign" of hypnotizability. He considers it a fixed biological marker related to the ability to dissociate. On a 0 to 4 scale, schizophrenics had an average eyeroll of 1.4. This is in contrast to MPDs, who averaged 3.4. No schizophrenic had an eyeroll score above 2. It is largely on the basis of this test that he has ranked diagnoses on the continuum of dissociation. The full test protocol is called the Hypnotic Induction Profile.

There were many unneeded enemas, twice the normal amount for a child. Sybil was forced to hold the cold water in, and walk about, which resulted in severe cramps. If she cried, or let the water out, her mother would beat her.

Hattie forced into Sybil's vagina a flashlight, a small bottle, a little silver box, the handle of a dinner knife, a little silver knife, a button hook, and often her finger (p. 160).

Hattie flung Sybil, dislocating one of Sybil's shoulders. She gave her a blow on the neck with the side of her hand, which fractured Sybil's larynx. She pressed a hot iron on Sybil's hand, causing a serious burn. She slammed a rolling pin on Sybil's hand, and closed a drawer on it. She tied a purple scarf around her daughter's neck, until she gasped for breath (p. 161).

Her mother filled Sybil's rectum or bladder with cold water. Then she tied her to a leg of the piano, while pounding out Bach, Beethoven, and Chopin to make painful vibrations in her child's head, bladder, and rectum.

As punishment for asking some innocent question, she would bind Sybil's face and eyes with dish towels. She would say "Anyone could see that who isn't blind ... I'll show you what it's like to be blind" (p. 162).

Hattie shoved a bead up Sybil's nose. She told the doctor, who finally removed it, that Sybil had pushed it up there ... (p. 167). She also closed Sybil up in a wheat crib, where she could have easily smothered. When confronted by her husband, she claimed the town bully did it (p. 168).

Sybil's psychoanalyst saw her (now adult) patient's multiple personalities as a "protective device for survival" (Schreiber, 1973, p. 158). She had no protection from her mother. Her father abdicated his protective role and never intervened, even though he knew his wife was schizophrenic. "I never dreamed a mother would hurt a child," he told Cornelia Wilbur, Sybil's analyst (Schreiber, 1973, pp. 200–201).

Hattie would often shake Sybil and call her a "bad girl" (Schreiber, 1973, p. 78). Any of Sybil's feelings of rage were turned into guilt, because her mother interspersed her tortures with brief periods of special attention, and told her what a lucky girl she was to have such nice parents and a nice home.

> What was most disturbing to Sybil was her feeling that she had no reason to be unhappy, and that, by being so, she was somehow betraying her parents. To assuage her feelings of guilt she prayed for forgiveness on three counts: for not being more grateful for all she had; for not being happy, as her mother thought she should be; and for what her mother termed 'not being like other youngsters.' (Schreiber, 1973, p. 94)

Gruen (1992) describes the pitiful attempts of children to continue to love their parents, despite the many parental sins of omission and commission. Here is Sybil, a child feeling guilty toward her mother, and thinking herself ungrateful because of all her parents' self-professed "love and protection." In fact, "On three occasions, Sybil's mother came close to killing her" (Schreiber, 1973, p. 200).

That is the crux of the argument. Sybil came as close to death, starting at the age of 6 months, as any baby or child could, without actually dying. She was taken to doctors again and again for various injuries. Even today much severe child abuse goes unnoticed and unreported, until the child finally dies or ends up acting out rather than withdrawing (which may bring him to the attention of the authorities). Sybil's creation of her 16 multiple personalities was her best way out of a prison and torture chamber and an escape from the many near-deaths created by her insane mother and her denying father. *She* was not enduring the pain and the rejection—her other selves were. Here is a dramatic case of the use of dissociation in coping with the fear of dying.

MPDs (now known as DIDs) are important to my thesis in this chapter, which is that dissociation is a defense or coping mechanism that can be invoked against the fear of death. Since MPDs are at the extreme of the dissociation continuum, they are crucial evidence of the connection between fear of death and dissociation. Of course, not all people react to trauma or abuse (which are linked to fear of death) with dissociation, which is a skill or aspect of the personality that varies widely in strength and is probably part of our natural endowment.

Sybil is not the only case to have several alters, to exhibit extreme dissociation, and to have experienced severe childhood physical, sexual, or psychological abuse.* To support the idea that MPDs do in fact exist, and that many of them have suffered some severe abuse or trauma, I will summarize several cases that illustrate their typical history. To avoid the possibility of collusion between a therapist seeking a "marketable" case and a suggestible patient trying to please the therapist, I have chosen some cases recorded years before "Sybil" and her attendant publicity hit the newspapers, bookstands, and the movie theaters. The dates (in boldface) I have given are for the time of publication or the approximate time the alters and amnesia appeared. The narrative is a combination of quotations and paraphrasing.

> Mary Reynolds (Kenny, 1986, a narrative based on quotes and paraphrasing of pp. 26–31) was reported in **1816** in the "Medical Repository" of New York. She fell into a profound sleep for quite a few hours. When she awoke she had amnesia for words and events. She had to relearn everything. In a few months she had another sleeping spell. On awaking, she had amnesia for all the events that had happened back to the time of her first sleeping spell. She had an "old state" and a "new state," with amnesia of one for the other. In the old, she could write well, but not in the new. At age nineteen she became unconscious while lying outdoors in a field. When she

---

* H. Spiegel does not think that high hypnotizability and childhood abuse are causal factors in MPD/DID. He says that they are often associated with MPD/DID. It is true that many children are abused, but only a very small proportion of them become MPD/DIDs. An association may often lead to the uncovering of a causal relationship, as in the case of tobacco and lung cancer. Our understanding of what makes an individual "choose" MPD, depression, antisocial behavior, or schizophrenia is very sketchy. Obviously both genetic and social/learning factors are involved. Whether these disorders are always a response to stress is not known, but they are *usually* associated with it. In my review of MPD cases in the literature, there is hardly one reported without some abuse or trauma. The dissociation itself makes it hard to obtain such material from the patient. Most MPDs are apt to deny abuse (at least initially).

regained consciousness, she was blind and deaf for a period of five to six weeks. (This
was before the "old and new states" appeared. She eventually developed into a third
or mature state.)(p. 36) "The above account...neglects to point out that the original
self that Mary Reynolds lost was conventional, pious, and according to the second self,
really quite dull. The second self that she acquired was gay, irresponsible, and mischievous." (p. 28)

(This "good/bad" duality is found in many of the cases of MPD/DID.)

At age twelve Mary had emigrated from Birmingham, England with her older brother
John, and *separately* from her parents. From a sheltered life the family had moved to
unbroken forest so her father could take up farming after his grocery business failed.
This was a life of severe privation. away from old friends, their church (they were Baptist
dissenters in England who fled after mob attacks), and civilized comforts. (pp. 30–31)

This early case showed dissociation, no permanent barrier between alters,
domination for a long time by a new alter, and early separation from her parents
at age 12 (she took a long sea voyage with only her brother as "family"). She suffered trauma due to the mob attacks on her family, and endured economic and
physical hardship.

Ansel Bourne (Kenny, 1986, the narrative and quotes are taken from pp. 66–78) was
born in 1826. In 1857 he set out for Westerly, Rhode Island from his home which was
near. He heard the voice of God tell him to go "To the Christian Chapel." He was in
conflict over this, and suddenly became "insensible," unable to see, hear, or speak.
During his trance-like state he felt that God had abandoned him—that his sins were
too great for forgiveness.

His hearing and speech returned. A month after the first episode he had another. A
vision commanded him to work for God, and he quit his trade of carpenter, and went to
"work for Him who was once known on earth as 'The Carpenter's Son.'" (quote on p. 66)

Twenty years later Bourne disappeared. He "had for a time lost his identity and
taken on that of an apparently fictitious person named Albert John Brown of Newton,
New Hampshire. One morning he had total amnesia for the entire period during
which he had been Brown, and asked 'Where am I?'" (p. 69) Bourne was brought to
William James, and hypnotized. The Brown alter was called out, and his steps
retraced. Bourne then disappeared again, and went to settle near Providence.

Was Bourne abused? His parents separated when his father "became dissi-
pated." He was then 7. The family fell into poverty. At 10 he was "sent to live with
another family for several years and later, after five years of factory work, was
apprenticed to the Olneyville carpenter. He was reported to be 'silent and stubborn'" (p. 77).

This was certainly not a pleasant childhood, but it is not a classic case of
"abuse." The early separation from his family may have been traumatic. Before
the 1900s, children were often "farmed out," and in Europe early apprenticeship
was the norm. There is evidence that under stress Ansel tended to dissociate. For
example:

When he became A. J. Brown he was sixty-one years old and going through a period
of distress correlated to economic loss, his second marriage, and abandonment of his

evangelistic career. William James asked the hypnotically resurrected Brown persona what he had undergone back home. "Passed through a great deal of trouble...Losses of friends...losses of property...Trouble way back yonder. All mixed up, confused. Don't like to think of it." (p. 78)

Ansel Bourne was dissociated, had at least one alter, had an amnesic barrier between his alters, was dominated for a long period by a new alter, suffered early separation from his parents, endured economic hardship, and evidenced poor self-esteem (which is typical of MPDs).

Christine Beauchamp (pronounced "Beecham") was treated by Morton Prince, starting in 1898. She is perhaps the most famous of all the MPDs. Her real name was Clara Fowler. (Prince, 1906)

Ms. B was 23 years old when first seen. She was a student in a New England college. She was an extreme neurasthenic. She had headaches, insomnia, bodily pains, persistent fatigue and poor nutrition. Her general appearance was that of an hysteric.

She was very suggestible, stubborn, and showed aboulia (an inhibition of the will, by which a person is unable to do what he actually wishes to do).

She had a limitation of the field of consciousness, and was dominated by certain ideas. These are the recognized psychical stigmata of hysteria. (p. 15)

In addition to her normal self, and the hypnotic state known as B II, Miss Beauchamp may be any one of three different persons who are known as BI, BIII and BIV.

BI is Ms. Beauchamp. BIII was Sally. Sally called BIV "the idiot." BI is the saint. BIV is the woman (frailties of temper, self-concentration, ambition, and self-interest "as in the average human being"). Sally is the devil—a mischievous imp'. (p. 16) Ms B felt "possessed" by Sally.

With the exception of Sally, all her alters had amnesia for what had gone before, and changed from moment to moment. Ms. B was very reticent to talk about her private life. She was well educated, had literary tastes, and was a bibliophile.

She was born in 1875 (based on subtracting her age when first seen, 23, from the year she was first seen, 1898). Her father had inherited the violent temper of his own father. Christine's parents were unhappily married.

"Ms. B was a nervous impressionable child, given to daydreaming and living in her imagination. Her mother exhibited a great dislike to her, and for no reason, apparently, excepting that the child resembled her father in looks...her presence having been ignored by her mother except on occasions of reprimand. On the other hand she herself idealized her mother, bestowing upon her an almost morbid affection; and believing that the fault was her own, and that her mother's lack of affection was due to her own imperfections, she gave herself up to introspection, and concluded that if she could only purify herself and make herself worthy, her mother's affection would be given her." (p. 12)

Her mother died when she was thirteen. "Prince records that Ms. Beauchamp received a violent shock when an infant brother died in her arms...This was only four days after her mother died of puerperal fever." (Kenny, 1986, p. 137) For several weeks she was half-delirious (disintegrated). The 3 years following her mother's death, when she lived with her father, were a period of successive mental shocks, nervous strains and frights. (Prince "can't give details, as this would lead to identification of the subject.") (p. 12)

She was a somnambulist. At 14 she wandered out in the street in her nightgown, and was brought home by a policeman. She also went into spontaneous trance-like states, lasting a few minutes.

At 16 she ran away from home. (Prince suggests that she was subjected to great emotional strain, but does not specify.) (p. 13)

"In 1893 (at age 18?) she had a shock, which played a principal role in the development of her MPD. Clara Fowler had a bad time of it in life, and, if her report to Prince is accepted, had a traumatic and apparently sexual encounter with an older man while engaged in nursing work, one that recurred during her time under medical care" (Kenny, 1986, p. 138) "Prince thought the crucial episode to have been the encounter with the enigmatic 'Jones' in Fall River." (Kenny, 1986, p. 145)

How well does Miss Beauchamp fit the various criteria for an MPD? She is dissociated, and has several alters, but one of them, Sally, knew about the others, so there is not a complete amnesic barrier between the alters. Sally dominated Ms. Beauchamp. She suffered emotional abuse from her mother, who was cold and rejecting, but she reported no sexual or physical abuse by her parents. At 13 she lost her mother and her infant brother within a few days, followed by several weeks of disintegration. Her somnambulism was further evidence of her dissociated state. A major sexual trauma (though apparently not abuse) occurred around age 18, during an encounter with an older man. She showed poor self-esteem, and blamed herself for her mother's lack of affection toward her. (This is a repeated pattern among MPDs.) There was no severe economic hardship. Miss B (Claire Fowler) fits the profile almost exactly, except she is not physically or sexually abused early on, and one alter knows the others. She is suggestible, and easily hypnotized (typical of MPDs). Her therapy took place before MPDs were in style, although those most critical of the MPD diagnosis might claim that Prince and his patient colluded in a scenario, or that she tried to please Prince with her various alters.

Eve White (Thigpen, 1957) famous through the publication of the book, *The Three Faces of Eve*, and a movie in which Joanne Woodward took the starring (multiple) role, Chris Sizemore lived in Georgia in the 1950s.

Eve (Chris) had migraines, blackouts and memory loss. Her doctor sent her to Colin Thigpen, a psychiatrist. Eve White was affectionate with her husband, but an alter, Eve Black, appeared. Eve Black bought and wore flashy clothes. (Cohen, 1996, p. 40)*

After going into a brief trance, Eve White "awoke" and said "Hi there, Doc!" This was the first (and spontaneous) appearance of Eve Black. Black was irritated by White's ladylike airs and her goody goody attitude. Black was also somewhat resentful of her child, four year old Bonnie. White didn't know about Black, but Black knew about White. White was conventional, conservative, and self-effacing. Black was a party girl, went out with men, hung around bars, and danced. (p. 40)

Later Jane appeared. She was warm, mature, a real woman. An electroencephalogram showed Jane and White to be closer to each other in brain wave pattern than they were to Black. Each alter took the semantic differential test. Jane turned out to be the healthiest. (p. 47)

---

* I have quoted or paraphrased Cohen's summary of Eve, which catches the essential points of her story. The extracted portion is all based on Cohen, *Alter Egos*, pp. 40–51.

> With Jane the childhood memories began to be unraveled. She eventually recalled being forced to touch the face of her dead grandmother at her funeral. It was her mother who made her do it. It made Eve feel very morbid and scared of death. (p. 49)
>
> Sizemore (Eve) also began to claim Eve's initial trauma started when she was only two, when she witnessed a grotesque accident at a sawmill. A man's arm was severed. There was blood all over. She had to escape the frightening blood. (p. 50)
>
> Ian Hacking and others criticize Eve—she didn't have enough alters, and she showed no signs of having been abused as a child. (p. 51) In fact, Eve later claimed that she had dozens of alters Thigpen had never uncovered. (p. 78)

As for abuse, its absence alone is no reason to throw out a diagnosis of MPD. A trauma or a series of traumatic incidents may substitute for sexual or physical abuse as a trigger for dissociation and MPD. Several authors have likened MPD to posttraumatic stress syndrome. Eve's being forced to touch her dead grandmother and her watching as a man's arm was severed might have been enough to trigger dissociation in a child already prone to that coping mode.

Eve meets many of the criteria for MPD. She was dissociated, and had several alters. She did not have amnesia across alters (a criterion notably absent in most of these famous cases). She was dominated by one alter, Eve Black, for a long time. Black caused a rift in her marriage and diminished her care of her child. Despite no evidence of abuse (unless forcing a child to touch a dead grandmother's face could be considered abuse in its current sense), at least two traumatic incidents were reported. The theme of the conventional versus the sexual and aggressive self is repeated in this case, as it is in "Lizzie," which follows, in Ms. Beauchamp and others. Low self-esteem was not evident in Eve, and clearly absent in Eve Black.

Sybil Isabel Dorsett (Schreiber, 1973) was described in detail earlier. She is inserted here chronologically (circa **1960–1970**) to illustrate the possible historical influence of her case and its attendant publicity on the later popularity of the MPD diagnosis. If she was not a true MPD, she was a close second—a "Dissociative Disorder, Not Specified"—according to H. Spiegel.

"Lizzie" is one of several MPDs described by David Cohen in his review of British and other multiples (Cohen, 1996, No. 192). She was born around 1966. Now in her 30s, she has been treated for 2 years **(circa 1990)** by her psychotherapist, "Trevor." He was always wary of being gulled by her.

> Lizzie had won scripture prizes. She had been good at Bible studies. Her father was an important figure in a local Baptist community. Since her teens she had been in and out of psychiatric hospitals. She had a serious depression, and slashed her wrists several times. Lizzie was very interested in fire and may have been a pyromaniac. She had electroconvulsive therapy and antidepressants. Trevor "fished for" memories of abuse. Lizzie for a long time denied any abuse. A second person (alter) appeared during therapy, named "Esther." Esther was a "witch who had been dead for 300 years. She had been burned at the stake in Faversham, and was called "Esther of Faversham." (p. 114)
>
> Lizzie's parents often sent her down to Margate, to stay with her grandmother (her father's mother) and her grandmother's boyfriend, 5 years younger than grandma.

Grandma had split with grandpa, who beat her when drunk. Lizzie often visited during the summer. Why did her parents send her away? *"Mum and Dad only liked me when I was being a Bible girl."* (p. 199)

   Victor, the grandmother's "fancy man," dried Lizzie off in the bathroom. Esther told the therapist that Victor "would have his hands on her while he read stories to her." The abuse became more intimate, involving masturbation, as he got her to touch his penis. Until Lizzie reached puberty, Victor did nothing else. Then he came into her bedroom one night, put a hand over her mouth and had intercourse with her. Esther did not object. Lizzie's reaction was very different *(the good versus the bad self)*. He made her touch his penis and rub it. She remembered when he had first come into her. She was terrified. She hated it. She hated Esther who seemed to like it. Esther hated and feared Lizzie because Lizzie could have told her parents. Lizzie didn't want to go back to Nan (grandma). (pp. 122–123) (Italics mine)

   When she was fifteen Lizzie got pregnant. Lizzie denied it. (Nan was onto this, and had "rows" with Victor.) Lizzie probably had an abortion.

   Lizzie was a "disgrace" to the family. They took her to a psychiatric hospital. There she started several fires. Lizzie walked out one day, without permission. She had a "third voice" (not really described in detail). "The third voice asked what could be done to rid her and Lizzie of Esther, who was still making their life miserable." (p. 127) The third voice is angry with Trevor, her therapist. She "has shared so much with him in the hope of getting Lizzie better and it seems to have got them nowhere." (p. 128)

How does Lizzie meet the criteria for MPD? She is clearly dissociated, and has two alters. She does not have amnesia for the alters, and in fact reports a struggle between herself and her third voice against Esther. She is strongly dominated by Esther, who is sexually aggressive and sets fires. She was sent to her grandmother's for the summer from her preteens on, which may be viewed as early separation. Lizzie says her parents, who were very religious, "only liked the Bible girl" (Lizzie the good), and rejected her for any other behavior. She was severely abused sexually by her grandmother's boyfriend, and emotionally abused by her strict religious parents. There is no evidence of economic hardship. Her suicide attempts and severe depression suggest very poor self-esteem. Her alters are at war, and the therapy thus far has failed. Cohen asks "How can you merge into one human being a formal, religious woman in her early thirties who keeps her small flat empty and spotless, a witch, and a much younger angry 'voice?'" (Cohen, 1996, p. 128)

   The use of dissociation to create Esther (the witch) seems to me to be a defense against the "fate worse than death" to which Lizzie had been exposed by Victor. If Lizzie is horrified, at least the Esther part of her not only survives the rape and continual sexual abuse, but even enjoys it. Once again, survival in the face of a series of death-like experiences has been accomplished through dissociation.

Jonah (**circa 1990**) (Cohen, 1996, pp. 98–110, paraphrased or quoted), a black man, was born in Kentucky. At age 21 while in the Army he went berserk when a friend of his was killed. He set fires. He was hospitalized. In Vietnam under fire, he cracked, and starting shooting wildly. He got a medical discharge. He beat up a girlfriend, and was hospitalized for two months. He served two short jail sentences. Then nine months later he was hospitalized again. He suffered amnesia at that time. Since age ten, or even before, he had a number of alters. "Sammy" was one who knew all the other alters. "King Young" was "streetwise and sex-smart." He reported that when he was six his mother stabbed his stepfather. His mother went to jail, which left him more or less abandoned. He said his mother dressed him in girl's clothes. When he was ten a gang of white boys beat him up. He was afraid he would die. He blanked out. At that time a third alter appeared. This was "Usoffa," an African warrior-king who was fearless and a super-hero. It is uncertain if he was abused (p. 112) but that he was subjected to various traumas is probably true. *"There is no evidence that these events were real, or fantasies, real alters during childhood, or later alters."* (p. 110). What is special about Jonah is that his various alters were each given an extensive battery of tests. The tests involving expression of emotion showed the greatest differences between alters…*"the results on the MMPI, the Adjective Check List, the Scale of Emotions and the ward observations all suggested clear differences between the alters."* (p. 110) *"In dealing with anything emotional, the four personalities were quite distinct."* (p. 111) His neurological response to pain varied between alters, especially his electroencephalogram (EEG).

How well does Jonah fit the criteria for MPD? These differences in test responses suggest that the alters are distinct from each other, and at a deep level of consciousness that Jonah was unable to control. It also makes me feel that his alters were not merely a histrionic display to convince his doctors of his illness, or to excuse his dangerous behavior. He had amnesia for his alters at times, but "Sammy" knew all of them. In almost every case there is not a complete amnesic barrier between alters, which suggests that this criterion is too strict, and would eliminate many cases that fit the profile of the MPD in most other respects. Jonah was dominated by "Usoffa" during his episodes of violence (for example, when he beat up his girlfriend). He suffered early separation from his mother, economic hardship, and trauma (being beaten for being Black and seeing his mother stab his stepfather). Information about emotional, physical, or sexual abuse is missing or uncertain. Self-esteem was notably high only in the alters "Usoffa" and "King Young." Several of the MPDs have set fires (including Jonah), which is noteworthy. "Usoffa" clearly shows the utility of an alter in a situation in which fear of dying is prominent. Becoming a superhero-alter in the face of possible death from a gang-beating is a good example of the utility of dissociation.

I am far from alone in thinking that some type of abuse or trauma is closely linked with the development of MPD or a dissociative disorder. D. Spiegel (1993, in Kluft, 1993; page numbers of the Spiegel quotes given in the text) makes this same connection repeatedly:

(MPD is a) "failure of self-integration in which individuals isolate or separate one component of memory from another, *usually for defensive purposes.*" (p. 99) [emphasis mine]

One MPD patient who was raped as a teenager dissociated to a new personality she called 'No One.' This enabled her to experience the rape as having happened to 'no one.'(p. 99)

Another MPD patient reported that the first time she dissociated was the first time her father took off his necktie, tied her to the bed, and raped her. The alter said to her "You don't want to be with that bastard. You come and be with me." (p. 89)

David Spiegel says that the evidence seems to support most of the reports of abuse as true (Spiegel, 1993, pp. 90–91). Cornelia Wilbur (Sybil's psychiatrist) was unequivocal about the connection between trauma and MPD:

> MPD is clearly a defense disorder against overwhelming emotional and physical trauma and is more closely related to [post] traumatic stress disorder than anything else. (Kluft, 1993, "Cornelia B. Wilbur in Her Own Words," p. xxx)

James Glass has written a very sophisticated book, which gives arguments pro and con MPD. He criticizes some authors who hold up the MPD as the hero of our postmodern world and as the symbol of a "nihilist awakening." He sees a lack of empathy and a "silence on how to heal or at least ameliorate intense physical and psychological pain" (Glass, 1993). He is referring to the pain of the MPD patient. Several times Glass states that MPD and dissociation constitute a defense against physical and sexual abuse, and the *horror* (my emphasis) that goes with repeated abuse:

> Protection of a traumatized and violated core takes the form of alter personalities that derive from repeated physical and sexual abuse. (Glass, 1993, p. 53)
>
> The origins of the multiple personalities I spoke with lay in the repeated violence of the father's incest and physical abuse. ... (p. 53)
>
> What saved these women from becoming totally mad, schizophrenically (*sic!*) fragmented, was the power of self-hypnosis (dissociation) and the capacity to forge alternative identities shielding, through language, the rape of the self and the experience of horror. (p. 56)

The use of language in the defense system is striking. Taking another name says in effect "This isn't happening to me, but to someone else." Lizzie isn't being raped, but her alter, Esther of Faversham (the witch), is. David Spiegel's example of the raped girl who developed an alter named "No One" again uses a trick of language as a defense. ("No One" was raped.)

There is no doubt that MPD (or DID) has lately been overdiagnosed. The reports of abuse by Satanic cults are now being largely discounted. We should not throw the baby out with the bath water. Abuse is still widespread, and our own study of 2000 families shows that parents willingly report physical (though not sexual) abuse in large numbers. Slapping, spanking, beating, and even burning were reported, even though these are considered "socially undesirable" by a good portion of the population. Cohen (Cohen, 1996, pp. 234–235) warns that abuse is not limited to the home. "Organized rings and gangs of pedophiles" exist.

In a case known to me, the parents lost a child to a pedophile ring in the United States. Detectives identified the "perpetrator" as a "chicken hawk," but were unable to obtain enough evidence to bring charges against him!

There is a fine line that has to be walked between believing all patients' reports of abuse and believing none of them. To say that it doesn't matter in therapy whether abuse really happened, since "the therapist and patient create a scenario" is to ignore and even abet a serious and protracted social and ethical problem. We don't know enough about the connections between abuse, trauma, and dissociation. Denial of a real problem by labeling all recall of abuse or trauma as fantasy is clearly as wrong as allowing a therapeutic cottage industry in recovered memory of abuse and Satanic cult fantasies to grow like a cancer.

MPDs are extremely dissociated, and have often been exposed to very severe stresses early in life. What about experiences less severe than physical or sexual abuse, and those that occur after childhood? Job loss for a skilled worker or executive or the limited job opportunities for slum-born Blacks can be experienced as mini-deaths. A slippery style can help, since it acts as a rationale for necessary multiple job shifts. Drugs and alcohol can "drown the sorrows" of those losing love or work (Freud's two *raisons d'etre*). MPD, fugues, and amnesia lie at the severe end of the consciousness-altering continuum. Not far from it lie drug addiction and alcoholism. The protean style and religious fervor and some "everyday dissociation" (discussed in the Summary of this chapter) lie at the milder end. Here are some of the ways in which dissociation, in its broadest sense, helps to diminish fear of death and dying.

Drugs and Alcohol

The use of hypnotic drugs to induce hallucinations or to stimulate is widespread.

> Amphetamines, stimulants, short-acting barbiturates and glutethimides are the most frequently used. Tranquilizers and anti-depressives must be viewed separately. They are different physiologically, can be prescribed medically, and probably don't cause addiction or habituation. (Farberow, 1980, Calvin J. Frederick, "Drug Abuse as Indirect Self-Destructive Behavior, p. 140)

The scope of drug abuse in the United States is tremendous. Frederick says that "twenty-five percent of the United States population use sedatives, stimulants, or tranquilizers" (Farberow, 1980, Calvin J. Frederick, op cit., p. 137). Research has shown a strong relationship between depression and drug and alcohol abuse. A circular relationship is involved, since many drugs, including alcohol, leave an aftermath of depression after the stimulating "high." However, it seems clear that drugs and alcohol are widely used to self-medicate against depression and anxiety states. Most drugs produce some variety of dissociation; a fragmenting of the conscious from the unconscious mind, and a shifting from affect (feelings) to cognition (information, ideas) or vice versa. Under the influence of drugs, one can behave in socially unacceptable ways without the usual feelings of guilt. How many men have hit their wives or abused their daughters under the influence of alcohol? The scenario is almost a bromide to the police and the social worker.

Drugs, then, put a damper on awareness of death and one's own mortality. They allow us to rise above our finitude. The bacchanal drowned sorrows in drink, and gave permission for uninhibited sex. "Eat, drink, and be merry" should probably have been rearranged as "Drink, eat, and be merry, for tomorrow we die," with heavy emphasis on the drinking. Fear of death is once again obliterated or temporarily weakened. There is also a strong element of time stopping, an adult (perhaps an adulterous) "gather ye rosebuds."

TRANCES, FUGUES, AND HYSTERICAL PARALYSES

Hypnotic trances can be self induced, and of course they can be induced by others. Hypnosis has found a great many uses in medicine. D. Spiegel cites absorption, dissociation, and suggestibility as defining characteristics of the hypnotic state (Farberow 1980, David Spiegel, "Hypnosis, Dissociation, and Trauma," p. 124). Some people have the ability to become completely absorbed in a film or a book, and they may even find themselves "in the picture," as did Mia Farrow in Woody Allen's film, "The Purple Rose of Cairo" (1985). This ability to focus on an object and to exclude all extraneous stimuli is surely a shield against fear of death.

In addition to what I already discussed about dissociation, (repression, multiple personality disorder, etc.), D. Spiegel mentions fugue states "...in which an individual experiences a discrete and reversible but rather profound change of personal identity" (Farberow, 1980, David Spiegel, op. cit., p. 137). In the typical "fugue state" movie scenario, the hero forgets who he is, wanders around, has a series of promiscuous or hair-raising escapades, and finally returns to his wife and to his former self. A physical injury or emotional stress can trigger such a state. It is a defense against extreme stress, just as dissociation in MPD is usually a defense against and preceded by various kinds of abuse. (See p. 128, D. Spiegel, in Farberow, 1980, for references to research that found that MPDs suffered "severe physical, sexual and emotional abuse.")

Suggestibility is probably a basic personality characteristic. H. Spiegel developed a well-known "eye roll" test, which can identify subjects who are easily hypnotized. Suggestibility is also felt to be due to a weak self-concept or self-esteem. Thus whatever the hypnotist suggests is accepted rather than challenged, because of these feelings of inferiority. (Farberow, 1980, see D. Spiegel, p. 137, under "Suggestibility.") This may be related to the concept of deep "enculturation" discussed earlier, in which the individual takes in the culture without any internal censor or criticism. This leaves little room for fear of death, since one is too busy with routine to notice approaching doom. The busyness is the defense. The automaton of the modern age is like the hypnotized patient, who does what he is told to do, but doesn't even recognize the source of his commands. He thinks they are coming from him, not from the hypnotist (read "leader" or "hero").

The metaphor of the ventriloquist and his puppet is similar. Many times the worm turns, as when Charlie McCarthy talked back to Edgar Bergen, or when the puppet bit Michael Redgrave, his schizophrenic ventriloquist, during a performance, and finally came to replace his human personality (Dead of Night, 1945). The popularity of defiant "Charlie" may have sprung from the fact that he represented a child struggling for independence and separation from the absolute control of his parent/hypnotist.

Hysterical paralyses, although less common than in the days of Charcot, Janet, or Freud, still contain a large element of dissociation. An arm or leg is paralyzed, and the patient is unable to move it. A "glove paralysis" of the hand is unrelated to the innervation of the hand and arm, but is shaped by the mind of the patient from what she knows about gloves and clothing. The paralysis usually acts as a defense against a sexual or aggressive impulse. (Left-handed individuals with bursitis typically have it in the left shoulder, or striking side, and vice versa for the right-handed. Bursitis may be associated with repressed anger.)

In the hysterical paralyses, the unacceptable sexual, aggressive, or other impulses are "displaced" onto a part of the body.

> In displacement, the avoided ideas and feelings are transferred to some other person, situation or object. For example, hypochondriacal patients may displace worry and ward off a concern that their minds are failing, focusing concern instead on a body part. (Mardi Horiwitz in Singer, 1990, p. 80)

Pain and Hunger to Induce Dissociation

Self-mutilation or mutilation by others is a worldwide phenomenon. The usual cosmetic mutilations, such as ear-piercing, nose-piercing, neck stretching, tattooing, the raising of keloid scars, and related mutilations, such as circumcision, subincision, and clitoridectomy, may be done for decoration, or for religious purposes during rites of passage. There are some instances in which mutilation was used to induce trance states. One example is among some of the U.S. Plains Indians. Strips of flesh were cut into the chest or shoulders of young men. To have a totem animal appear to them, they had to achieve a trance state. They were hung, often for days, until weak with pain and hunger. In this semiconscious state they were dissociated, and usually saw or talked to a bear, otter, eagle, raven, or other totem animal.

The pain inflicted in sado-masochistic sexual practices often involves bondage, pinching male or female nipples, whipping, hanging, and other means of inflicting pain. It is possible that some sexual inhibitions are overcome by the dissociation created by this pain. A not incompatible interpretation is that such masochistic practices are adaptive:

> For all of them (masochists) however, the perversion was an effort to get some sexual pleasure in a world that seemed empty of living people. The perversions functioned

as defenses against depression and were an effort to hold their personalities together. (Farberow, 1980, p. 34, "Psychodynamics of Indirect Self-Destructive Behavior," Robert E. Litman)

While the motivation of masochists is complex and varies greatly, one major element is the attempt to "feel alive," to enhance feelings—sexual and otherwise. The depressed and suicidal histories of bondage practitioners suggests that the various procedures are a way of combating death anxiety and the feeling of being more dead than alive. Another major element is the desire for humiliation. It may be that this is the only form of "love" that they ever received in childhood, a hunch that is supported by several studies.

The symptomatology of self-mutilators varies widely, with mood instability being predominant. Diagnoses are varied, running from hysteria to schizophrenia, but borderline schizophrenia seems to be the best fit (Farberow, 1980, Litman, op. cit., p. 262). Again dissociation is strongly suggested.

Self-mutilators have suffered cold, distant, cruel, or domineering parenting. They exhibit a fear of abandonment (Farberow, 1980, Litman, op. cit., p. 266). This suggests a strong link with fear of dying, which I believe is evidenced in children by fear of abandonment. As stated in the section "Probable Causes of the Fear of Dying," fear of abandonment is the child's equivalent of fear of death and dying, since early helplessness makes them equivalent.

While the average masochist actually seeks pain, the typical "cutter" (wrist, vagina, testicles) does *not* feel pain during the actual wounding. The anesthesia wears off after a while, and the pain then ensues. The difference between the whipped–pinched–squeezed–stretched masochist and the "cutter" type is challenging, for it suggests very different motivations.

Hunger is another means of bringing on dissociation. There are many tales of shipwrecked sailors or passengers who have hallucinations while adrift on the sea without food. Thirst is famous for producing mirages in the desert (visual hallucinations, indicating dissociation). Anorexia is sometimes seen as a way of controlling parents and others:

...the anorexia nervosa patient who, maintaining herself at a just-viable weight, literally puts her life on the line for the sake of her independence. (Farberow, 1980, p. 236, "Hyperobesity as Indirect Self-Destructive Behavior," Christopher V. Rowland, Jr.)

However, anorexia and the bulimia that often accompanies it may also induce some dissociation. Again, the underlying dynamic is fear of abandonment. The anorexic is sometimes described as a "poor little rich girl" syndrome, in that the patient is "rich" in having her physical needs taken care of, but parental love and warmth are lacking.

Epileptics have traditionally been religious leaders (shamans) among Siberian tribes. The dissociated states and accompanying seizures seem to be attractive to worshippers, and are interpreted by them as evidence of divine inspiration. Many charismatic religious leaders have been epileptics. Not a few have been dissociated enough to hear voices and have visual hallucinations as well. (Joan of Arc heard voices in her teens telling her to support Charles VII of France. She was also a cross-dresser!) Some religious followers are equally capable of self-induced dissociation. Several Southern sects in the United States are known to "speak in tongues." These are foreign languages of which they purportedly have no previous conscious knowledge, and that they employ only during religion-inspired trances.

The oracle at Delphi supposedly sat on a stool over a fissure in the rocks from which natural gas issued. This probably caused a state of mild dissociation, which enabled her to prophesy the future. Of course, the use of inhalants is not limited to Greek oracles. Many drug addicts also inhale gases to produce dissociated states.

> Inhalants are volatile substances which, while never intended to be used as drugs, are abused because of their mind-altering effects…The inhalants include solvents like gasoline, cleaning fluids, liquid shoe polish, lacquer, nail polish remover, and airplane glue; aerosols like spray paint, insecticides, and hair spray; and anesthetics like nitrous oxide…also abused are amyl nitrate…(and) butyl nitrate. Inhalants temporarily stimulate before they depress the central nervous system. Their immediate effects include a *dreamy euphoria … mental confusion … hallucinations*, dizziness, nausea, lack of coordination, fatigue, loss of appetite and blackouts. (italics mine) (Josephson, 1985, p. 357)

It seems that almost anything volatile will eventually be "sniffed." The desire for "transcendence," in the form of relief by rising above (transcending) the fear, anxiety, and depression caused by the stresses of everyday life, is probably the main motivation for the use of inhalants and other drugs. Teenagers are the primary users of inhalants, and their stage of life is known for its *Sturm und Drang*. The emphasis on the transcendental in religion centers on the concept of the unknowable, the obscure, and the unintelligible aspects of the universe, or that which is beyond common experience and *control*—the supernatural. This state of transcendence is second cousin to dissociation. It can be achieved by meditation (as described later), through prayer and religious ceremonies, or through inhalants and other drug use. By blotting out the stimuli of the conscious world and its cares, dissociation by most means can produce pleasant states of relief.

THE DOUBLE, THE SHADOW SELF, AND DISSOCIATION

There are two parts of the self that we recognize in everyday speech as our angel and devil, or good and evil self, or the light and the dark side of the self. These selves also go by the names of the Ego and the Id, or the Conscious and the Unconscious. The familiarity of these names testifies to the presence of dissociation in all of us.

Like all criminals, the dark side has further special aliases, a.k.a. (also known as) the demonic and the shadow self. When this shadow self is projected onto a mythical figure, the aliases proliferate: Satan, Beelzebub, Asmodeus, Mammon, Moloch, Diabolus, Azazel, Ahriman, Eblis, Belial, Baal, Samael, Hades, Abaddon, Apollyon, Lucifer, Set, Mephistopheles, or, more colloquially, the Deuce, the Old Boy, Harry, Old Nick, the Tempter, the Old One, the Wicked One, Prince of Darkness, Foul Fiend and the Evil One (Laird, 1985, revised edition, pp. 104–105). Could the preponderance of projected figures over names that show recognition of the dark side of one's *own* self be a sign that most people would rather "put the blame on Mame," or say "the butler did it?"

The shadow self is the part of us that is dissociated from central awareness. It is the repressed sexual, aggressive, selfish, domineering or submissive, lazy, and stupid part of us that is socially undesirable. It shows itself in our dreams, in slips of the tongue, and when we call others *Schweinhund*, bitch, or jerk (see "Animalization," discussed in a later chapter). Molly Tuby suggests other ways the shadow shows itself:

> In our exaggerated feelings about others ... In negative feedback from others...(When we) have the same troubling effect on several different people ... In our impulsive and inadvertent acts ... In situations in which we are humiliated ... In our exaggerated anger about other people's faults. (Zweig, 1991, pp. xviii–xix, Introduction)

Harville Hendrix takes dissociation one step further, dividing the self into the "lost self" ("those parts of your being that you had to repress because of the demands of society" — especially the demands of your parents as the agents of society); the "false self" ("the facade that you erected in order to fill the void created by this repression and by a lack of adequate nurturing) and the "disowned self" ("the negative parts of your false self that met with disapproval and were therefore denied") (Zweig, 1991, p. 51, Harville Hendrix, "Creating the False Self") (and especially the demands of your parents as the agents of society). Where the "true self" lies is still a mystery, and may present a philosophical as well as a psychological problem.

Arno Gruen describes the process whereby the child's original self is lost, a false self created, and some of the self disowned, although he does not use those exact terms. To get love, the child surrenders autonomy by submission to the parents' will. The child sees her submissiveness as a bargain, forcing the parents to take care of her. There are consequences of this arrangement:

> First, children accept their parents' evaluation of them without reservation; introjection is therefore a process of collaboration through submission. Second, this means that children begin to hate everything in themselves that could bring them into conflict with parental expectations (*false self created*). And third, out of this self-hatred grows a readiness for even more submission. (italics my comment) (Gruen, 1992, p. 4)

Gruen feels that the child recognizes the loss of love, as the parents exert their power and demand that the child's autonomous self be given up. Thus the parents create the child's "lost self." Children cannot bear the feeling that their needs (love) are denied, and thus make basic changes in their psychic structure:

> To deny their inner needs, children must either completely or partially split them off. This *dissociation* involves a basic shift: in order not to be forced to perceive that father and mother are causing them pain, children will search in themselves for the cause of their despair. This tragedy, leading to children's surrender of self, consists not only in the dissociation of their inner world but, also, in the fact that—in order to maintain the life-giving bond with mother and father—they must see the lack of parental love as the result of a defect in themselves. (italics and parentheses mine) (Gruen, 1992, p. 19)

In Gruen's view, the "disowned self" (as labeled by Hendrix) is created by the child, struggling to blame himself for his parents' rejection and abandonment of him. In effect, it is an attempt to preserve the illusion of parental love. It results, however, in a negative self-image, "self-hatred and self contempt," a state of perceived weakness that can be overcome only by striving for power. Gruen sees this as the basis for the development of the authoritarian character.

The disowned self is the evil part of us. Most people deny that part of themselves through repression and dissociation. The existence of evil as a permanent fixture of the world and an innate feature of mankind is also widely denied. Gruen, as explained previously, sees the disowned self (and by the same logic sees evil) as the result of a learned (not innate) compromise—that is, formed by giving up the autonomous self. Becker and Jung take the dim view (evil as innate and ever present) while Delbanco deplores the downsizing of the concept of evil, without going into psychodynamics. He wants to call a spade a "goddamn shovel," and not pussyfoot around. St. Augustine saw evil as merely the absence of good, and Alice Miller criticizes Jung for seeing evil as inevitable and innate. There is a brief but excellent discussion of these views in Zweig and Abrams (Zweig, 1991, see Part 7, "Devils, Demons, and Scapegoats: A Psychology of Evil," pp. 165–189). My take on this is that evil behavior is clearly learned, and learned early in infancy and childhood. It is not innate. The neo-Lombrosians would have us believe that genetics is the key to criminality, but there is stronger evidence for social learning and modeling on parental figures (and especially on older brothers, as we found in our child study of 2000 families).

The shadow self concept was preceded by the term Double or "Doppelgänger," in literature and in psychology. Robert Jay Lifton has revived and refined the concept of the double by coining the term "doubling." He uses it to describe the process by which Nazi doctors were able to function as killers (selecting victims to be gassed) while still maintaining their self-image as healers adhering to the Hippocratic Oath. He criticizes the terms "splitting" (typically used to describe dissociation in schizophrenics) and "dissociation" as not being applicable to the doctors, because of their "continuous routine of killing, over a year or two or more" (Lifton, 1986, p. 219).

I think his distinction seems to fade a bit if we consider the position of "doubling" on a continuum of dissociation.

> Yet doubling does not include the radical dissociation and sustained separateness characteristic of multiple or "dual personality." In the latter condition, the two selves are more profoundly distinct and autonomous, and tend either not to know about each other or else to see each other as alien. (Lifton, 1986, p. 222)

It is clear to me that "doubling" is another name for dissociation, albeit in milder form. It may lie somewhere between MPD and the Dissociative Personality Style so prevalent nowadays. The early onset of MPD stems from its origins in childhood trauma, which also accounts for its relative persistence throughout the life of the patient. Lifton further points out the *similarities* between MPD and doubling, such as "intense psychic or physical trauma ... extreme ambivalence, and severe conflict and confusion over identifications, all of which can also be instrumental in doubling" (Lifton, 1986, p. 222). Doubling "occurs as part of a larger institutional structure." Lifton compares it to the Mafia, death squads, and delinquent gangs. Later I will take up the issue of "Institutionalized Dissociation," and show that *all dissociation is clearly institutionalized*, except for the extreme states such as MPD, fugue states, and amnesia. Dissociation is built into the very roots of our modern society. Thus doubling is not unique or demonstrably different from dissociation, but may be considered a special subtype when applied to the Nazi doctors.

For us, the crucial question is, "How did dissociation save the Nazi doctors from fear of death?" Lifton explains this ingeniously. He quotes Otto Rank as saying that the "opposing self" (the double) can be equated with a form of evil which represents the perishable and mortal part of the personality.

> *The double* is evil in that it *represents one's own death*. The Auschwitz self of the Nazi doctor similarly assumed the death issue for him but at the same time used its evil project as a way of staving off awareness of his own "perishable and mortal part." It does the "dirty work" for the entire self by rendering work "proper" and in that way protects the entire self from awareness of its own guilt *and its own death*. (italics mine) (Lifton, 1986, p. 221)

The sort of "psychic numbing" (a term used by Lifton), the lack of feeling, and the elaborate rationalizations of the Nazi or similar killers are described in Chapter 18. This is more evidence for the protection that dissociation affords the aggressor. Allowing himself to realize that he is not killing an animal, but a human being, and allowing himself to feel empathy for his victim, could trigger a mini-death (severe cognitive dissonance). It could cause a total disintegration of his self, if the two parts of the self—the shadow and the light—actually confronted each other. Thus the "opposing" or "disowned" self is kept under wraps, separated from the everyday or "good" self, and fear of death (disintegration of the self) is avoided.

Dissociative Personality Style

Having discussed the use of drugs, alcohol, trances, fugue states, hysterical paralyses, and the use of pain and hunger to produce dissociation, I would like to turn to what might be considered less severe types of dissociation. Here is evidence for a continuum of dissociation, from amnesia through the double-talk of politicians. These milder forms can also be considered less "self-destructive" types of dissociation, since they do not involve loss of identity or loss of contact with reality. (The "lesser destructiveness" and "lesser severity" of such types of dissociation apply only to *self*-destruction. In reality, the "mildest" dissociation, which is a widespread personality style, is the most destructive of other people, making such abominations as genocide and war more easily accepted by each individual's conscience.)

Meditation

The first of these "less self-destructive" (or more adaptive) types of dissociation is meditation, which has historically been connected with religion. Medieval monks and nuns spent hours in prayer and meditation. Buddhist monks still devote long hours to deep meditation, obliterating all the stimuli of the outside world. I can't begin to do justice to these practices which are found worldwide, but came to us principally through Buddhism. My sole source is *The Tibetan Book of Living and Dying*, by Sogyal Rinpoche (1994), which has been widely read in the United States. Despite a denial that meditation is "a trance-like experience of an altered state of consciousness" (Rinpoche, 1994, p. 67), every description of meditation and its induction is consonant with a mild state of dissociation. These descriptions document the fact that it is a skill that is possessed by everyone, but can be greatly enhanced by learning and by the teaching of a master. The dissociative quality of meditation is beautifully expressed time and again.

> What then, should we "do" with the mind in meditation? Nothing at all. Just leave it, simply, as it is. One master described meditation as "mind, suspended in space, nowhere." (Rinpoche, 1994, p. 72)

My impression is that meditation does not involve a conscious attempt at suppression of conflicting emotions and thoughts, or even a therapeutic repression. (Repression is now seen by some therapists as natural, adaptive, and symptom-reducing. Forgetting is seen as functional, and excessive uncovering or interfering with "natural amnesia" may be dysfunctional for the patient) (Singer, 1990; see "Repression, Reconstruction and Defense," p. 19). Meditation is like a deep relaxation technique. The methods of inducing this state of relaxation are complex:

> *To bring your mind home* is to turn your mind inward...To *release* means to release the mind from its prison of grasping, since you recognize that all pain and fear and distress arise from the craving of a grasping mind...To *relax* (means) letting all thoughts and emotions naturally subside. (Rinpoche, 1994, p. 62)

Three meditation techniques (out of 84,000 taught by Buddha!) are stressed by Sogyal Rinpoche:

> *Watching the breath* ... When you breathe out, just flow out with the outbreath. Each time you breathe out, you are letting go ... *Using an Object* ... an object of natural beauty, such as a flower or crystal...an image of the Buddha, or Christ, or particularly your master, is even more powerful ... *Reciting a mantra* ... When you are nervous, disoriented, or emotionally fragile, chanting or reciting a mantra inspiringly can change the state of your mind completely. ... (Rinpoche, 1994, pp. 68–71)

The various states of mind that can be achieved with meditation give clues to exactly what is being dissociated and is (temporarily) banished from conscious awareness. In addition to the old bugbears of desire (sex, venality, greed) and aggression, the sin of ignorance is also halted. At times this sounds almost Freudian:

> When you experience bliss, it's a sign that desire has temporarily dissolved. When you experience real clarity, it's a sign that aggression has temporarily ceased. When you experience a state of absence of thought, it's a sign that your ignorance has temporarily died. (Rinpoche, 1994, p. 75)

It is in the goal of Buddhist meditation that the striking difference between it and modern psychotherapy comes to light. The control of anxiety and depression, the search for peace of mind, and the focus on inner change rather than on action against societal problems are all common to Buddhist meditation and most psychotherapy. The contrast is between the goal of awareness of life as illusion, and the (partial) stripping away of illusion so longed for by Freud (1957).

> Meditation awakens in you the realization of how the nature of everything is illusory and dream-like; maintain that awareness even in the thick of samsara.* One great master has said: "After meditation practice, one should become a child of illusion." (Rinpoche, 1994)

Clearly, meditation is closely allied to dissociation. It is a mode of controlling conscious awareness of disturbing thoughts, sexual and aggressive drives, and the anomie of continual unlimited desire. (Unlimited desire was Durkheim's original concept in anomic suicide.) Buddhism originated in India, and is practiced in Sri Lanka, China, Korea, Burma, Japan, and in Tibet (when it is not suppressed by Chinese troops). Zen Buddhism is popular in the United States. Thus dissociation, via meditation, is institutionalized through one of the

---

* Samsara is the belief that life is full of an ocean of suffering caused by desire and that humans are in bondage to an endless sequence of births and deaths. The way to end this suffering and birth/death cycle is through enlightenment.

Samsara is defined as "the uncontrolled cycle of birth and death in which sentient beings, driven by unskillful actions and destructive emotions, repeatedly perpetuate their own suffering. Nirvana is a state beyond suffering, the realization of the ultimate truth, or Bhuddahood." (Rinpoche, 1994, p. 393, footnote 5). It is not clear that all masters recommend the perpetuation of illusion, or a view of the world and life as illusory.

major religions, and is encouraged in many other religious ceremonies, not necessarily in the form of meditation.

Dissociation has historically been thought of as psychopathological, yet it is really a universal human capacity that can be used for health or illness. Rieber, in preparation for a discussion of the dissociation necessary to wage war and to engage in "enmification," points out the healthy or adaptive functions of dissociation. Note that this type of dissociation is not brought on by some external agent (such as a drug or a hypnotist).

> Because dissociation is so intimately related to the breakdown of the integrative mechanisms of the mind, it is often confused with psychoanalytic concepts like repression and regression. By and large, dissociation can be thought of as potentially normal. In the healthy organism the dissociative processes are part and parcel of the overall capacity for selective adaptation, just as in the individual they contribute to the ability to live in terms of different systems of values at different times. (Rieber, 1997, p. 70)

Rieber distinguished two types of "dehumanization," by which the subject protects himself against emotional involvement or empathy with others. "Self-directed dehumanization" is found in the aloofness and indifference of doctors and the police to patients or offenders. In "object dehumanization" the subject depersonalizes another individual. Rieber uses the term "enmification" when the object is reduced to a "thing" (see Rieber, 1997, p. 74). I use an additional term, "animalization," in Chapter 18, since terms such as "pig," "rat," "skunk," "dog," "goat," "bitch," "camel," "donkey," or "snake," are commonly used in many cultures when reducing a person to an inhuman state. Selfishness, extreme sexuality, nastiness, dirtiness, stupidity, betrayal, sneakiness, and other sins are portrayed by different animals, with some overlap. The German *Schweinhund*, literally "pig-dog," combining the sloppiness of the pig with the aggressiveness and sexuality of the dog, is an especially choice epithet.

What both types of dehumanization and enmification have in common is dissociation. They vary only in the direction and degree of the dissociation. In dehumanization, animalization, and enmification, the goal is to reduce cognitive dissonance through a form of dissociation. When the neo-Nazi (see Chapter 18) tries to bomb and kill innocent victims, he makes them into nonpersons, enemies, or simply has a blank spell during which he "forgets" everything except his mission—to destroy others. If he killed or mauled someone who was human, and also a "good person," it would create anxiety (dissonance) within him. Making him or her nonhuman solves the problem. You can kill animals with impunity and without guilt. Thus Jews, Communists, and Gypsies in Germany were viewed as animals.

Like many of the so-called "defense mechanisms," dissociation may be either adaptive or maladaptive for the individual who uses it. Singer looks at dissociation as a skill or ability that can have negative or positive results for the subject and for those in his environment.

> If dissociation is a basic skill or capacity, then it is possible that some persons use it more adaptively or effectively, while others use it for avoidant (*or worse*) purposes. Once crystallized into a habitual pattern, a dissociative trend may lead to acting *skill*, to the ability for self-distraction or self-entertainment, and to absorption skills that permit one to become deeply engaged in the enjoyment of reading, films, music or other aesthetic experiences. Conversely … dissociative ability may develop into the classic hysterical symptoms of amnesia, fugue, multiple personality … states of confusion … (and) excessive reactivity to drugs or alcohol. (Singer, 1990, p. 487)* (Parentheses and comment in italics mine.)

I feel that we can call a "crystallized habitual dissociative pattern" a Dissociative Personality Style. The evidence for the prevalence of this style is growing. The concept of "Protean Style" did not come out of thin air. The "recreation or reinvention of the self," the multiple careers, the widespread use of drugs and alcohol, the popularity of meditation, the attraction of cross-dressers, the fascination with homosexuality, and the growing disparity between stated morals and values and actual behavior all seem to point to the development and spread of the Dissociative Style in Western culture. This may be an age-old human failing, since Barbara Tuchman (Tuchman, 1978) documents the great chasm between chivalrous and religious principles and actual behavior in the Middle Ages. Robert Browning said, "A man's reach should exceed his grasp, or what's a heaven for?" The question still remains, *How far behind* should his grasp be? *How great* is the gap between ideals and behavior: an inch or a mile?

INSTITUTIONALIZED DISSOCIATION

A Dissociative Personality Style must be supported by the society in which it is found. What supports are there for such a style? What kinds of structures encourage it? I already mentioned the influence of the institution of religion, especially Buddhism, in spreading dissociative styles.

Robert K. Merton, in his landmark essay "Social Structure and Anomie," (Merton, 1968; see especially the fourfold table on p. 140) notes that in U.S. culture, large groups of people separate the goals of society and the legitimate means of attaining those goals. In a fourfold table (two cells across and two cells down) called "Typology of Modes of Individual Adaptation," he classifies people who do or do not internalize approved societal *goals* and who do or do not internalize approved societal means of attaining those goals. Those who

---

* I have inserted the italicized "or worse," because Singer has not considered here the incredible damage that this "skill" of dissociation has inflicted on the human race since the beginning of history. While it is adaptive from the standpoint of the individual, or even the society, in the long run it is the basis for war, race prejudice, and class conflict—and it facilitates killing or depriving others who are seen as worthless undeserving animals.

internalize both goals and *means* he calls "conformists."* Those who internalize neither goals nor means are "retreatists." There are two "cross-cells" left. One of these contains those types who internalize the goals, but not the approved means of attaining those goals. He calls them "innovators." Criminals, especially those in organized crime, fit into this cell. The Mafia member is likely to insist that "We're just ordinary businessmen, trying to make a living." Yet the way they make their living is by extortion and killing. Those are not acceptable means, although "success" is an acceptable goal that they have internalized.

During the 1990s the tobacco companies showed that they fall into the same innovator's cell. They said "We are just trying to run a business" or "make a living" or "satisfy our stockholders," but they did so over the bodies of hundreds of thousands of dead and disabled who suffered lung cancer and emphysema. They suppressed their own studies showing that tobacco was carcinogenic. Evidence has come to light, via a whistle-blower and former executive officer of the Liggett Group, that the cigarette companies got together to discuss how to add nicotine to tobacco to make it more addictive. They also discussed how to target teenagers so as to ensure profits in the future. The same type of "innovative" behavior might be attributed to Dow Chemical, Ciba-Geigy, DuPont, and Monsanto, among other giant chemical corporations. Their carcinogenic products, such as alachlor, atrazine, formaldehyde, and perchloroethylene, used in farming, building materials, and dry cleaning, have been indicted in hundreds of studies. Now a book, *Toxic Deception* (Fagin, 1996; see especially p. x, "Science for Sale," and "The PR Juggernaut"), shows how public relations campaigns, political contributions, and corporate-sponsored "scientific" studies have managed to keep these dangerous products on the market, in our food, in our clothing, and worst of all in the tissues and organs of our bodies. The goals of "making a living" and "financial success" are legitimate, but in these cases the legitimate means to those ends have clearly not been internalized. This is obviously the dissociation of means and ends, in the broadest sense of fragmentation (H. Spiegel), or nonassociation.

The routinized life of the bureaucrat and the obsessive–compulsive quality of most working lives illustrates the institutionalization of the opposite or second cross cell, the "ritualists," those who have forgotten the goals, and are focusing only on the means. Merton cites the petty bureaucrat as an example. The "ritualist from hell" works in the postoffice. You can't get your package mailed, because you didn't use brown wrapping paper, or you used tape where the

---

* Merton does not use the term "conformists" in his table, but calls that cell "conformity." That is because he is describing modes of adaptation rather than people. I think it is easier to comprehend if we think of actual people populating these cells, but it is not true to Merton's original table. The cells would be labeled Conformity, Retreatism, Innovation, and Ritualism. A fifth cell is called Rebellion, and involves a rejection of both goals and the means of achieving societally approved goals.

stamps should go, or your package is just oversized. You filled out your insurance or return receipt form incorrectly. Come back another day!

"Zero tolerance" rules concerning drugs or weapons in schools have resulted in exposing the ritualists in our midst. A young child brought in a family heirloom to "show and tell" at school. It had a tiny knife attached by a chain. She was temporarily suspended from school. Teenage girls who take ibuprofen in school for their menstrual cramps now risk expulsion! The ritualist type of dissociation was discussed in Chapter 8, "Obsessive–Compulsive Behavior." Kenneth Burke characterized such bureaucratic personality types as being "fit in an unfit fitness" (Burke, 1954).

Rieber (1997; see Note 16, pp. 189–192. References on anomie are made to R. K. Merton, and to Srole, Langner et al., 1962) discusses the relationship of anomie (Durkheim's state of normlessness or deregulation) to psychopathy. He sees dissociation as an innate disposition, which can lead to greater disinhibition of antisocial behavior in both psychopaths and normal individuals. While there is great *individual* (and probably innate) variability in the tendency or ability to dissociate, this emphasis on the individual tends to diminish the importance of the institutionalization of the dissociation of goals and means. Merton's "innovators" and "ritualists" may have been born with the ability to ignore or split off means or goals, respectively, but they are also entrenched in their Mafias, their gangs, their corporations, or their bureaucracies, which encourage and support that splitting.

The point here is that dissociation is institutionalized in the business world, the legal world, in organized crime, and in bureaucracies. Where else but in the institution of government do we see it so clearly? The dissociation of Richard Nixon, Ronald Reagan, George Bush, and Newt Gingrich on the right was clear cut. While harping on "family values," they were busy trying to cut the heart out of 50 years of social support legislation. While claiming to protect the environment and the public's health, they were busy selling out our forests, rivers, air quality, and freedom from chemical pollution.

What about William Jefferson Clinton, merging toward center, promising Hillary Rodham Clinton's "village" (Clinton, 1996) to support children, but in reality cutting Welfare and other maintenance for children, especially children of legal immigrants? The test of association between promise and behavior might have come during his second term. Instead, the attacks on the President during the Monica Lewinsky scandal and the impeachment attempt may have forced him even further toward the center-right. Can these giveaways to the right wing, presumably to win reelection, ever be recouped or "corrected?" Peter B. Edelman, who said that "Signing the new welfare law is the worst thing Bill Clinton has done," thinks that "the measure cannot easily be fixed" (Pear, 1997, p. 39).

Perhaps we judge politicians too harshly. Maybe it is naive to think that politicians should not be bought and paid for by the different interest groups that give them campaign money.* What politician will dare to give up his chances of reelection to promote strong legislation that would limit campaign fund contributions? In my view, the Nixon–Reagan–Bush–Dole–Gingrich–Lott–Lamar Smith–Christian Coalition array is so far right that it is hard to imagine that there is any internal conflict in their psyches over these human rights issues. I know that Bush personally believed in abortion rights, as did his wife Barbara (outspokenly), but he showed no conflict, at least not publicly, when it came to siding with the "right-to-lifers" (anti-abortion activists) while campaigning.

Alas, it is easier to see some hints of dissociative personality in Bill Clinton, because he at least *tried* to be a "good guy," although he so often failed through compromise. Here's what Bob Herbert said about him:

> Bill Clinton is one of the great masters of the art of politics, which in its essence is the art of the con—the ability to convincingly declare that day is night, that up is down, that what is so is not…To move people from welfare to work there has to be enough work. Right now there is not nearly enough. Mr. Clinton knows that. But he goes on the radio and speaks as if he didn't. The art of the con. (Herbert, 1997, p. A15)

You are torn between thinking that such behavior is conscious outrageous lying, and that it might be the result of some form of "cognitive dissonance," a conflict of values, as described before. The President knew that the new Welfare job rules were ludicrous, since there were then few real full-time jobs to be had. Why not let the government set an example by providing full-time government jobs to former Welfare recipients? It turns out that there are very few such job openings. Well, why not ignore that unfortunate fact for a while? Then Clinton becomes a "true believer." (See Chapter 18.) He is not a charlatan, for he has convinced *himself* that those jobs exist in adequate numbers. This scenario (true or not) is evidence of dissociation.

In 1997 Clinton was defending himself against accusations that he had solicited contributions from the White House, and "sold" overnight visits to the Lincoln Bedroom in the White house to big contributors to his election campaign. Walter Goodman said:

> One didn't know whether to howl in laughter or embarrassment at the repeated straight-faced assurances to viewers of Jim Lehrer's "Newshour" by Ann Lewis, the

---

* Leonard Garment, in "Scandals Past and Present," an Op Ed article in *The New York Times*, 3/13/97, says, "After all, one thing America takes for granted about its politicians is that by hook or crook they get and spend as much cash as they can to gain office and stay there." This statement by a former counsel to President Richard Nixon shows how deeply accepted and institutionalized crooked (by hook or crook) fund raising actually is.

appointed White House defender, that all those rich overnighters were old pals with
whom the friendly current resident liked to chat. (Goodman, 1997, p. B12)*

In this case, where a paid public relations person is engaged in defending
the President's integrity, it would seem to be a clear-cut case of professional lying.
No dissociation in the usual sense is involved, since the spokeswoman/defender
was not the same person as the accused. You could say that it is dissociation by
proxy, or once removed.

Clinton escaped impeachment, and regained much of his popularity.
Because his behavior during "Monicagate" was so clearly dissociated (the media
called it "compartmentalized"), it is an excellent example of the survival value
of this coping mode. Perhaps the majority of Americans view the attempt to
impeach President Clinton as clearly orchestrated by the right wing of the
Republican Party, and as financed mainly by Richard Mellon Scaife, who
donated millions to foundations that paid the lawyers for Paula Jones. Jones was
the woman who originally sued Clinton, claiming that he crudely propositioned
her while he was Governor of Arkansas. The Jones case put Clinton on the spot.
If he told the truth about his affair with Lewinsky, a young White House intern,
he would expose her and himself to public ridicule and slander, and further hurt
his family. If he lied, he might save face.

When Linda Tripp tape-recorded Lewinsky's phone calls to her in all their
sexual detail, she was urged by Lucianne Goldberg, a long-time Clinton hater,
to get in touch with Kenneth Starr, the Independent Counsel. The information
was apparently passed on from Starr's office (via a triumvirate of three conservative lawyers with ties to Starr) to the lawyers for Paula Jones. This set up a "perjury trap" for Clinton, who when testifying did not know of Tripp's tapes, while
Jones' lawyers already had the tape transcripts. Clinton denied "having sex with
that woman," when in fact the telephone tapes clearly showed he did.

Despite the illegality of this entrapment (it is against Maryland law to tape
someone's phone conversation without his or her knowledge) Clinton's responses
made him seem equally criminal. His hair-splitting definitions of the word "is"
and "sex" (oral sex is not sex) were enraging to some of the public, and laughable
to the rest. These responses probably lay somewhere between "true belief" and
out-and-out lying. After 7 months of pressure, when it seemed that the business of
running the country might come to a halt, he confessed to a "relationship with
that woman" which he had denied to all but his closest confidants.

---

* Goodman thinks that Vice President Gore, faced with the same accusations of selling White
House access to raise funds, and soliciting from his office, was "graceless in his on-camera performance" compared to Mr. Clinton, and that that was a sign of grace, (i.e., he didn't cover up). Of
course, Clinton was busy consoling flood-stricken residents of Arkansas, so it was easy to be graceful.
He was very cool in his responses to questions about selling the White House bedroom, but didn't
exactly deny it.

The media consistently marveled at Clinton's ability to "compartmentalize." How was he able to conduct the nation's business at the same time he was defending himself against charges of perjury and obstruction of justice? This same extraordinary ability was exemplified by his taking a telephone call from a United States Senator while Miss Lewinsky was administering oral sex. Perhaps one of the qualities by which leaders are self-selected is that very same ease of dissociation or compartmentalization. This allows for periodic intense concentration on a war in Bosnia or Kosovo, on gun control legislation, or on trade problems with China, while in the midst of a painful and career-threatening nationally televised legal battle. In addition, there must have been a severe marital crisis. Whether we are on the left, right, or center, I think we can't help admire Clinton's continuing ability to function under extreme pressure. Dissociation is a large part of the secret of his survival.

The concept of "deniability" so popular in recent administrations could be called preparation for lying to the public, but it is also a form of dissociation. Nixon excelled in this. He also almost "reinvented" himself as an elder statesman, after losing his job and his face via Watergate and the tapes. This reinvention is easier in the age of fluid identities.

What about parents, who still say, "Do as I say, not as I do!" That's about as dissociative in style as you can get. Children model on how their parents behave, not on what they preach. Blaming the kids for all their misbehavior is like the old immigrant who said to the manufacturer, "Take back this tape recorder. It speaks with an accent!"

Dissociation is an American way of life. It is ingrained. Religious institutions sometimes encourage it. There is the hypnotic effect of chanting, still used in the Catholic Mass and in Jewish ceremonies. Incense is widely used to speed communication with God all over the world. In Bali, incense is inhaled. Censers are used during the Mass.

Values are dissociated, which makes for institutionalized value conflicts. This automatically puts the individual in a state of cognitive dissonance, since the culture itself has not "made up its mind." Competition versus Brotherhood, Faith versus Inquisitiveness (as in science), Love versus Aggression, Sharing versus Acquisition, Masculine Macho versus Feminine Supportiveness, Intimacy versus Independence; the list is endless. In traditional (associated) cultures these value-conflicts are still found, but they are much diminished in power. The price of their reduction is extreme social control.

DISSOCIATION IN LITERATURE AND MYTH

Myth

The gods have almost always come in pairs—one good, one evil. In Christianity, Judaism, and Islam, Satan is depicted as the adversary of God.

Ahriman was balanced by Ahura Mazda, the god of light. Set (who represented the desert and was often depicted with a donkey-head) murdered his brother, Osiris, but was killed by Horus (who was a sun-god and was portrayed by a falcon or falcon head). Loki, among the Norse gods, represented evil. With his protean ability, he was able to be a fish, or the Midgard serpent, among many disguises. He murdered Balder (or Baldur). This slippery quality is a characteristic of the subconscious, which shows itself only in dreams and slips of the tongue. Odin (Woden or Wotan) was the supreme Norse god, the creator of man and woman, and the laws of the universe. The splitting of the gods is a projection of the dissociated self. You might say that the various Satans represent the "disowned self," the destructive unacceptable impulses, while the gods of light represent the ego or consciousness, creation, and creativity.

Literature

Siblings and twins in literature symbolize the "divided self." Cain and Abel of biblical fame were one of the earliest good/bad pairs. Anyone who asks, "Am I my brother's keeper?"* bears the "mark of Cain," a killer. Dissociation is discovered in another biblical character, Moses, and seen as contributing to creative potential, which is the adaptive aspect of dissociation discussed earlier.

> In his book *Moses*, Leopold Szondi demonstrates how the truly creative individuals also possess pronouncedly destructive sides. Szondi introduces his argument with the case of Moses, whose 'case history' begins with the murder of an Egyptian overseer and ends with his becoming the father of his nation, leader and law-giver in one. (Zweig, 1991; see p. 224, "Why Psychopaths Do Not Rule the World," Adolf Guggenböhl-Craig)

In discussing plagiarism, Schwartz mentions two tales by famous authors of the mid-1800s with dissociated main characters:

> Hawthorne's 'Howe's Masquerade' (1838) was supposed to have been taken from none other than Poe's 'William Wilson' (1839), whose agonist finds in another of the same name a haunting double, '*and his singular whisper, it grew the very echo of my own.*' (Schwartz, 1996, p. 311)†

> William Wilson can't escape from the whispered exhortations of his double. One William is the conscience to the other. (Schwartz, 1996, p. 65)

Hillel Schwartz (1996)†† reports that the case of William Brodie of Edinburgh was a living model for Robert Louis Stevenson's *The Strange Case of*

---

* A cartoon appeared in *The New Yorker* that showed two monkeys talking in their cage at the zoo. One asks the other, "Am I my keeper's brother?"

† Note that an echo comes back as the identical twin of your voice, while the dissociated self is not an identical twin pair, but perhaps fraternal or dizygotic twins—one evil, and good. Tweedledum and Tweedledee are not a dissociated pair, though they are twins.

†† *The Culture of the Copy* is an excellent source for literary references to doubles, twins, double identity and multiple personality.

Dr. Jekyll and Mr. Hyde (1886). Brodie was a "deacon of the Wrights (cabinet and coffin makers) *and* a gamester, cheat, bigamist, and chieftain of a gang of thieves. He was hanged in 1788." He belongs right up there with Dave Beck and Jimmy Hoffa of the (U.S.) Teamsters Union, who were both imprisoned on charges of corruption. Hoffa disappeared, and his body has never been found.

The tale of the "pillar of society" who turns out to be a crook is all too familiar.

> "Though so profound a double-dealer," Jekyll stated, "I was in no sense a hypocrite; both sides of me were in dead earnest"—and had long been. Hyde, pleasure-loving, corrupt, was fully half of Jekyll. in the "toils of a moral weakness," Jekyll had to face "that truth by whose partial discovery I have been doomed to such a dreadful shipwreck: that man is not truly one, but truly two" (Schwartz, 1996, p. 80)

Another description of a double that smacks of dissociation is Joseph Conrad's "Secret Sharer," a short story. A ship's captain (the narrator) finds the naked body of a man (Legatt) lying in the water, and clinging to a rung of the ship's ladder. The man climbs aboard. The captain gets him some of his own clothes, which fit him perfectly. He hides Legatt in his cabin for days. To his astonishment, this man is his alter ego. He hides Legatt from the crew and from the visiting captain of Legatt's former ship. At the end of the story he says:

> Walking to the taffrail ... I was in time to catch an evanescent glimpse of my white hat left behind to mark the spot where the secret sharer of my cabin and of my thoughts as though he were my second self, had lowered himself into the water to take his punishment: a free man, a proud swimmer striking out for a new destiny. (Conrad, 1962, p. 36)

Interestingly, the captain seems to be the good self, and Legatt, his double, a man in trouble. As first mate of another ship, Legatt strangled a surly disobedient man in the midst of a gale, but did it as his duty to save the ship. He is instinctive, rather than evil, while the Captain is cerebral, like dizygotic twins.

> ... the narrator of Joseph Conrad's *The Secret Sharer* is a double for the protagonist, that actions and gestures of this newly-appointed captain are reflected in the movements and behavior of the recently escaped Leggatt, and that each man echoes the most private thoughts and sentiments of the other. (Conrad, 1962, commentary by a critic)

The captain in Conrad's *Outcast of the Islands* is similarly a "good self." He is a stern judge of the moral disintegration of the "outcast," as well as a defender of white civilization against the debauchery of the primitives. Yet Conrad also criticized the role of white colonials, which was unusual for that period.

Doubles, twins, and other dissociated types abound in literature, but few are as famous as Jekyll and Hyde and the Captain and Legatt.

Alice of *Alice in Wonderland* [Carroll, 1865 (original publication), Reprint 1996] also dissociates. After Alice has fallen down the rabbit hole, and has taken a drink from a bottle labeled "Drink Me," she shrinks to 10 inches in height.

Because of this she can't reach the key to unlock the door to go back out to the garden. She starts to cry.

> 'Come, there's no use in crying like that!' said Alice to herself rather sharply; 'I advise you to leave off this minute!' She generally gave herself very good advice (though she very seldom followed it), and sometimes she scolded herself so severely as to bring tears into her eyes, and once she remembered trying to box her own ears for having cheated herself in a game of croquet she was playing against herself, for this curious child was very fond of pretending to be two people. 'But it's no use now,' thought poor Alice, 'to pretend to be two people! Why, there's hardly enough of me left to make *one* respectable person!' [Carroll, 1865 (original publication), Reprint 1996, p. 9]

Movies

"Seconds," starring Rock Hudson (1966), deals with identity problems. It is somewhat different from the standard plot. A middle-aged suburban business man, tiring of his wife and stultifying life, is remade through plastic surgery by a secret corporation. Since the new body (Hudson's) and new artist's role call for promiscuous sexuality and high lifestyle, while the old self is still pedestrian, middle-class, and loyal to his former wife, a massive conflict ensues. He is finally killed, because of the conflict between his old conscious self and his old shadow self (now fulfilled and made conscious). While the "Company" that did the operation and placement has him killed, so as not to reveal its murderous replacement system, he is also killed because he publicly confesses his internal conflict. The movie asks: "What if your shadow self suddenly became dominant, your subconscious sexual wishes were all fulfilled, and you were living in a perpetual orgy?" This is a twist on the Faust tale.

"A Double Life," with Ronald Colman and Signe Hasso (1947), tells the story of an actor (a dissociative profession to begin with), who in real life becomes Othello, the part he has been playing to great acclaim. He eventually kills his wife in real life, mistaking her for Desdemona. The actor "plays a part," and the playing or taking on a role other than the self is enhanced by an ability to dissociate. In this movie, dissociation gone too far ends in tragedy.

"The Dark Mirror" (1946) with Olivia De Havilland tells the story of identical twin sisters, one good and one evil. A doctor (Lew Ayres) finds out which sister is the murderer, by using the Rorschach ink-blot test! At the climax, the evil twin tries to kill the good twin. Identical twins in psychological dramas can be seen as representing the good and evil halves of a single person. Again, the suspenseful appeal of ambiguity is strong, since the killer-twin's identity is not revealed until almost the end of the film.

"The Three Faces of Eve" (1957) starred Joanne Woodward as the MPD patient, and Lee J. Cobb as her psychiatrist. Woodward won an academy award for her role(s).

Social Change

J. H. van den Berg (Schwartz, 1996, p. 81)* has pointed out that fascination with doubles seems to increase at times of social change (the 1790s and 1890s). This fits in with my list of interests and fads near the end of the 20th century, the 1990s. I said as much under "Dissociative Personality Style," and pointed out the recent fascination with ambiguity in general, and specifically with cross-dressing, homosexuality, and meditation. Dissociation through the wide use of drugs and alcohol is a growing national problem, and teen drug abuse is on the upswing. Twins seem to be increasingly interesting to the public. With the announcement of the first cloning of a sheep in 1997, mankind became capable of deliberately producing a second self. Will the most severely divided selves be the first to get cloned, thus making four selves in all?

Rapid social change increases the need to avoid value conflict by dissociating (since values are changing so rapidly, as evidenced by post-modernism, multiculturalism, and deconstruction).

Irony is the natural twin of value conflict. It is a type of mild dissociation. When used as a figure of speech, irony is "the use of words to convey a meaning that is the opposite of its literal meaning ... as in the comment 'Beautiful weather, isn't it?' made when it is raining ... Ironic literature ... stress(es) the paradoxical nature of reality or the contrast between an ideal and actual condition ..." (Flexner, 1987, p. 1009). The separation of speech or writing from its true meaning can be a positive adaptation, which can facilitate social criticism. It can also be maladaptive, since you can hide behind the sarcasm and satire of your words, and distance yourself from any strong feelings or value-commitments. "Hip" and "Camp" are ironic styles, which developed in the counter-culture (Delbanco, 1995).†

---

* Schwartz has a brilliant discussion of twins and Doppelgängers in pp. 19–87. He relates the fascination with twins and the divided self to a general culture of copying, xeroxing, plagiarism, and duplicity. This book is as entertaining as it is informative.

† Delbanco discusses irony in pp. 187–92, 202, 205, 208–14, 216, 220, 223, and 234. He sees irony as a villain, destroying fundamental values. He is especially concerned that irony weakened the concept of evil, and that it was not until World War II and the Holocaust that the awareness of evil was reawakened. His strange mixtue of liberalism and conservatism (arising from his attempt to conserve the concept of evil) makes irony his enemy, since it derides such permanent values, and questions the independent existence of good and evil, except as points of view. I have discussed his interesting ideas in Chapter 18. I think his desire to avoid psychological explanations of evil (such as dissociation) stems from the fact that Freud and the psychoanalytic schools that followed him tended to debunk evil, and see it as the product of bad parenting, mental disorder, or some type of early emotional or economic deprivation. This can be viewed as a "watering down" of evil. I refer again to the Pirates of Penzance, who excuse their murdering and plundering by saying that they are all orphans. Certainly the "early victim" role diminishes evil. The sense of responsibility for one's actions is Emersonian and somewhat old-fashioned. One can empathize with Delbanco's position, to a point.

He refers to Hip and Camp styles as other evidence of irony on p. 203.

The attraction of the sexually ambiguous figure is growing, and is becoming more acceptable. Even the Mayor of New York City, Rudolph Giuliani, once dressed in drag at a political dinner-cum-amateur-theatrics.

Ads for hair bleaches used to ask, "Does she or doesn't she?" with the implication that she might indulge in sex. Nowadays most everybody "does," and the more likely question is, "Is she or isn't she a 'she?'" The rule for gay men in the armed services is, "Don't ask, don't tell." Again ambiguity is encouraged. Dissociation on the part of politicians and our society is clear; we pretend to accept homosexuals in the armed services, but at the same time we tell them not to "come out of the closet"—not to go public.

SUMMARY

Dissociation can be seen as an adaptive skill, or it can be viewed as pathological and maladaptive. The reason is partly because dissociation lies on a continuum of severity. At one end lie multiple identity disorder, fugue states, and amnesia. In the middle are drug- and alcohol-induced dissociated states. Less extreme dissociation, with a greater degree of control, is found in meditation. There is dissociation of conflicting values, and dissociation of goals (ends) and means of achieving those goals.

The world in which we live has institutionalized dissociation. The best examples of this are the Mafia and delinquent or drug-dealing gangs, large or multinational corporations, the legal profession, politicians, to a great extent academics, parenting by dictum rather than example, and bureaucrats, to mention a few. The stock market (whose wares are often priced by rumor rather than true value) and "managed care," which purportedly has a goal of providing proper medical care to the public, but whose all too apparent motive is the "bottom line" of profit, can be added to our list of the "Dirty Dissociated Dozen."

At the end of the dissociative continuum which is least injurious to the self and others, there are a number of what we could call "alterations of consciousness in everyday life," or *everyday dissociation.* I will review these briefly. Many people get a feeling of relief from stress by staring at a vast landscape. In the Rorschach (ink-blot) test, there are several blots that can be seen as a landscape, perhaps two mountains with a river or valley running down the middle, to a faraway point in the distance (partly the result of folding the paper to make the blot). This is called a "vista" response. I was trained (in classes with E. G. Schachtel) to think of this type of response as an attempt of the subject to distance herself from some emotion stirred up by the blot. The vista response is linked with certain types of verbal responses to the blots:

> Examples of words or phrases which connote this spatial relationship (distance between the observer and the percept) are 'distant,' 'very far away,' 'bird's eye view,' 'looking down into the depths,' 'far into the background', 'extending into the water'…Mountains, valleys, canals are typical. There must be perspective (Phillips, 1953, p. 97).

It is interesting that we use the word "perspective" to describe spatial relationships in drawing or architecture, but we also use it to mean the ability to see all the facts in a situation and to put them together in a sensible way. Having perspective on one's life or one's current situation means *standing back* a bit to get an overview. This is exactly what the "vista" experience means. It is a standing back, away from the strong emotional content of a situation, to try to gain intellectual control and understanding. The *pointilliste* painting is a paradigm for the need to distance oneself, to stand back so that the dots of paint can become a whole picture. If you are too close to the dots (emotionally involved?), nothing makes sense—nothing comes together.

The "vista" seen in the ink-blots is a form of dissociation. So is the pleasant trance-like state induced when actually looking out over a river, or the ocean, or looking at a sunset against distant hills. Gazing at the sky can be soothing. Astronomy, or even amateur night-viewing of the stars and planets, is like a "vista" experience, but it involves even greater distancing between the eye and the heavenly object, without the intervention of earthly objects.

It is easy to "get lost" when listening to one's favorite music. There may be some conscious associations with loved ones, or with the past, but a sort of reverie is very common. This can become a frenzy if the music is hard or "acid" rock, or is mainly composed of drumbeats. The loud beat of the "boom box"* may cause some splitting—mainly ear-splitting. Prolonged dancing can increase the dissociation.†

Daydreaming is supposedly confined to adolescents, but all adults know this is a fiction. Mooning about (in its older, not current, meaning), letting your mind wander, musing, wool-gathering, and fantasizing are all synonyms for a type of mild and primarily pleasant dissociation.

Watching television, and particularly movies, involves distancing from the usual stimuli. Movies are shown in the dark, which allows for greater absorption and less external stimulation or distraction than television.

TV has become an addiction, partly because it costs little compared with moviegoing. McLuhan said that, "The medium is the message." Given the poor quality of much TV fare, it is very likely that the hypnotic effect of the "boob tube"

---

* For those who have been fortunate enough to have never heard a boom box, it is a large portable radio, usually carried by a teenager, with its volume turned up all the way, and usually playing music devoid of harmony, counterpoint, development, or anything other than just booming uninteresting rhythm. The drumbeats of Africa are a thousand times more sophisticated.

† The dangers of dancing are expressed in a curious joke. A liberal priest (rabbi, or minister) is counseling a young couple about to be married. They ask, "Can we have sex before marriage?" "Of course!" "Well, can we have them play our favorite song at the wedding, and dance to it?" "No, dancing is *absolutely forbidden!*" "Oh, well, can we have sex swinging from a chandelier?" "Of course, feel free!" "One last question, can we have sex standing up?" "*Absolutely not! That is forbidden!*" "But why?" "*Because that could lead to dancing!*"

itself is its main attraction. TV, then, acts much like the drugs and alcohol that we consider to be so dangerous. What, then, must be the effect on some children of this generation, who are watching as much as 6 to 8 hours of television daily?

Photography and using binoculars in bird and game watching may be other ways of distancing oneself from reality, and from the cares and fears of the everyday world. What you see through the lens is what is happening, and all else is irrelevant. It is common for the tourist to experience his trip "through the lens," rather than through direct contact with the people or objects of the countries he visits. He brings back his photos as trophies from the safari. He is a safe distance from the ideas and emotions (and often the poverty and hunger) of the people he visits.

Everyday objects, especially natural ones, are recommended by Sogyal Rinpoche to induce meditation (Rinpoche, 1994, pp. 80–81). These can be a flower; a candle (focusing on the flame); a stream or waterfall; moonlight; or the hypnotic effect of sight, sound, and touch (wind on the skin, especially the face). A focal point of attention is helpful, but some individuals can easily dissociate without the aid of a point of convergence. Certainly we all recognize the soothing and pleasant effect of these objects and experiences. One has to be a robot not to feel some joy and a certain calmness in contact with nature.

I can't help but think that there is a distinct survival value inherent in the ability to dissociate. Stress reduction, and the control of anxiety (which in itself certainly has survival value as a preparatory response, *up to a point*) are necessary to balance the terrors of this world. Dissociation can give us respite from our worries and cares. This brings us back to the whole thrust of this chapter.

Dissociation at all points on its continuum of severity seems to be a means of controlling fear of death, and its related forms, anxiety and depression, and fear of abandonment in young children. Severe sexual, physical, or emotional trauma usually precede multiple identity disorder, fugues, and amnesia. These are "near-death" experiences (not in the usual sense), during which the child is attacked by the very source of her life—her mother or father. The dissociated soldier or policeman is protecting himself from a terrible moral conflict when he has to kill to do his duty. Even the criminal dissociates to protect himself from whatever scruples he may still have. The Mafia Don and the CEO (chief executive officer) avoid depression or even dissolution of the self by claiming bottom-line (monetary) goals as the sole legitimate goals, and so escape mini-deaths of the self. Cognitive dissonance is a threatening condition. It has to be resolved. The politician may take graft and illegitimate campaign money, but does it "only to get re-elected," and thus saves his good image of himself. All of us meditate, pray, commune with nature, and calm ourselves for a few precious moments by means of various types of mild dissociation. Job loss, divorce, death of loved ones, illness, starvation, war—a thousand threatening life events (or conditions such as "non-events"—no promotions, no loved ones, no friends, permanent unemployment, no shelter)* prey on our minds. Any one of these is tantamount to a brush with death for us. We need "time out" from fear. This "time out," this communing with nature, music, good books, TV, and movies, is a way of fighting fear of dying, for that is what these losses feel like—a loss of the self, of a "piece of me," gone forever.

Whether on an individual level or an institutional one, our lives are suffused with dissociation of varying intensities. We go from one state of consciousness into another, in what seem like quantum leaps. We go from various levels of sleep to waking, and from reverie to the work-a-day state on the job. During sex some (lucky ones) pass into states bordering on unconsciousness, known in France as petit morte (those wonderful French)! We have states of arousal during fights or arguments, when we are superconscious. We may be hyperesthetic, or supersensitive to outside stimuli. Our hormones are constantly at work, changing our degree and type of consciousness.

Dissociation not only keeps us from fear of death. It governs the degree to which we are "in the world" or out of it. If it is moderate, it actually keeps us from dying, because it is one of our main methods of stress reduction. Excess anxiety and depression kill, and we now know that the immune system is closely tied to these states. Far from being a subject for psychopathologists alone, dissociation should be meat for all behavioral scientists, for educators, for parents, for the general practitioner, and for the average human who wants to know more about how to conquer fear of dying.†

---

* Studies of life events typically overlook some of the worst "events," the "non-events." One might be wishing for an event— a baby, a marriage, a job, or a promotion. The barren woman, the spinster (this is not a term for a female public relations expert), the person (often a woman or minority member) in a dead-end job with a "glass ceiling," are all experiencing "non-events." They can be fully as stressful as events. This may be why "life events" correlated only about 0.20 with various types of functional impairment in our longitudinal studies. This would let life events account for only 4% of the variance in impairment and/or psychopathology! Inclusion of non-events could improve the correlation. Early experiences, such as bad parenting, were much more predictive of poor outcomes than later events.

† Of course, the proper uses of dissociation should be taught to the Dissociated Dirty Dozen. The politicians, lawyers, CEOs, stockbrokers, bankers, serial killers, and many others could use some insight into their own mechanisms. Naturally this wouldn't work for the Army or the police, for how could they kill once they became conscious of the process that allows them to kill? We would have to educate the "enemy" and the criminals too, about their dissociation! What a colossal job! Maybe we should start with all the children?

16

REPRESSION/DENIAL

In the introductory section I have already described the equivalence of denial and repression. For all intents and purposes we can use these terms interchangeably. There is no doubt that denial (and illusion) are absolutely necessary to carry out the business of living. We are always striving to be "realistic," but in truth, reality is paralyzing. Death, disease, and destruction are everywhere, if one cares to look. So are cruelty, depravity, and selfishness. The crucial role of denial in keeping our sanity (blind though it may be) cannot be "denied."

> It can't be over stressed, one final time, that to see the world as it really is, is devastating and terrifying. It achieves the very result that the child has built his character over the years in order to avoid: *it makes routine, automatic, secure, self-confident activity impossible.* It makes thoughtless living in the world of men an impossibility.... (Becker, 1973, p. 60)

The evidence for denial is hard to find, since repression has as its goal the hiding of disturbing information from consciousness. We have to look to indirect measures, when repressed unconscious material breaks through into consciousness. Such breakthroughs are found in the very areas that first made Freud aware of the unconscious: dreams, slips of the tongue, and humor. We have no statistics of how many people dream of death or dying, nor how frequent these dreams are, but everyone has probably had at least one such dream.* There are numerous jokes about death, which I have discussed previously in the chapter on humor.

Another place to find evidence of repression is in euphemisms. If you want to avoid thinking about slums, you can use the term "inner city." George Carlin, the humorist and social critic, points out that if you can't stand to think of crippled people, you use the phrase "the physically challenged." He says "shell shock" has been replaced by the mild term "posttraumatic stress syndrome." How we avoid the words "dead" and "dying" is shown in the language of obituaries and funeral eulogies.

---

* Freud pointed out that dreams about rushing to get on a train, plane or boat that is about to "depart" are disguises for fear of dying (as in "dear departed," or "departing this world").

Feifel mentions that in Western culture you seldom "die"—you "pass on," or "end your days" (Feifel, 1959, p. 115). Other camouflaging terms come to mind, such as "he bought it," she "kicked the bucket," he "passed away," she "met her Maker." Other synonyms for dying are "fade away, perish, expire, meet your fate," and "curtains" (of the stage or the hearse?). For the term death we have "demise" and "fate." For the dead person we have "the deceased" and "the departed." For burial we have "interred" and "laid to rest." There are many other terms that avoid the horror of death. Among the more interesting of these are "come to naught, be taken, go to glory, fade away, RIP, go belly up, join the choir invisible, cross the Styx, give up the ghost, shuffle off this mortal coil, return to dust, hand in one's chips, go west, push up daisies, bite the dust, croak, check out, kick off." There are no fewer than 76 synonyms for the word "die" in Webster's thesaurus! (Laird, 1985, revised edition, p. 196). This seems in itself evidence of the importance of denial of death and avoidance of the word "die." One of the largest American industries is the insurance business, built on a euphemism—"life insurance," which is really death insurance. Who would want to buy death when they can buy life? It has been suggested that as belief in the afterlife waned, so avoidance of the topic of death grew. Our culture is heavily youth oriented, and this means that death and aging get short shrift. It has been said that death today is as tabooed a subject as sex was to the Victorians.

What is taboo is also intriguing, and murder, disease (especially AIDS, with its connection with sex), and war are constantly in the news. There is an audience for the gory details of the death of Nicole Simpson—hours of media discussion of her stab wounds (although photographs are shown only to the jury, not on television). Escape from almost certain death fascinates. This is what makes the hero.

When a U.S. jet pilot was shot down over Bosnia recently, he survived on insects and rainwater for 6 days, hiding by day and moving only at night. After being rescued, he became an overnight hero. He appeared on television with President Clinton, and made a short speech to the American public. He had cheated death, which is what everyone wants to do. The death or near escape of a hero or victim is not taboo, but our own inevitable death, or that of our loved ones, certainly is.

If we are so preoccupied with death, then how can we manage to live our daily lives without deep depression and fear? First, the death of others (not oneself) is a palliative. The *other* guy is slipping on a banana peel, but not I! Second, repression of thoughts about one's own death allows us to function.

> The answer is that men do not actually live stretched openly on a rack of cowardice and terror; if they did, they couldn't continue on with such apparent equanimity and thoughtlessness. Men's fears are buried deeply by repression, which gives to everyday life its tranquil facade; only occasionally does the desperation show through, and only for some people. (Becker, 1976, p. 92)

An interesting slant on what we are calling denial or repression is given by Rue (1994). He is a professor of religion and philosophy, and comes to this subject with a somewhat different approach, which I discussed briefly in Chapter 11 on religion. He is well aware of the role of denial. He quotes Mandi Horowitz' catalog of the forms of denial (avoided associations, numbness, flattened response, dimming of attention, daze, constricted thought, memory failure, and disavowal) (Rue, 1994, p. 170). While his description of the deceptions used by plants and animals (especially insects) to get their food is fascinating, the leap to "self-deception" as a means of survival for humans is somewhat less convincing.

If we view the human condition in the same manner that Becker or Freud does (a terrifying world) then we can accept Rue's formulations too. He contends that self-deception (in the form of a "myth" which he clearly equates with denial and illusion) is necessary for our survival. We fabricate facts and distort reality, to bolster our self-esteem. He says, and I quote him again, that the "noble lie'... would introduce a third voice, one which first agrees with the nihilists that universal myths are pretentious lies, but then insists, against the nihilists, that without such lies humanity cannot survive" (Rue, 1994, flap copy).

How similar this is to Becker's argument! He sees denial of death (a "lie" in Rue's words) as necessary for human functioning. How similar too, to Freud's idea that man must have an illusion (lie) like religion, and that if you take it away from him he will replace it with some political religion or some rigid system for sustaining the individual who is so threatened in this terrifying world (Freud, 1957).

I would like to discuss at length the battle of the relativists and the universalists, but that would fill another book. They are opponents in the "culture wars." To my mind, both camps are driven by a fear of death, one by the shakiness of values and the uncertainty of the universe as they come face to face with "reality," and the other by the threat that the "multiculturalists" might initiate social change and destroy their carefully preserved "Western white male" philosophy and way of life.

All in all, then, Rue's equating of denial with self-deceit does not add phylogenetic continuity to this argument. The deceit used by snapping turtles to lure a fish by wiggling its tongue, or by a human liar to cheat someone out of money, bears little on the problem of *self*-deceit among humans. What is of value here is the further elaboration of the survival value of self-deceit.

Denial is seen as a temporary defense by Elizabeth Kubler-Ross (Kubler-Ross, 1969). She is famous for identifying five stages that terminal patients go through upon being informed that they are terminally ill. These are Denial and Isolation, Anger, Bargaining, Depression, and Acceptance. It is commonly accepted that not all patients go through all of these stages, nor do they necessarily occur in any sequence. I mention it here because denial, which has been so well hidden when there is no immediate threat to life, comes very much to the fore upon the announcement of the patient's imminent death. Seeking other doctors to get a different diagnosis, or walking away from the medical profession entirely, are just two of the possible methods of denial. The major point to make here is that denial of death is not temporary, nor does it apply only to terminal patients (Kubler-Ross, 1969, p. 35, "Denial is usually a temporary defense ..."). It is ever present, and starts in childhood. It is not just a stage in attitude. The possible origins of the fear of death have been discussed previously. The origin of denial is probably both learned and instinctive.

Fear of death has a primary role of physical self-preservation. Denial of death has a self-protective function for humans, who possess the capacity for constantly dwelling on the subject of death. To permit normal psychological functioning, denial/repression puts the fear of death on a back burner. A constant state of arousal is thus avoided, but can be called upon in times of emergency. This is well expressed by Zilboorg:

> Therefore in normal times we move about actually without ever believing in our own death, as if we fully believed in our own corporeal immortality. We are intent on mastering death ... A man will say, of course, that he knows he will die some day, but that he does not really care. He is having a good time living, and he does not think about death and does not care to bother about it—but this is a purely intellectual, verbal admission. The affect of fear is repressed. (Zilboorg, 1943, pp. 468–471)

Is there less denial of death today in the United States? There is no clear-cut answer to this. Denial of death certainly decreases with age, and we have a rapidly aging population. In Kakutani's review of *The Afterlife and Other Stories*, by John Updike, there is the sense of repressed death fear breaking through:

> For Mr. Updike's people, perched on the margins of old age, life has divided itself into a then and now, a before and after. They are constantly measuring the dangerous and perplexing present against their memories of a simpler time ... Lurking behind their memories, of course, is the ghost of illness and mortality, an unwelcome emissary from the near future. 'More and more you see your contemporaries in the Globe obituaries.' One character observes 'The Big Guy is getting our range.' (Updike, 1994, quoted by M. Kakutani, 1994)

In preparation for the 50th reunion of my undergraduate class at Harvard, I estimated that 29% of my class had died. This came as a shock, and my denial mechanism immediately set in. First, I thought, a large number of my classmates were killed in World War II, so the 29% figure should be revised downward. I realized later that I had carefully avoided checking to see just how many had died during that war, although it would have taken only about an hour to do so. I didn't really want to know! My second denial was more elaborate. I had read that preselection bias would take out (another euphemism for 'kill') all those with physical disabilities and congenital heart or other serious defects. Those who had lived into their 60s and 70s were therefore healthier than the average, and their life expectancy would be increased. This gave some comfort, but again,

I studiously avoided looking up the actual expectancies for my cohort, which would have been the appropriate step for someone trained in epidemiology. I have spells of reading the obituaries in *The New York Times*, and this surely makes denial more difficult. Writing this book has decreased my denial, but increased my intellectualization of death, so that I feel somewhat protected by using this more time-consuming mechanism.

The increasing focus on death (or the lack of "sublimation" or transformation of death fear into transcendent art forms) is a major point of Arlene Croce's much disputed attack on "victim art," and the use of videotapes of dying AIDS patients in a dance recital. Although she comes across as ultra-conservative by criticizing dancers who present their victimized selves as "dissed blacks, abused women, or disfranchised homosexuals," she makes a major point about art as a way of transforming sorrow and death, citing Keats, Chopin, and Schumann.

> Personal despondency is not so easily sublimated today, nor do we look to sublimate it. Instead, it's disease and death that are taking over and running the show. As in the old woodcuts of Famine and Plague, a collective nightmare descends from which no one may be spared. And the end of twentieth-century collectivism is the AIDS quilt. (Croce, 1995, pp. 59–60)

She seems to be making a strong case for the shrinking of the denial of death, and says that this has had a terrible effect on the arts. She uses the term "sublimation," but I would prefer to use the term "transformation" to describe how the artist turns his despondency over impending death into great art. Croce says that "Keats wrote no 'Ode to Consumption.'" Yet he did write a famous sonnet, "When I have fears that I may cease to be," which I described earlier in relation to his own tuberculosis and his brother's recent death from the same disease. He doesn't say "I am dying, pity me." Croce is right in pointing out how art must transcend or transform death fear, or else it is not art.

> After two world wars and the other unspeakable terrors of our century, death is no longer the nameless one; we have unmasked death. But we have also created an art with no power of transcendence, no way of assuring us that the grandeur of the individual spirit is more worth celebrating that the political clout of the group. (Croce, 1995, p. 59)

It is obvious that she prefers creativity to group membership as a way of dealing with death fear. This is probably natural, since she is a famous dance critic. There are, however, many who derive their strength from their group membership, and many who, by reason of poor education or poverty, cannot find emotional support in creativity or the arts. Her point about the "unmasking of death" is relevant here. Perhaps death is becoming less tabooed, and the raw presentation of death or dying figures in plays, movies, television, and dance is evidence of this shift. Whether it is "art" remains for the critics of the future to decide.

17

SUICIDE

Suicide is defined as "the intentional taking of one's own life" (Flexner, 1987, p. 1902). How can suicide be included as a means of coping with the fear of death and dying? Isn't taking one's own life a submission to the very juggernaut of death that so terrifies you? As with many of the poor coping behaviors, suicide looks like a complete failure to deal with life's problems, for it brings on the end of life itself. Yet to the actor, his or her decision will end those apparently insoluble problems.* It is another "final solution," but unlike the Holocaust, it puts to death only one individual, not millions.

Suicide also involves a kind of empowerment, since it allows one to gain some sort of control over death, illusory although it may be. It is active, rather than passive. It is a choice, and offers a mirage of freedom.

Suicide in some ways is like counterphobic behavior. You seek out that which you fear the most—death. The difference is that counterphobia doesn't have as high a risk of death as suicide. The "death ratio" (completed suicides over attempted suicides) for female suicide is usually one in six. The death ratio for males is about one in two. In contrast, the death ratio for dangerous sports can be lower than 1 in 1000.

The motivation for suicide cannot easily be categorized. It varies widely between individuals and cultures. A better feel for the terrible stresses and depression that lead up to the suicides most common in our culture can be best seen in the history of one person's suicide. The statistics are faceless and voiceless.

Let me give an example. A woman, aged 30, threw herself out the tenth story window of her parents' apartment, and plunged to the pavement in New York City.

What could lead a woman in the prime of life, a woman who was a talented artist and scenic designer, who was good looking, who had a college education

---

* The "tunnel vision" of suicidal persons has been noted. They have restricted cognition. They see only two choices—the disgrace, bankruptcy, jail, or whatever fate awaits them, or death by suicide. They are unable to see alternate solutions.

and the financial support of her parents and grandparents, to kill herself? Sally, according to her mother, was a "difficult birth," with a labor lasting 48 hours. From early childhood, comparisons with her older brother were always negative. Although early on she received love from her mother, there was a growing competition between mother and daughter during Sally's adolescence. Once she dated a French sailor. Her mother "took over," since she was an accomplished linguist and had translated many plays from German and French, which were produced on Broadway. Sally was left out of the French conversation completely. This scenario happened many times.

During childhood she had numerous problems. She stuttered from an early age. Around age 12, she had an operation to correct "walleye" that involved both eyes. The operation lasted for many hours.

School was difficult. Alhough she had some friends, her grades were never very good. Sally later went to a small mid-Western college. After college, she seemed to find lovers who were artists and musicians. Some were very creative, but they were a motley lot. At least twice Sally became pregnant, and had to seek an abortion. In those days it was a criminal offense, and only the bravest or shadiest of doctors would perform it. Once her mother held the anesthetic during the procedure.

Her father felt he had been abandoned by his mother. He never really loved a woman because of this. He certainly withheld love from Sally, and was very critical of her. It was to be expected that Sally would choose boyfriends and lovers who were cruel to her. The problem she was trying to resolve with her father made for an "object choice" that mirrored her earliest experience with a man.

Her mother, in contrast, was an only child from a sheltering and loving family. She was, however, dominated by her own mother, who kept trying to force her to be more famous and productive than she could be. Her mother's sorrow over her husband's philandering made her withdrawn, and may have caused her to be jealous of her young, pretty, and sexually active daughter.

At age 14, Sally had a psychotic episode. She cried out in the night. She sobbed that someone was putting poison gas under her door. In truth, she was being poisoned by a lack of love.

At around that age she entered psychotherapy with a well-known psychoanalyst. She did not improve with this treatment. Sally loved playing the classical guitar. She was fond of flamenco music and dancing. She met a Spanish guitarist, Rinaldo, who was very handsome, and clearly a psychopath. He had been one of Generalissimo Franco's bodyguards in Spain. He was married. He went to jail for statutory rape, for he had sex with his 13-year-old stepdaughter. Apparently he had been giving drugs to Sally for some time. He took nude photographs of her, and now was blackmailing her from jail. He threatened to expose her, and ruin her life. For Sally, this was the end of the line. She would be ashamed before her whole world.

Sally came uptown from her apartment in Greenwich Village, and told her mother that she was being pursued by the FBI. They were going to jail her on drug charges. She would be exposed by Rinaldo, who would spread her nude pictures all over. Her mother, at her wit's end, tried to call Sally's current therapist. As she picked up the phone to call for help, Sally ran out of the bedroom to the kitchen, flung open the window, and leaped out.

What led Sally to such a terrible end? First was the lack of love she experienced in childhood. Rinaldo was someone she chose, but he was 10 times more overtly destructive than her parents. Her self-esteem was extremely low. She was always made to feel inferior. Her eye operation must have been traumatic. Her stuttering was an early symptom of the problems to come. Freud hypothesized that in committing suicide, the subject is killing an introjected image of a rejecting love-object. This fits Sally perfectly. She even acted out the killing on a statue she had made of Rinaldo. She plunged a knife into the forehead of the plastilene bust shortly before she killed herself.

Sally suffered from a "narrow cognitive style." This is often a contributing factor in suicide. She saw no alternatives. It was either disgrace or death. Jumping was her solution to what she imagined was an insoluble problem. At least one option would have been to move away from the city for a while, so that blackmail wouldn't work. Her parents would have given her the money she needed. She was probably on drugs at the time she killed herself. These may have produced some of the paranoid ideas she had. At 14, she also had a paranoid episode, so this was very much her style of response to stress.

Sally killed herself to escape a living death. Bereft of the love of her parents, persecuted by her lover, she was terribly lonely and fearful. Her act was also a murder of her lover. In addition, drugs and a possible psychotic episode at the time of her suicide contributed. Her motivation was complex, as any individual suicide appears when it is closely examined. The "why" question is answered by onionlike layers of motivation. As you look at her life, one level of explanation yields to another deeper layer of explanation.

Let's look at some of the attempts to classify and explain suicide, along with a few brief examples. Individuals, not groups, (with some exceptions) commit suicide.* We can look at their motives first. Later we can review briefly what sociologists, psychiatrists, and other behavioral scientists have said about why some groups have higher rates of suicide than other groups.

---

* This is not entirely true. For example, the use of the atomic bomb might be called group suicide, since a whole species, namely humans, have exposed themselves to a destructive force that they can now hardly control. The lemmings are an example of animal mass suicide, although their jumping off cliffs into the sea seems to be prompted by food shortages, which would aid the survivors. The constant wars between or within nations suggest some form of group suicide, although we always seem to find some justification for them, be it race, religion, or property. Several group suicides in cults have taken place in the past decade.

One of the leading suicidologists has reduced the motivations and causes of suicide to a single common cause.

> Suicide is caused by psychache. Psychache refers to the hurt, anguish, soreness, aching, psychological pain ... in the psyche, the mind. It is intrinsically psychological — the pain of excessively felt shame, or guilt, or humiliation, or loneliness, or fear, or angst, or dread of growing old and dying badly, or whatever ... Suicide occurs when the psychache is deemed by that person to be unbearable. (Shneidman, 1993, p. 369)

To me, psychache cannot be exclusively psychological in origin (nor exclusively sociological, psychiatric, or genetic) as Shneidman claims. It clearly is affected by sociological factors. For example, the fear of growing old varies greatly among cultures. Depression, as discovered by psychiatry, has many physiological and genetic correlates, and can certainly trigger suicide, by increasing "psychache" to the point where it is unbearable. Psychosis may lead to paranoid fantasies, which involve intense fear (psychache). This end state of unbearable pain may be common to most suicides, but its origins are quite diverse.

The motivations, rationales, and fantasies of suicidal patients, those who attempted suicide and those who completed it, give clues to the complexity of "psychache." We risk going from a reductionist statement, which explains suicide in one word, to a bewildering array of motives. Shneidman sees the forest, but we must also look at the trees. Two sources, Hendin (1965) and Meerloo (1962), dispel the idea that suicide can be summed up in one phrase. I have tried to combine their categories, and have abbreviated their lists.

Suicide as being magically killed: Surrender to a destructive god (as in the juggernaut), homosexual panic with merging which obliterates identity, after transgressing a magic taboo, magic fantasy of rescue by superparent or god, you're only loved when you're dead.

Suicide as contagion: A cry for help, mental contagion, as in panic.

Suicide as revenge: Retaliatory abandonment, punishment of those who rejected, power over survivors by haunting.

Suicide as retroflexed murder: Killing the internalized tormentor (parent, lover, or leader), killing the world (Samson complex and omnipotent mastery).

Suicide as unconscious flight: Self-punishment (killing the defeated self, "I cannot bear myself"), escape from confusion and guilt, escape from extreme anxiety, flight from feelings of deadness (flattened affect, inner decay, "death in life" or "living death"), flight from disease, avoidance of feelings of sexual inadequacy.

Egoistic suicide: Loss of control of external world, loss of control of inner world (fear of own rage), boredom (lack of incentive), incurable disease, pain or mutilation, lack of dignity and privacy, cheating death or the gallows.

Suicide as conscious flight (anomic suicide): Suicide due to unlimited aspiration or lack of societal limitation as in sudden wealth or power (pure Durkheimian anomie; see later), to escape "slow and messy death" (Hemingway), flight from decline of life, crisis, disease, addiction, expiation, fear of punishment (the law), avoiding dependency, flight from overintellectualization, flight from inability to love, escape from rejection.

Suicide as magic revival: Death and rebirth fantasy (somewhat similar to classic religions!), search for a rescuing prince or knight in shining armor, suicide as reunion or joining the lost love object, belief in reincarnation.

Altruistic suicide (one of Durkheim's types): Sacrifice to the code, as in suicide of military officers, hara-kiri, and the kamikaze (dive bomber suicide).

Many of these fantasies and motivations have become part of the classics of literature. When Tom Sawyer and Huck Finn are believed to have drowned, and come back to their own funeral, they represent two motives for suicide: the belief in reincarnation and the punishment of their tormentors. Children sometimes say "You'll be sorry when I'm dead," and many adults act out this scenario through suicide, unconsciously thinking they will return to view and savor their survivors' suffering.

This book attempts to show how various coping behaviors and defense mechanisms can ward off or diminish the fear of death and dying. Which of the above motives for suicide seem related to the fear of death and dying?

A distinction between fear of death and fear of dying may help at this point. Meerloo thinks fear of dying is more common in old age:

> Especially during the decline of life, the involution, when some life processes slow up and adaptations become more and more difficult, one can observe this form of suicide ... (passive surrender to fate, giving up the will to live) ... rooted in changed vital feelings. People have made, as it were, a pact with death. For them, old age is equal to mutilation. They are not afraid of death, but much more of the transition toward death, of the *disease of dying*. (Meerloo, 1962, p. 41) (italics mine.)

Suicide in the elderly, then, can be considered as a mode of coping with the fear of *dying* , of a flight from bodily deterioration, reduced vitality, or the downward path of addiction. It is an escape from the specter of terminal cancer or congestive heart failure, which involves intractable pain, prohibitive expense for medical care, and separation from loved ones.

Suicide as a mode of coping with fear of death (in contrast to fear of dying) is more likely to cover all age ranges. Death is inevitable, and essentially out of our control. Benjamin Franklin told us that "In this world nothing can be said to be certain, except death and taxes" (Cohen, 1978, p. 162, No. 15). Suicide offers control to people of all ages. It offers a choice to the terminal cancer patient: either commit suicide or suffering protracted pain while dying. It offers control to the "living dead," who suffer from lack of emotion ("flattened affect"). They escape a living death through suicide.

Life is full of near-deaths and mini-deaths. The fear of a living death after job loss, the end of a career, or the loss of a loved one may be a motive for suicide. We can call it separation fear, depression, trauma, or damage, but the feeling state after such major negative life events is often of being dead. It is to escape this "death-in-life" feeling that many suicides are undertaken. Psychic numbing is in itself a defense against the "psychache" of loss or defeat. While the pain stops, the feeling of deadness is just as bad, if not worse.

Let's look at a few more suicides or attempted suicides to put some of these motives and fantasies in the context of an individual's life. Ernest Hemingway has been mentioned as motivated to suicide by a wish to avoid slow deterioration due to a terminal illness. He committed suicide by gunshot, a method chosen by his father before him.

James Michener, the author, died when he decided to stop his kidney dialysis treatment. This was apparently a rational decision for a person faced with gradual deterioration due to kidney failure. Dialysis must be performed several times a week. It takes several hours, during which time the patient is hooked up to a dialysis machine. As a National Institutes of Health reviewer on a grant proposal for the study of the "quality of life" of dialysis patients, I was impressed by the poor quality of the dialysis patient's life described by the researchers. There is often severe nausea. Parts of the procedure can be painful. Getting to and from a dialysis center is difficult for those patients not hospitalized. For many patients it is one more type of "living death."

One of the most discussed suicides of recent years was that of Sylvia Plath, the poet and author of *The Bell Jar*. In his brilliant book, *The Savage God*, A. Alvarez, a professor of English literature, analyzes the path that led to Plath's suicide. He also describes his own suicide attempt, the attitudes toward suicide over the centuries, and suicide as it appears in literature. Alvarez helped Plath to publish some of her poems, and was a frequent visitor. She often read her poems to him. From these contacts, and from an analysis of her poetry, he was able to come up with a convincing picture of the dynamics leading to her death.

Sylvia's father died when she was a young girl. *The Bell Jar*, which is autobiographical, tells how the heroine weeps at her father's grave, and then swallows 50 sleeping pills. Alvarez says that:

> In 'Daddy' (*one of her better known poems*) describing the same episode, she hammers home her reasons with repetitions:
>
>> 'At twenty I tried to die
>> And get back, back, back to you.
>> I thought even the bones would do'
>> (Alvarez, 1973, Bantam Books, original 1971, p. 20) (italics mine)

Sylvia's husband, Ted Hughes, had left her. She was severely depressed, and was expecting a reply from a psychotherapist whom friends had recommended. The plumbing in her house froze solid. She had bad sinus trouble. She had to care for two small children. She put her head in the oven and turned on the gas. A note to a babysitter who couldn't enter the locked building asked someone to call the doctor, but the *au pair* girl arrived too late. Alvarez asks:

> Why, then, did she kill herself? In part, I suppose, it was 'a cry for help' which fatally misfired. But it was also a last desperate attempt to exorcise the death she had summed up in her poems. I have already suggested that she began to write obsessively about death … when she and her husband separated, however mutual the arrangement, she again went through the same piercing grief and bereavement she had felt as a child when her father, by his death, seemed to abandon her. (Alvarez, 1973, Bantam Books, original 1971, p. 36)

In Sylvia Plath's suicide, the motives of rejoining a lost loved one, and the reinforcement by marital separation of an early loss of a parent, are most prominent. The flight from the rejection by her husband added to the original loss of her father, which she felt (as many children do) as a rejection and abandonment. In her poems, her father appears as a Nazi and a vampire, indicating her ambivalence toward him—a mixture of love and hatred.* The suicide attempt in her 20s (described in *The Bell Jar*), foreshadowed her later death, and illustrates her great vulnerability.

The dilemma of Vince Foster, the deputy White house counsel who committed suicide by firing a gun into his mouth on July 20, 1993, seemed to be strongly work related. He wrote shortly before his death that he was "not meant for the job or the spotlight of public life in Washington. Here ruining people is considered sport" (Starr, 1997, p. A8, *The New York Times*, 10/11/97). Foster had been busy defending the Clintons on various fronts, including the Whitewater investigation, the appearance of pressure to replace the presidential travel officials with Clinton's friends, and possibly the President's brushes with various ladies claiming sexual advances. Foster told his mother, 2 days before his death, that he was unhappy because his work was a "grind." He was considering resignation. He cried at dinner with his wife 4 days before killing himself.

Perhaps a less self-critical person could have weathered the vicious tactics of Washington politics. A suicide expert quoted in Starr's report said: Mr. Foster was:

> … under an increasing burden of intense external stress, a loss of security, a painful scanning of his environment for negative judgments regarding his performance, a rigid hold of perfectionistic self-demands, a breakdown in and the absence of his usual ability to handle that stress primarily due to the impact of a mental disorder which was undertreated. (Labaton, 1997, p. A8)

Foster's suicide seems to be a "conscious flight from an unbearable crisis." This might be called a anomic suicide. However, there is the slight possibility (and Clinton's enemies would certainly favor this interpretation) that Vince Foster killed himself to protect what he knew about Bill Clinton's activities. They were close friends, and he and Hillary Clinton had worked in the same law

---

* See Alvarez (1973, Bantam Books, original 1971, p. 37), for a description of Plath's fantasy of the struggle between her "Jewish mother and Nazi father."

office. He was privy to the family secrets. Could he have killed himself to avoid being forced to testify against his friends? If so, his would be an altruistic suicide, another of Durkheim's types (see later). We'll never know if he was really a kamikaze from Arkansas.

Suicide attempts often differ in their motivation from completed suicides. Some of them are meant to fail, and to coerce or punish others without losing one's own life. One great advantage of suicide attempts is that they offer a chance to interview the survivor. (To study them in an attempt to understand completed suicides may involve the reasoning of the oft-quoted drunk who was on all fours in the street. A cop came along and asked him what he was looking for. "My watch." "Where did you lose it?" "Over there" "Then why are you looking here?" "Because at least there's a street lamp over here.") Perhaps one day computer scientists will "download" the brains of completed suicides, and we will find out if there is a disparity between attempts and completions. Until then, a pair of suicide attempts described by verbally gifted suicidal writers may help in understanding this sad and puzzling behavior.

Kay Redfield Jamison, a clinical psychologist, is a Professor of Psychiatry at Johns Hopkins School of Medicine. She has written a standard text on manic–depressive psychosis, and is in fact manic–depressive herself. Her book, *An Unquiet Mind*, is exquisitely written, and gives deep insight into the terrible mood swings of this illness. Her family dynamics don't point clearly to the development of the disorder. Her father, however, suffered violent mood swings, and there is a strong genetic component to manic–depression. Starting in high school, she had severe manic and depressed periods. She struggled through her clinical training, She was treated with lithium, and responded to it. However, she longed for her manic moods, which gave her transcendence. She was grandiose during those periods, and enjoyed the affairs she went through and her heightened work-related inspirations during her highs. She would stop taking her medication, hoping for more highs. Instead the black moods would descend upon her.

> The morbidity of my mind was astonishing. Death and its kin were constant companions. I saw Death everywhere, and I saw winding sheets and toe tags and body bags in my mind's eye. Everything was a reminder that everything ended at the charnel house. (Jamison, 1995, p. 111)

While in therapy three times a week, she bought a gun, and lingered at the top of the hospital stairwell, wanting to jump. She refused to be committed, couldn't sleep for days on end, and avoided others for fear of being a "burden." She decided to kill herself with an overdose of lithium, the very drug that had helped her. She even got a prescription for an anti-emetic drug to keep from vomiting the lithium. She lay on her bed, waiting to die. The phone rang. It was her brother, who was indeed his sister's keeper. She answered, and her slurred speech alerted him that she was dying. He called her psychiatrist. She was semicomatose for several days. Her psychiatrist, her friends, and her mother nursed her back to life. She finally became persuaded that she would die without lithium, even though it meant giving up her manic periods which she so loved.

Jamison's suicide attempt was another flight from an unbearable depression. Her obsession with death was in fact a living death. The genesis of her moods may have been partly psychological, yet she pictures her mother as a loving Rock of Gibraltar, and her father as loving but moody. Her positive response to lithium was clearly pathognomonic; it identified manic–depressive psychosis with its strong genetic component as the primary cause of her illness. The "psychache" of her black moods is like a peek into hell. Even in high school she felt "deeply tired, bored, indifferent to life ... Then a gray, bleak preoccupation with death, dying, decaying, that everything was born but to die, best to die now and save the pain while waiting" (Jamison, 1995, p. 39). The key word here is *pain*, that drives so many to kill themselves. Schneidman is right. If one word (however inadequately) can sum up much of suicidal motivation, it is "psychache," or its simpler country cousin, "pain."

Alvarez was no doubt inspired to write *The Savage God* by his own lifelong preoccupation with death, and his almost fatal suicide attempt as an adult. Again, his expressive skills as a professor of English, like the writing skills of Sylvia Plath and Kay Jamison, help us to understand his feelings about and motivation for suicide. We know little about his childhood, but one fact stands out. Both his parents claimed to have put their heads in the gas oven, although "half-heartedly." This suggests two very negative models for a growing boy, and a possible genetic tendency to depression as well.

Alvarez had many squabbles with his wife. After one of these fights, he realized the meaning of one of his favorite phrases, which he repeated like a mantra: "I wish I were dead." It was like an "aha-experience," an epiphany. He knew from then on that he didn't want to live. When the family moved from England to New England, where he had a teaching job, his wife was isolated and miserable. She packed up after 2 months and went back to England with their 3-year-old boy. During the Christmas break, he returned to England. It was disastrous. They started fighting again, and he drank heavily. When his wife departed for a dingy flat, and left him alone once more, it "seemed like the final nail. More likely, it was the unequivocal excuse I had been waiting for. I went upstairs to the bathroom and swallowed forty-five sleeping pills" (Alvarez, 1973, p. 263).

The description of his symptoms and recovery is harrowing but written in crystalline-cold objective sentences. He was unconscious, deeply cyanosed, and vomit had clogged his lungs and bronchial tubes. His doctors had to perform a bronchoscopy, and put an air pipe in his throat. He suffered from double vision. Despite all this he left the hospital against medical advice. Alvarez recovered at home, and returned to the United States to finish his term. The marriage lasted only a few months more.

Alvarez sees his attempted suicide as stemming from a failure to grow up:

> The truth is, in some way *I had* died. The over-intensity, the tiresome excess of sensitivity and self-consciousness, of arrogance and idealism, which came in adolescence and stayed on and on beyond their due time, like some visiting bore, had not survived the coma. (Alvarez, 1973, p. 268)

Alvarez clearly mourns the death of his youthful self. In a strange parallel, he exhibits the same ambivalence about his adolescent self as Jamison does about her beloved manic self, which she finally had to give up to avoid death.

> ... after all, the youth who swallowed the sleeping pills and the man who survived are so utterly different that someone or something must have died ... Before the pills was another life, another person altogether, whom I scarcely recognized and don't much like—although *I suspect that he was, in his priggish way, far more likable than I could ever be*. (Alvarez, 1973, p. 272) (italics mine)

Like so many suicidal people, Alvarez thought death would be a solution. It was a bust—not a "moment of cathartic truth." If he had succeeded in killing himself, it would have been, indeed, a final solution to his "despair ... pure and unadulterated, like the final unanswerable despair a child feels, with no before or after" (Alvarez, 1973, Bantam Books, original 1971, p. 271) (Is this both psychache and cognitive narrowing?)

> Above all, I was disappointed. Somehow, I felt, death had let me down; I expected more of it. I had looked for something overwhelming, an experience which would clarify all my confusions. But it turned out to be simply a denial of experience ...
>
> Once I had accepted that there weren't going to be any answers, even in death, I found to my surprise that I didn't much care whether I was happy or unhappy; 'problems' and 'the problem of problems' no longer existed. And that in itself is already the beginning of happiness ... It seems ludicrous now to have learned something so obvious in such a hard way, to have had to go almost the whole way to death in order to grow up. (Alvarez, 1973, pp. 269 and 271)

This belated acceptance of the travails of life sounds much like a deathbed religious conversion, yet we must respect it. While it smacks of denial, it is surely a way out of the tortures of seeking a solution to life's insoluble problems. Alvarez is antipsychoanalytic, at least where his own motivations are concerned. He gives short shrift* to his early childhood experiences and his parents' character. What he does tell us, in brilliant prose, is the terrible pain that drives some people, especially intellectuals, to suicide. In addition, he illustrates how suicide can *seem* to be a solution to a person in such severe psychic pain. The problems of a person of his type—a highly gifted professor, with the ability to earn a reasonably good living—are not those of the ghetto dweller, the refugee, or the victim of natural disaster. His depression is clearly endogenous, the result of his internal

---

* Not in the sense of confession, but in the sense now common, of writing. This is consonant with the origin of the word, shrift, from the German, *schreiben*, "to write."

conflicts, rather than the exogenous depression caused by current external events. True, his wife's leaving triggered the suicide attempt, but he states that he intended to kill himself long before that.

DURKHEIM: A SOCIOLOGICAL ANALYSIS OF SUICIDE

After reviewing several suicides and suicide attempts, it is probably clear that while they show a common element of pain or "psychache," the individual motivations are strikingly different. The case history or individual approach (also known as the ideographic method) is in sharp contrast to the nomothetic approach, best illustrated by sociology. The nomothetic method involves the "study or formulation of general or universal laws." Other than Freud's writings on depression, his theory of the death instinct, and psychoanalytic writings building on his work, the largest body of theory bearing on suicide stems from the work of Emile Durkheim, who has been mentioned before. Durkheim was looking for a general theory of social cohesion and social control, to illustrate his ideas on "the rules of sociological method." His work is heavily nomothetic, since it relies on group statistics. He seized on suicide to demonstrate how marital status, religion, and other demographic variables influence the rates of suicide. His overall conclusion was that for the most part, social cohesion prevented suicide, except in subcultures where suicide was required in particular circumstances. Most people in most societies were *regulated* enough to keep them from suicide. If they were underregulated or overregulated, suicide could occur.

Remarkably, Durkheim's classification of suicide into anomic, altruistic, egoistic, and fatalistic categories has not been greatly improved upon since its publication just about 100 years before the year I am writing this chapter (Durkheim, 1897). The *anomic* suicide, he said, was the result of sudden societal deregulation of the individual, a lack of limits. An example would be the suicide of someone who wins a lottery, becomes a millionaire, and loses his roots. There are now no limits on his behavior, and his life may become unstructured or "deregulated." The person living in a society that is anomic, or in a state of anomie, is "overwhelmed by his good fortune." He suffers from *too little societal regulation*.

The *altruistic* suicide is demanded by society. It is the result of *too much regulation*. It is typically illustrated by the Japanese *kamikase* pilot who plunges his plane onto a battleship for the sake of the emperor and his country. An American World War II soldier's joke expresses amazement at such altruism, as well as contempt for the enemy.

A Japanese Colonel is delivering a graduation speech to a class of *kamikase* pilots. As he ends his speech, he shouts, "Now you are *kamikaze* graduates. You dive-bomb the

American warships! You die for the Emperor! You die for Japan! *Banzai!* Are there any questions?"* A small voice from the back row of cadets asks "Are you out of your fucking mind?"

Perhaps this illustrates the incomprehensibility of altruistic suicide to the average American soldier. Certainly by the end of the Vietnam War, young men were even less willing than during World War II to die for God and Country. Letters home from Civil War soldiers showed that honor and duty were strong motives for staying in combat, despite the high casualty rate. Similar sentiments were expressed by British, French, and German warriors, among others, including those involved in World War I.

Another form of altruistic suicide is seen in hara-kiri, although this is a bit more of a mixed bag than the kamikaze. This is a way to die with honor, and it is accepted as a way out of financial or interpersonal wrongdoing. The suicide of the sergeant or lieutenant who failed to keep his men out of danger or failed to take an enemy position was quite frequent in countries such as France and Germany, which had longstanding military elites with their own traditions. These soldierly suicides were usually accomplished by blowing one's brains out. From the standpoint of the observer, the *altruistic suicide is clearly the result of societal overregulation.*

The *egoistic* suicide is one in which self-absorption dominates. The individual is not properly bonded to his society. It is not due to societal problems (a societal state of anomie) or to societal rules governing behavior after some type of failure (altruistic). Nowadays we might consider it more associated with endogenous depression.

The *fatalistic* suicide occurs when the individual is totally overregulated by society, and has no escape routes. The suicides of slaves, prisoners, and concentration camp inmates are typical. Interestingly, Durkheim stuck this type into a footnote!

We tend to think of death as always unwelcome, but when it is inevitable, it may be a blessing. The suicides of Hemingway and Michener, when they were faced with painful and prolonged terminal illness, seem to me to belong in Durkheim's "fatalistic" category. The overlapping of these suicide types becomes clear when even experts lump them together. For example, Meerloo puts "incurable disease" under "Egoistic suicide," and this overlaps with his category "Suicide as unconscious flight" in which he places "flight from disease." The terminally ill in great pain may be likened to people undergoing torture.

---

* U.S. Army officers, including myself, were taught to ask "Are there any questions?" regardless of the lesson being taught. It was to be spoken rapidly, and in most cases was immediately followed by bellowing "Section Marcher!" or some other command, so that no questions could possibly be asked by the G.I.'s (another word for soldiers, and an abbreviation of General Issue, which described all clothing and equipment of the ordinary soldier).

Slaves and prisoners have historically been victims of torture. Even today, people are being crucified in some way all over the world. There are many examples: in the Bosnian–Serbian–Croatian conflict, or in the "dirty war" in Argentina from 1976 to 1983 (previously referred to) in which thousands were tortured, and many drugged and dropped naked from airplanes into the sea (Sims, 1995, "Argentina Tells of Dumping of Captives at Sea," *The New York Times*, 3/13/95). People have been tortured since the beginning of history, but some instances stand out, such as the "experiments" that Nazi doctors (led by Dr. Mengele) inflicted on Jews, Gypsies, and political prisoners; the torture of early Christians by the Romans; and the horrors of the Spanish Inquisition. How these victims must have longed for death. They were powerless to escape their torturers.

The inventive sadism of the torturers denies the label of "banality" accorded them by Hannah Arendt (see also Chapter 18). Jeffrey Benzien worked in the security branch of the South African police during the era of apartheid. Some of his surviving victims confronted him before the commission that decided on whether to grant amnesty. Should anyone doubt that torture victims might want to die, let me briefly recount some of Benzien's torture methods:

> ... he admitted that he had used electric shocks as well (to the nose, genitals, and in the rectum). One victim said Mr. Benzien had shoved a broomstick up his rectum. There were beatings too, and some people were hung for hours by handcuffs attached to the window bars in their cells.
>
> Mr. Benzien was particularly adept at the use of the 'wet bag' in which a cloth placed over victims' heads took them to the brink of asphyxiation, over and over again. Few withstood more than half an hour.
>
> (A victim says) 'Do you remember saying that you are going to break my nose and then putting both your thumbs into my nostrils and pulling it until the blood came out of my nose?' (Parentheses mine) (Daley, 1997, pp. 1 and 12)*

In situations in which one is faced with inevitable death (fatalistic) suicide can be a blessing. Sandor Ferenczi recounted an event told him by a hunter, who was watching a small bird trembling with fear in front of a falcon with open beak. The bird shivered, and flew directly into the maw of the raptor. Ferenczi concluded:

> The anticipation of certain death appears to be such torment that by comparison actual death is a relief. (Ferenczi, *The Clinical Diary of Sandor Ferenczi*, edited by Judith Dupont, Harvard University Press, Cambridge, MA, p. 179)

---

* Mr. Benzien is unusual, in that he came forward to ask for amnesty. None of the other police officers in his unit have. There is nothing "banal" about his behavior, and he certainly doesn't suffer from a "lack of imagination," as Delbanco describes torturers and killers. Benzien even says to a victim, "I can treat you like an animal or a human being," suggesting that he had not unconsciously "animalized" his prey.

It is true that Durkheim often injected individual psychological explanations into his sociological analyses when describing the motives and feeling states of various types of suicide. We can't really understand what rates of behavior mean unless we look at possible individual motives behind each rate. True understanding demands a blending of the social and psychological into a social psychology of behavior, be it suicidal or any other behavior.

What Durkheim found 100 years ago still generally holds true today, depending on the culture being studied. For example, married men have much lower rates of suicide than unmarried males. They "benefit" from marriage. Unmarried men lack ties to a wife and child, so generally have "less to live for." They are also more isolated, and can't satisfy their normal dependency needs. Because they are men, they have usually not been brought up to run a household, or nurse themselves. As sons they were used to "being taken care of" by their mothers. In depressed states, the thought of leaving dependent wife and children behind cannot act as a deterrent for single men against taking their lives. In a word, they have few "roots."

Women, in contrast, are less likely to "benefit" from marriage, and the suicide rates for married and unmarried women do not differ as widely as those for married and unmarried men. There is no necessary conflict between individual and group approaches to suicide. Society underregulates unmarried men. If anything, society still tends to overregulate women, married or unmarried. With women's liberation, we might have expected major anomie (deregulation) for them. Instead, they now have the overregulation of the family and child care, plus the overregulation of the workplace for less pay, on average, than men doing the same work without the household duties! This is certainly no argument for going back to the days of the *Haustyrann* husband of the classical authoritarian German family. Does this overregulation of women help to account for the fact that U.S. women have three or more times the rate of depression of U.S. men? Is it possible that women are more prone to egoism? Not likely, for they are more strongly bonded to family and society than men. Perhaps they fall more into the Fatalistic category, a state of slavery, with few or no escape routes? Several studies suggest that the self-esteem of girls drops precipitously after age 9. Girls "gradually lost their prepubescent strength, independence, spirit and lucidity and become riveted to the issue of how they look. Boys, in contrast, seem to develop greater self-esteem as they grow older" (Brody, 1997, p. F9).*

In the discussion of differential rates of depression and self-esteem between boys and girls, or men and women, the interaction of psychological variables with those rates helps us to understand what is happening. This is also true of sociological rates and psychological descriptions in the study of suicide.

---

* Brody makes reference to several studies, especially one by Dr. Emily Hancock, *The Girl Within*, Ballantine, 1990.

Suicide is always an individual event, but (or *and*) it always occurs in an individual who, willy-nilly, holds one or more citizenships* in one or more cultures…The emphasis on the individual does not at all preclude interest and concern with social (and economic) and especially cultural forces as they reside or swirl within the individual psyche. (Shneidman, 1985, p. 210)

The psychological, psychiatric, and sociological approaches to suicide have only been briefly covered here, and they are only a few ways of looking at this elephant. Shneidman lists 13 approaches to suicide; theological (Augustine, Aquinas), philosophical (especially existentialism), demographic, sociological (Durkheim), psychodynamic (Freud, Karl Menninger, Zilboorg), psychological (Shneidman), cognitive (Kasanin, Arieti, Beck), biological-evolutionary (Pepper, Dawkins), constitutional (Kretschmer, Sheldon), biochemical (writings on depression), preventional (Shneidman, Farberow, and Litman), and last but not least global, political, supranational (Shneidman, 1985, pp. 30–40).† I have only touched briefly, if at all, on these approaches.

MASS SUICIDE

The last approach (global or supranational) seems to me of such critical importance that I must mention it briefly. It was only a few years ago that the threat of a "nuclear holocaust" was on everyone's mind. While the selling of nuclear components or weapons to smaller but aggressive countries, especially sales by demoralized segments of former Soviet Russia, is still possible, new threats to humanity in general are on the horizon. Saddam Hussein of Iraq has denied access to United Nations inspectors searching for biological weapons such as anthrax, and chemical poisons similar to sarin. These weapons can kill up to 60 million people at a time, and can be delivered by artillery.

---

* The sociologist in me would add here the various roles the individual holds in those cultures and societies. The excessive role demands of some age–sex and marital statuses within and across cultures are crucial to an understanding of differential suicide rates. The role conflicts are equally important. For example, a current favorite is motherhood versus career, yet the same might be said of fatherhood. When a British au pair recently shook to death the little boy she was supposed to be guarding, she was convicted of second-degree murder. More amazingly, hate mail poured in to the family, accusing the mother of neglecting her child, since she worked as a doctor! We ask women to perform two conflicting roles, and then blame them for the death of a baby for whom they provided what they thought was more than adequate care.

† I have included only a few of the references, but you are encouraged to look at this fine list of "approaches," each of which has a voluminous literature behind it. I refer to the story of men of different nationalities and their treatises on the elephant. If ever there was a large animal, it is suicide. Worse yet is the subject of this book, for "choices in living" covers all of life. Fear of dying is just a springboard for covering love, hate, killing, and everything else in between.

As if that were not enough of a threat to life on earth, the issue of global warming has been up for international discussion in Kyoto, Japan. The United States has hesitated to cut down rapidly on carbon dioxide emissions, since it is felt that this would hurt industry and raise the cost of all products. President Clinton suggested, and President George W. Bush agrees, that we postpone cutting emissions drastically for another 10 years. Since the United States is the greatest polluter and contributor to the "greenhouse effect," how much we cut back emissions will strongly influence what other nations are willing to do. It may have been political suicide for Clinton and Bush to work for stronger cuts. Yet it is also possible that they and the leaders of the developed nations are presiding over the death of the planet!

Computer modeling of weather predictions has been improving to the point where it is probably only making mistakes by region, but not in global estimates of warming. What are the models telling us?

> A doubling of carbon dioxide concentrations is expected late in the next century if the world pursues business as usual ... a doubling of carbon dioxide concentrations in the atmosphere would raise the earth's average surface temperature by three to eight degrees Fahrenheit. (Stevens, 1979 p. F6)

Are these climatologists really Chicken Little in disguise? Not likely. Since the world is 5 to 9 degrees warmer now than during the last Ice Age, imagine what another 8 degrees might do to this island Earth. Most tropical areas would become desert, just as the Sahara has spread as a result of interglacial warming. As ice caps melt, sea levels would rise, and inundate many islands and low-lying coastal areas that are even now subject to occasional flooding. Food shortages would be disastrous, since even as coastal agricultural land is lost, population growth will continue due to medical innovation. Rehydration of infants suffering from diarrhea is starting to save countless millions who previously died. Vaccinations may save millions more. Food shortages will then ensue, with more mouths to feed and less land upon which to grow crops. Are we about to commit mass suicide through a lack of will to distribute birth control materials worldwide, and a short-sighted "penny-wise and pound foolish" policy of snail-paced control of carbon dioxide emissions from fossil fuels (coal and oil) and sulfate aerosols? Since we are not in the middle of a major world war, it gives us a little time to plan for the future of the planet and the human race. Individual fear of dying may soon be projected onto global warming, as it once was on the hydrogen bomb. These fears, unfortunately, are not unwarranted. As for overpopulation, Joost Merloo, a Dutch psychiatrist who narrowly escaped the Nazis, had strong words of warning:

> The population explosion anticipates a future for human rivalry such as been unheard of until this day. When will mankind take this phenomenon and its history in hand?

> Birth control is an absolute essential if famine and war are not to regulate population growth. How to persuade mankind to restraint is one of the most tremendous problems of our time. Failure to regulate the population explosion will be inadvertent surrender to a form of mass suicide. (Meerloo, 1962, p. 92)

Meerloo wrote in 1962. The world's population has more than doubled since then!

ASSISTED SUICIDE

Whether to allow assisted suicide has become not just a medical, but a political and moral issue. There is a bitter struggle going on, and the state of Oregon will apparently be the first to allow doctors to help terminally ill patients kill themselves. Assisted suicide is really a special variety of "fatalistic suicide." It is not crucial to my thesis (that suicide is one of many modes of coping with fear of dying), for it is a special case. In fact, for the terminally ill, fear of dying (in pain) is probably much greater than the fear of death (nonbeing). Rather than "psychache," the person who wants assisted suicide fears just plain "ache"—that is, excruciating* physical pain during the process of dying.

SUBINTENTIONED DEATHS: ARE UNINTENTIONAL "SELF-DESTRUCTIVE" BEHAVIORS REALLY SUICIDES?

Suicide, as stated previously, is defined as "the *intentional* taking of one's own life" (italics mine) (Flexner, 1987, p. 1902). The same word "suicide" is often used to describe the *unintentional* "self-destructive" behaviors, which may be found only by looking at the unconscious level. Karl Menninger wrote about such behaviors as addiction and polysurgery (seeking out repeated surgical procedures, often for organs that are not diseased) (Menninger, 1938). His book became a model for Norman Farberow, who edited a book called *The Many Faces of Suicide* (Farberow, 1980). He included in his list of "Indirect Self-Destructive Behaviors" or ISDB's, physical illness used against the self (ignoring symptoms, not taking medication, or being an uncooperative patient), drug abuse, alcohol abuse, hyperobesity, smoking, self-mutilation, auto accidents, gambling, criminal activity (delinquency, prostitution), altruism (intervening in violent events), and high-risk sports.

---

* I have chosen this word on purpose. It is derived from the Latin excruciare, "to torture," which in turn refers to crucifixion and the cross. There are few symbols of suffering as powerful as that of Christ on the cross. We also speak of being "racked" with pain. The rack was a common form of torture in times past.

Jack R. Ewalt (then Director of Mental Health Services for the Veterans Administration) wrote in his Foreword that:

> There may be some who will disagree about the activities which have been included ... the authors of two of the chapters disclaim or at least question whether their areas are most appropriately conceptualized as indirectly self-destructive. Lichtenstein and Bernstein believe that cigarette smoking, at least in its milder phases, is better explained with other concepts. Geis and Huston find their Good Samaritan interveners acting in a self-enhancing, socially lauded, although recognizedly high risk way, when they rush to the aid of an unknown victim of a crime. (Farberow, 1980, pp. xiii–xiv)

I have discussed many of these behaviors in the chapters on counterphobic behavior and gambling. Since many, or perhaps all of the behaviors, have as their motivation the solution of some human problem, they cannot be viewed only from the viewpoint of the outsider, or the society. Suicide, in particular, is often a solution to a problem that is truly insoluble, or that is seemingly insoluble, due to the restricted or "tunnel" vision of the actor. Gambling surely has rewards for those who win. At this point about half the nation has invested in stock market mutual funds. Everyone knows that there are risks, and that the market crashed in 1929, slipped in 1987, and dipped in 1997 and 2000, yet we don't call these investors "self-destructive." Even homicide has its psychological (as well as monetary) rewards, as Becker so brilliantly pointed out (Becker, 1973). Drug use and abuse is found at every level of our society. For those who get their drugs on the street, the self-destruction may realistically be greater than for the wealthy who get their tranquilizers and stimulants through their private physician's prescriptions. Fear and anxiety know no social class boundaries. The counterphobic may be self-destructive when he takes on the risks of skydiving or scuba diving, but he enjoys the kudos of his companions, and is admired for his bravery. In each chapter that deals with potentially self-destructive behavior, I have tried to show how the same actions can be self-enhancing, and may be adaptive.

Confirming my strong convictions about restricting the use of the word "suicide" to intentional deaths, Shneidman says:

> My own view is that all these deleterious outcomes (drug abuse, alcohol abuse, obesity, drunk driving, and high risk sports) are more meaningfully called *subintentioned deaths* than one or another kind of suicide. (Shneidman, 1985, p. 21)

To keep unintentional deaths out of the realm of suicide (intentional deaths) I have written separate chapters on counterphobic behavior, gambling, and killing (all of which are high-risk activities often resulting in death).

Love of Life: An Endnote

I feel sorrow for the Sallys of this world, the Kay Jamisons, the Sylvia Plaths, and the thousands of talented (and not so talented) people who kill or try to kill themselves every year. Not having "been there," I find it strange and tragic that they have lost the will to live and the love of life. I hope I never completely understand that depth of despair. I can only look on with sympathy, from a distance.

Projection, Killing, and the Problem of Evil

This chapter is so complex that it may be helpful to have a brief summary of its contents here:

Death is the greatest natural evil. Killing (especially homicide) is the greatest man-made evil (among many others). Killing offers illusory immortality. Projection allows the killer to project his (unacceptable) desire to kill (torture, rape, steal, dominate, etc.) onto some target group or person. This demonizes *his target, making it even more acceptable to kill. Dissociation (splitting or doubling) allows the killer to kill without the psychological damage that guilt or remorse would normally inflict.*

We seem to be able to define degrees of evil. There may be mitigating circumstances or motives.

The sources of man-made evil are still in dispute, whether biological, hormonal, genetic, social or familial, historical, or economic.

The search for fixed values against which we can judge evil seems to end up as a longing for "community." This nostalgia for "Gemeinschaft," shared by liberals and conservatives alike, brings us close to the emotional state that made Germany ripe for the Nazi takeover.

Becker's thesis, that killing others offers a kind of illusory immortality, and is a major aspect of the denial of death, was the inspiration for my starting to write this book. While he focused on killing others as a way of gaining some control over death, there are obviously many other pathways to achieve control. Given our limited life span, all these methods are somewhat illusory, but it is the illusion that so often allows us to function. Kings from time immemorial have had slaves and servants killed and buried with them. Becker and later Lasch, (1979) have pointed to the role of (secondary) narcissism in the genesis of the sado-masochistic killer. Rank pointed it out early on in discussing human and animal sacrifice (Rank, 1932, pp. 300–324). I must put this mode of coping with death at the very bottom of the list. *It is evil.* It is destructive of the self and others. It has caused the greatest misery of mankind. So many human leaders, through the ages, have been killers—Attila the Hun, Hitler, Mussolini, Stalin. We have often elected generals to be our leaders, even though generals are trained in killing, and obliviousness to the death of others.

Stalin said, "A single death is a tragedy, a million deaths is a statistic" (Seldes, 1967).* Presidents Grant, Jackson, and Eisenhower were all generals. We sometimes get a glimpse of what generals really think about killing. General Sherman certainly didn't show much compassion for his own men (much less the enemy).

> I begin to regard the death and mangling of a couple thousand men as a small affair, a kind of morning dash—and it may be well that we become so hardened. (Seldes, 1967, quoting William T. Sherman, in a Letter to his wife, July 1864, in *The Great Quotations*, p. 254)

The armed service and war record of candidates for public office is often cited as evidence pro or con their abilities to govern! We still worship the war hero, while we secretly recognize the fact that he is the consummate killer. Until he got Grant, Lincoln couldn't seem to get his generals to attack. Not all generals have the ability. Not all generals cut a swath of death and destruction such as Sherman and Attila did. It seems there are degrees of slaughter!

Are there then degrees of evil? One might say that evil, like beauty, is in the eye of the beholder. Yet there are certain areas of agreement on what constitutes evil, and I think these may even be cross-cultural. The most basic idea is that taking a life is evil. In some cultures killing a fly or a grasshopper would be considered evil. but in Western societies, only the killing of higher mammals is considered evil. Even this belief is not consistent, since there are groups who still hunt, or believe that "lower" forms of life can be killed with impunity. The conflict generated over the protection of the spotted owl in the U.S. Northwest, for example, has pitted the forest industry against the conservationists.

The animal rights activists are seen as a threat by the Christian Right. This may have something to do with the fundamentalist belief that we are not descended from animals. Phylogenetic continuity is frightening to all humans, when they confront their individual rapacity. Some writers (Norman Brown, for one) have suggested that man is a tube stuffed at one end with thousands of living things, which all come out excrement, and that this is our Achilles' Heel.

It is hard to define evil, but by breaking it down as a concept we may be able to get a better grip on it. Evil can be seen as an outside force, or it can be viewed as internally generated. If viewed as an outside force, it can be either a projection of the individual's inner socially unacceptable impulses, or simply as a force of nature (with or without personification).

---

* Quoted by Anne Fremantle, *The New York* Book Review, Sept. 28, 1958, in *The Great Quotations* compiled by George Seldes, Pocket Books, New York, p. 255.

The projection of internal evil onto such figures as the Devil, Satan, Beelzebub, Mephistopheles, or Old Scratch is older than the Bible. While Satan didn't appear in Christian theology until about 300 A.D., such evil gods as Ahriman (the Zoroastrian dark side of Ahura Mazda) and the Egyptian deity Set had been around for thousands of years (Pagels, 1995). Angry or punitive gods appear in almost all mythologies, and it is not too much of a conjecture to say that the bad feelings of mankind have been projected onto these bad gods since time immemorial.

However, these gods also represent the destructive forces of nature, and to that extent are not projections. The personification of wind, water, and fire is common. We need explanations for these evil forces that will drown us, burn us, freeze us, and in the final instance kill us (Death as the grim reaper). Such Gods as Poseidon (the sea god) and Haephestus (fire) were powerful but not basically evil. A god such as Loki, Siva, or Ahriman would be closer to Satan, because of the threat of death and the guile of the trickster. In numerous stories, Satan tricks people into giving up their souls (as in *The Devil and Daniel Webster*). Loki could change himself into various forms, often dangerous or poisonous ones, such as the Midgard Serpent. These gods who represent the exogenous evils of nature can be propitiated, and with prayer, sacrifice, and good luck one can possibly escape those seemingly uncontrollable forces in the natural world.

What about endogenous evil? This inner evil, the dark side of ourselves, or "shadow self," can be labeled variously as the Devil, "the unconscious," the "id," "aggressive impulses," or "sinful thoughts." This inner evil has been handled by religions through human sacrifice, then animal sacrifice, and through confession. There are also various forms of exorcism, such as inducing vomiting, which help to rid the body of evil. The sickness or poison is often sucked out by the shaman. He then spits out arrowheads or other objects to demonstrate what was causing the problem. The shaman and curandero lie halfway between religion and modern medicine. The modern Western healing professions have handled inner evil (and the conflict it sometimes causes) through psychotherapy and drug therapy. It was not very long ago that hydrotherapy (hosing with alternately hot and cold water, and baths in cold water) was used in the United States, and frontal lobe surgery and electroconvulsive shock therapy are still in use to some extent.

Unfortunately, a much more common method of dealing with endogenous evil is to project it onto living targets or scapegoats. For example, in the Serbian–Bosnian conflict, if you are feeling "dirty" inside, then you "cleanse" yourself by projecting filth onto your neighbors, who are then easier to rape or kill. (While this ignores the conscious political manipulation involved in the "ethnic cleansing" of this particular war, the element of "demonization" is still clearly present.) Cleansing suggests washing away your own sins by sacrificing others.

Becker has made killing (and secondarily sacrifice) the central thesis of his book, *Denial of Death*. He emphasizes the human striving for immortality. Since killing others seems to imply the power over life and death, the killer assumes a sort of pseudo-immortality. Less emphasized in Becker's writing is the role of projection in alleviating one's bad feelings. The link between the striving for immortality and projection is found in part by Becker's concepts of righteousness and perfectionism.

A general theory of the origins of human evil is that it is caused by "man's hunger for righteous self-expansion and perpetuation" (Becker, 1976, p. 135). Again, "Evil comes from man's urge to heroic victory over evil" (Becker, 1976, p. 136). In his vulnerability (against eventual death) and in his perfectionism, Becker sees a "second evil." "In proving his worth, he destroys others."

If one's self-esteem, or worth, is central to one's feeling right (and righteous), then getting rid of one's "bad" self by projection onto some imaginary figure, such as the Devil or Lady Luck or Fate is one method of preserving self-esteem ("Born to Be Bad," "The Bad Seed," "My father was an alcoholic," etc.). A more extreme method is through projection onto a living enemy (through the process of "enmification" (Rieber, 1997) or demonization. If the Devil did it, then no human need be hurt. But if the "Red Devils," or the "Great Satan" (the United States as seen by Saddam Hussein of Iraq) did it, then they must die.

"Cleansing" appears as a theme in Hitler's *Mein Kampf*, and in the writings of Julius Streicher and Paul Goebbels. Lady Macbeth wanted to wash away the murders she committed, but the "damned spot" would not come out despite her somnambulatory hand washing. Perhaps she should have demonized some ethnic group, and then she could have cleansed herself and Macbeth too. You can "wash away" your sins by the sacrifice of others. We still believe in this principle. Jesus died on the cross for us—to redeem our sins. Saint Sebastian and other martyrs become holy through their redemption of the sins of ordinary humans. By crucifixion, or with arrows, the victim of sacrifice cleanses the victimizers, and at the same time the society to which they belong.

Sacrifice is also a convenient way to get rid of your enemy, at the same time making this killing into a "holy" cause. Thus the Germans in World War I had the motto "Gott mit uns." The British and Americans have killed "for King and Country," or "God and Country." The Japanese kamikase pilot dies for the Emperor and Japan. The call to combat always has an evangelical tone. The Arab "jihad" is translated as a "holy war."

Before you can kill or harm with impunity, you must demonize or animalize to make your targets inhuman. This makes it permissible to kill them, since they are now a lower order of being. Blacks have been called monkeys and apes. The Nazis depicted Jews as bestial rapists, lusting for Aryan women, and sacrificing Gentile children in secret religious ceremonies. This was certainly a projection of their own bestiality, for this is just what they did to Jewish and Gypsy women and children. (This is not to deny that there was conscious manipulation of imagery on the part of the Nazi propaganda machine, but even those images had to come from somewhere.) Once demonized, these victims could more easily be sacrificed.

Demonization is frequently used by fundamentalist preachers, such as Pat Robertson. He makes references to the "international (European) bankers" who control the world through their money. The unwritten connection is to the Rothschild family, and to Jewish bankers. Sometimes these accusations are not so indirect.

Demonization and scapegoating are becoming more open in the war against the "little people" in the United States. Welfare families have recently been compared to dependent alligators and wolves that were unable to forage for themselves in the wild. They had become "dependent" on humans to feed them. The obvious implication is that we should abolish Welfare, since it makes these "animals" too dependent, and forces us to pay taxes to support them. If rabbits or mice had been chosen as the dependent animal models, there would have been little demonization, but alligators and wolves are already seen as hungry and rapacious.

Racism, sexism, and homophobia make demons who then must be sacrificed. Blacks are pictured as killers or Welfare cheats. A notorious example is the publicity given to the release of Willie Horton, a Black who murdered while on parole. His release played a large part in George Bush's presidential campaign against Michael Dukakis, who was Governor of Massachusetts at the time of Horton's release. That may have cost Dukakis the presidential election, yet he was not personally responsible for reviewing the parole board's decisions. Again, the element of conscious manipulation of scapegoat symbols was used to call forth the latent (if not unconscious) racism of the general population.

A specialized form of demonization could be called "animalization." In an imaginative list of epithets applied to criminals, Fjerkenstad includes "Animals, perverts, dogs, mongrels, coyotes" (Fjerkenstad, 1990, in Zweig, 1991, p. 226). To this list might be added the label of "pig," commonly applied to the police in the United States during the 1960s. The French are known to apply the name "camel" to their worst enemies. The Germans (as mentioned before) at one time preferred the term "Schweinhund" (pig-dog). The origins of "animalization" can be found in the extreme and uninhibited sexual and aggressive behavior of animals, and their "dirtiness." Becker wrote about Wilhelm Reich's explanation of the source of (human) evil.

At about the same time that Rank wrote (*about the fear of life and death being the main source of human misery*) Wilhelm Reich, in a few wonderful pages in *The Mass Psychology of Fascism*, laid bare the dynamic of human misery on this planet. It all stems from man trying to be other than he is, trying to deny his animal nature. This, says Reich, is the cause of all psychic illness, sadism, and war. The guiding principles of the formation of all human ideology "harp on the same monotonous tune: 'We are not animals'" (Becker, 1976, pp. 92–93, referring to Wilhelm Reich, *The Mass Psychology of Facism*, 1933, Farrar, Strauss, New York, 1970, pp. 334ff.) (In quoting Reich's early work, I am not supporting his later work on the orgone, which was probably the result of his developing mental illness.)

The opposite side of his animality is man's morality, his striving for perfection, purity, and righteousness. These terms, unfortunately, are often used by politicians and propagandists, to promote the very "animal" behavior that they decry in others. A good example is the "Moral Majority" movement in the United States, or the sudden emphasis on "family values" by the right wing in politics. The recent book of William Bennett, a collection of stories whose object is to promote ethics and morality, and the writing of Gertrude Himmelfarb (*The De-Moralization of Society: From Victorian Virtues to Modern Values*) are examples of a wave of concern about multiculturalism, Welfare, and similar worries of the right wing. A loss of values and of concern for one's fellow man is surely a problem that worries everyone. It is the age-old plaintive cry for more Gemeinschaft, and less Gesellschaft. What one *does* to increase the warmth and consensus of "community" and decrease the coldness, lack of consensus (read multicultural), and legalistic approach of "society" is what makes the difference between the political right, left, and center. The Clinton administration was concerned with "communitarianism," but did not favor cutting basic services and "safety nets" in order to achieve that end. In a period of rapid social change, the cry for more "community" is like a rush backward to some form of revivalistic nativism. The exhumation of myths, the glorification of the past and national history—particularly of war—and the search for universal and unchanging values are symptoms of a dying or at least a rapidly changing culture.

Further insights about the concept of evil, and the mechanisms that encourage it, can be gleaned from an article in *The New Yorker* magazine, "Explaining Hitler," by Ron Rosenbaum (1995). Rosenbaum's main thesis is that our explanations of Hitler's evil vary widely, and tell as much about us as they do about him. In the process of making this point, he offers some fascinating discussion of the difference between what I would call two types of endogenous evil. One is the conscious manipulation by a politician or leader who orders killing to achieve political ends. The other is also an "inner" type of evil (since it is not an external force of nature—it is man-made evil). Yet it comes from the "true believer," who kills or orders killings because of a strong belief system. We might label these two types as the psychopath (manipulator) and the schizoid (true believer, who may even hallucinate). This would be doing an injustice to the concepts, however, since psychopathological labels may obscure the differences rather than clarify them. We tend to view the conscious manipulator as more evil than the true believer, but the consequences for his victim are the same.

We also tend to think of leaders as more likely to be manipulators, while followers are more often true believers. The true believer may have a "socially patterned defect," the term coined by Erich Fromm for a character trait that is so generally accepted in the culture that it has no negative social consequences for the individual. Quite the opposite, it may enhance his acceptance and self-esteem, for he is surrounded by others with the same defect. The "authoritarian personality" is a patterned defect, and we find it not only in Germany in the Hitler era, but widespread in the United States, and perhaps in Japan, Russia, and other countries. The blind obedience to a higher authority can involve killing, racial prejudice, and religious or political fanaticism. Rosenbaum (1995) contrasts the view of Hitler held by two British historians. One, Hugh Trevor-Roper, thought Hitler was a "true believer." "The development of a coherent philosophy in his book, *Mein Kampf*, showed that Hitler was sincere" (Rosenbaum, 1995, p. 61). This was almost perceived as a virtue. He called Hitler a "wizard," and "enchanter" (Rosenbaum, 1995, p. 58). Rosenbaum says that Trevor-Roper (at least initially) couldn't believe that a human being could be so depraved as to commit Hitler's crimes without being "convinced of his own rectitude." In contrast, Alan Bullock (and to some extent, Emil Fackenheim), saw Hitler as an "opportunist, a mountebank." Rosenbaum defines a mountebank as a public figure who is on a grander scale than the con man or charlatan—"a person who is both cynical and manipulative" (Rosenbaum, 1995, p. 61). The word "rectitude" seems to echo Becker's concept of "righteousness." Becker sees the main source of evil in "man's hunger for righteous self-expansion and perpetration." As long as man has the feeling of righteousness, of the correctness of his cause, he can do evil things without guilt or remorse. When killing or torture go against his early moral training, he is able to invoke his righteousness, "true belief" system. This needs the assistance of dissociation, however. The process of splitting off the bad part of the self, so it can seemingly act on its own, is assisted by the strong belief system. The term "schitomatization" has been used to describe this mechanism. A related mechanism is called "doubling" by Robert Jay Lifton.

He describes how the Nazi doctors who tortured prisoners and even performed vivisections without anesthetics could behave in ways so opposed to their roles as doctors, as healers. He uses the term "doubling" to mean "...the division of the self into two functioning wholes, so that a part-self acts as an entire self" (Lifton, 1986, p. 218, in Zweig, 1991). He distinguishes between "doubling" and other types of splitting, or dissociation, as follows; the term splitting can describe the "psychic numbing" or suppression of feeling that the Nazi doctors underwent, but it cannot account for the autonomous functioning of a "divided self" (actually two virtually independent selves) over long periods of time. The term "shadow self" is somewhat similar to Freud's term, "the unconscious," but it is seen as a more autonomous set of "elements repressed from consciousness" (Whitmont, 1991, p. 15, in Zweig, 1991).

Projection, a mechanism related to doubling, has been discussed previously. The "evil" elements in the unconscious mind, usually sexual or aggressive, are dealt with by projecting them, primarily onto a human target or victim. For example, if you are stingy, then you rail against "stingy Jews" (or in the Orient outside China, against "stingy Chinese.") If you have unacceptable sexual fantasies, the Blacks, Gypsies, and in Nazi Germany, the Jews, become "sexual beasts" who rape your "pure, Aryan" women. Note how the ideas of purity and cleansing keep coming up (as in "ethnic cleansing" in Bosnia). Doubling and projection often go hand in hand, but they need not necessarily appear simultaneously. They are really independent ways of handling internal conflict. But what if there is no conflict? What if what we, as observers, consider to be "evil behavior" is actually institutionalized in a particular society or subgroup? Homicide, torture, rape, and arson can be acceptable behavior when the society condones it, or under special conditions. This behavior is usually viewed as psychopathy. It could also occur in a person diagnosed as having a "character disorder." When it is widely condoned or even encouraged, in what Erich Fromm called a "socially patterned defect," the rates of such behavior go up. It may become a way of life. Again, if the racist or killer is surrounded by others of his ilk, he is not ostracized, and eventually he feels no guilt. His need for projection diminishes. The internal conflict is alleviated. (What happens after he has killed all his targets for projection is another story. He may turn on himself or family members in his need to cleanse himself. The institutionalization of violence alleviates guilt. An example is the "My Lai" incident, in which an American officer, Lieutenant Calley, led his men in a massacre of Vietnamese women and children in an undefended village. The authority of the Army sanctions killing. The very purpose of war (at least in the view of the Armed Forces) is to kill the enemy. We use the euphemism "Department of Defense" to describe the directors of our armed forces. Only a short while ago, the same department was called the War Department. Now it seems we must appear to be attacked, (defense) but never appear to be the attacker (war).

You might develop three types of homicide to parallel Durkheim's three types of suicide (Durkheim, 1897). The egoistic homicide would be one in which the killer kills for personal purposes—for revenge, for personal gain, or in a fit of rage. The anomic homicide would occur when society is so deregulated that killing occurs without social encouragement or disparagement. It is like the killing of mice by their fellow mice in cramped quarters, where all the rules of mouse society have been abolished. The altruistic homicide (if such a concept is not an oxymoron) occurs in an Army, where soldiers are expected to kill for the sake of society (not for personal gain, and because they are regulated, not because of deregulation). Assisted suicide might also be considered a type of altruistic homicide.

Now these pure "ideal types" are never found in real life. Living human beings always show a mixture of these extreme constructs. One example of the mixed quality of what at first appeared to be an "altruistic homicide" is the case of Myrna Lebov, 52, and her husband, George Delury, 62. Myrna was dying a slow death, progressively crippled by multiple sclerosis. She wrote her sister a letter, saying:

> I've been trapped in my life, with no escape except suicide. My life is over, It's time to end it. (I'm) tired of bodily functions being my major concern. And how helpless I have become! I can't do much for myself anymore. Can't cut my food, touch type. (James, 1995)

Unfortunately for him, George wrote a diary, in which he alternately grieved for his wife and raged against her and against his fate in having to take care of her night and day. He was near the end of his rope.

At one point, for example, he wrote in the diary that he wanted to say to Ms. Lebov:

> 'You are sucking my life out of me like a vampire and nobody cares. In fact, it would appear that I am about to be cast in the role of a villain because I no longer believe in you.' (Belluck, 1996, see also Goldberg, 1995)

George was arraigned on charges of second-degree manslaughter, pleaded guilty to second-degree attempted manslaughter, and served several months in prison.

Was this an altruistic homicide, an assisted suicide, or a selfish egoistic homicide? George says that his diary showed "the complex tortured feelings associated with taking care of a loved one who is so ill." Though this was bad for the individuals, it was helpful to the process of justice. If a lesson can be drawn from this sad tale, it is "Never keep a diary or make a tape!" Richard Nixon and Senator Bob Packwood are examples of politicians who were ruined when their private thoughts and conversations were made public. Detective Mark Fuhrmann, a prosecution witness in the O. J. Simpson trial, should never have made a tape revealing his racist sentiments. However much it influenced the outcome of the trial, it almost destroyed his own career.

As another example, real-life "altruistic homicide" (killing for God and country) is never clear-cut. The phrase, "I was only obeying orders" is often mixed with words of guilt, remorse, or regret (in descending order). This excuse for killing must be as old as mankind. A horrifying example comes from Argentina. A former officer confesses after 10 years that he dumped drugged victims into the ocean from airplanes after stripping them naked. They were the "desaparecidos," the disappeared ones, who were killed by the Argentine dictatorship. At first there was some guilt about this act, and there are still feelings of remorse 10 years later that brought this officer to voluntarily confess his crimes (for which he has not been punished)! Yet he overcame his bad feelings (his loss of self-esteem and righteousness?) soon enough, and made several murderous trips. He was, after all, "only following orders." His ambivalence is evident when he talks:

> At first it didn't bother me that I was dumping these bodies into the ocean because as far as I was concerned, they were war prisoners. There were men and women, and I had no idea who they were or what they had done. I was following orders. I did not get too close to the prisoners, and they had no idea what was going to happen to them. But I would be a hypocrite if I said that I am repentant for what I did. I don't repent because I am convinced that I was acting under orders and that we were fighting a war ... I have spent many nights sleeping in the plazas of Buenos Aires with a bottle of wine, trying to forget ... I have ruined my life. I have to have the radio or television on at all times or something to distract me. Sometimes I am afraid to be alone with my thoughts. (Sims, 1995)

In 1999 notebooks of Eichmann were found, in which he claimed that he was "only following orders" when he zealously pursued the goal of killing millions. He blamed his authoritarian Germanic upbringing for his adherence to orders. He even said that while living in Argentina, where he fled after the war, he longed to return to a stricter society where everyone was told what to do. This strongly supports Erich Fromm's thesis that the authoritarian society offers an "escape from freedom."

In the narrowest sense, killing during war is "altruistic," since it is being done ostensibly not for one's own gratification, but out of a sense of duty to one's country, to God, or to some political credo. The "true believer" is more altruistic, since he is convinced of the righteousness of his behavior and his cause. Yet Navy Commander Adolfo Francisco Scilingo, who estimates that the flights killed 2000 people, was the first Argentine officer to describe the killings (voluntarily), and he is obviously suffering from the after-effects of his participation. He is clearly not a "true believer"; he knows that what he did was wrong, and against the tenets of the Catholic Church. He is depressed, but the magic words "I was acting under orders" seem to preserve his last bit of self-esteem. If there can be degrees of altruism, this is certainly near the bottom of the scale!

When leaders order killings, they cannot claim they were following orders. They *give* the orders. It is their responsibility. Rosenbaum (1995, p. 64) tells of an incident related by Hitler's secretary. After Hitler ordered his S. A. Generals killed in the "Night of the Long Knives," he said to her, "So ... now I have had a bath and I am as clean as a newborn babe again." Rosenbaum sees this as documenting Hitler's cynicism as a cruel joke. "Rather than being convinced of his own rectitude, he is making an obscene joke about it." One could also argue that this is evidence of dissociation. In such a dissociated state, one can really believe that a bath will wash away the sins and the blood. In such states, the true believer and the charlatan can coexist. The argument of whether Hitler was a true believer or a charlatan is not resolved.

Rosenbaum recognizes the problem when he says that at some point even the charlatan begins to believe in his facade, his public face (which is a lie) (Rosenbaum, 1995, p. 67). The private dark "shadow self" can live side by side with the public *persona* or mask. Rosenbaum also shows how Bullock changed his position. Initially he saw Hitler as "a man of shrewdly rational calculation; a human scale schemer." He quotes Aristotle: "Men become tyrants because they wish to exercise power." Later he saw Hitler's ideology as armor against remorse (Rosenbaum, 1995, p. 67).

In our search for the role of the fear of death and dying in molding our lives, we have focused on many patterns and mechanisms, such as obsessive behavior, creativity (which is often related), counterphobic behavior, reproduction, religion, etc. The mechanism of projection is used in everyday life, but it is especially common in killing and prejudice. To understand evil, we ought to examine the details of projection further.

Gustav Ichheiser (1944) said that the stereotypes of target groups were actually a projection of the unconscious itself, not just its contents. The very qualities of the unconscious, its sneakiness, the way it worked behind the scenes, its uncontrollability (all as shown by slips of the tongue and by dreams), and its dark and mysterious aspect, he saw projected onto minorities in Germany, particularly onto Jews and Gypsies. He asked his subjects whether they feared swindlers or gangsters more. The swindlers could cheat you, the gangsters might kill you. He found that prejudiced people feared swindlers more than gangsters. The sneaky, hidden, and uncontrollable attack was seen as more dangerous than the concrete, open, but life-threatening assault. This fear of the unstructured, the abstract, seems related to Erich Fromm's ideas in *Escape from Freedom*.

Again, the authoritarian personality demands direction and structure, and finds "freedom" frightening. Independence implies isolation and loneliness, and for some, this is worse than death. Being at the mercy of your sneaky unconscious also implies loss of control. (This comes out so clearly in the case of the Argentinean officer, who had to have the TV or the radio on constantly after he had slaughtered thirty "desaparecidos.") The willingness to lose some control, to free your associations, and to be a little isolated from society constitute some of the requirements for creativity and innovation.

It is a truism that sexual and economic stereotypes are based on repressed material. Ichheiser pointed out that in the United States, Blacks bore the "sexual beast" stereotype, while Jews bore the cheating-lying-penny-pinching economic stereotype. In Nazi Germany, he noted, the Jews were labeled "sexual beasts" (by Julius Streicher) as well as being called "international bankers." There were not enough Blacks in Germany at that time to transform them into a sexual enemy.

While the enemies created by racial and religious prejudice have provided a steady stream of alleviation for "bad feelings," the most effective pain reliever is war, in one form of another. Becker (1976, p. 137) explains how people, through their leaders, gain "self-expansion in righteousness." This is achieved through religious rites, worship of the economy, contracts, and covenants (read Gingrich Republicans' "Contract with America" versus Clinton Democrats' "Covenant") and through waging war. The war that is waged against a foreign country is the best type of war (if there is any such thing), for it has the function of producing cohesion in the society of the attacker and the attacked. It is also a great opportunity to be righteous, even self-righteous. Our "Desert Storm" war on Iraq was righteous, and so was our venture in Somalia. Our war in Vietnam started out "righteous," and later became a source of social conflict, rather than social cohesion.

War is used as a metaphor, and it always seems to stir the emotions. We now have a virtual war on Welfare clients, minorities, and homosexuals, a "war on crime," a "war on drugs," and we even had a "war on poverty" a while back. At least the "war on poverty" had clear goals of alleviating suffering, rather than producing it. People seem to be aroused by the war metaphor, no matter what the goal. Fighting seems to make for cohesion, as long as you can identify an enemy. It is a rallying cry. A joke is told about a conference of experts at a meeting of various groups fighting race prejudice. The chairman said "We need a new motto; not some namby-pamby phrase like 'Speak out against Bigots.' One eager young man shouted 'I've got it! How about "Fuck Hate?"'" What is funny about this joke (if anything) is the self-righteous anger suggested. One has to "hate hate," which seems contradictory, to say the least. (I looked up the origin of "oxymoron," which certainly fits "hate hate." It comes from "oxy" meaning sharp or acid, and "moros," meaning dull. This word should be used sparingly!)

The need for righteous self-expansion is not the only prerequisite for the creation of evil (endogenous evil, as we distinguish it from natural or exogenous evil). Becker outlines some of these prerequisites in *Escape from Evil* (Becker, 1976, p. 134). First is "unselfish devotion." This may be coupled with "hyper-dependence." He sees Evil (aggression) as not innate, but as a function of child rearing. I can say that my own research showed that "cold" parents and "punitive" parents had children who years later were more antisocial, more likely to get into trouble with police, and were more assaultive. Becker sees independence, initiative, stability, and self-reliance (via Ralph Waldo Emerson) as qualities that enable mankind to avoid ("sado-masochistic") scapegoating. He leans heavily on Fromm's concept of "autonomy." The autonomous individual has no need for scapegoating or killing (evil).

At various places we have talked about the importance of the fear of death in creating our choices of life patterns. Here is the key to linking fear of death to endogenous man-made evil. As Becker so brilliantly puts it "... evil comes from man's urge to heroic victory over evil." Using our breakdown of evil to clarify this statement, endogenous (man-made) evil comes from man's desire for a victory over exogenous (natural evil), as manifested primarily by death. What Becker is really saying is that DEATH ITSELF IS THE GREAT NATURAL EVIL, AND TO ESCAPE IT, MAN SEEKS IMMORTALITY IN SOME FORM. IN SEEKING IMMORTALITY THROUGH FOLLOWING POLITICAL OR RELIGIOUS "CAUSES," HE CREATES THE GREAT MAN-MADE EVILS OF KILLING AND OTHER AGGRESSIONS.

What struck me so forcibly when reading *Escape from Evil* was that Becker gave very little credit to death (the greatest exogenous or natural evil) for driving us on *positive* life paths. He does mention that the great religions (whose genesis is generally considered to be found in an attempt to deal with death) have all preached brotherly love in some form. (This love sometimes did not extend to those outside one's tribe or family, but love of siblings, family, clan, and tribe was generally supported.) Yet Becker sees this as an exception to his basic theme that the search for immortality leads ultimately to the destruction of others. (To paraphrase "The paths of glory lead but to the grave," we might say "The paths of glory lead but to someone else's grave.")

It struck my mind so sharply that man has many ways of achieving some semblance of immortality (and by boosting his self-esteem and his feeling "right," achieves a state of grace that will be to his advantage in heaven too, should he still be a believer). Some of these negative (evil) mechanisms and behaviors fall short of murder: for example, prejudice, economic selfishness, monopolization of power or worldly goods, counterphobic behavior, gambling, control of others through memorials and wills, and so on. I felt that artistic or scientific creativity, charity, and love (caring for others, especially strangers, and the protection of the helpless), humor, and religion (when not used as a rallying cry for slaughtering an outgroup) and some forms of obsessional behavior (which has given us our museums and much of our science) are just as important as homicide, and are just as surely connected to our striving for immortality and to our fight against death.

Most of these behaviors make a person feel good, feel "right." Some of them are more simplistically related to our quest for immortality, such as creativity that is the striving for immortality through literature, art, music, and science. The link between having children and the fight against death couldn't be clearer. The King always wants a child to bear the family name and ascend to the throne. "The King is dead, long live the King."

Of special interest is charitable behavior. I might call this the Good Samaritan complex. In these times of rampant self-interest (at least in our culture) it may be hard to understand why people go out of their way to help others, even sacrificing their lives at times. Sociobiologists (creatures of our time) would try to explain away this altruistic behavior by various biological mechanisms. A mother nursing her own child is responding to the size of its eyes, the unbearable piercing tone of its cries, or the pressure of her milk, all of which can be stopped only by nursing or strangling.

We are shocked by the mother of 6-year-old Elisa Izquierdo, who punished her child for defecating on the floor by pushing a hairbrush handle up her rectum, and grinding the child's face in her own feces. She finally beat the child to death. For weeks the news columns obsessed over this tragedy (Haberman, 1995).

Three weeks later, another mother, Debbie Dwyer, slashed her 10-year-old daughter's throat, and then cut her own throat (*The New York Times*, 12/21/95, P. B7).

A few days later Judith Frade brought her unconscious son, age 3, to an emergency room and said he had accidentally drunk her supply of methadone. The doctors found he had black eyes, burn marks on his buttocks, and scars from numerous assaults (Cooper, 1995, p. 43).

Only months before, the two Smith boys were strapped into car seats by their mother, who then shoved the car into a lake and reported them missing.

How can such behavior be explained by evolutionary psychology or sociobiology? How does a mother's infanticide promote the welfare of the species, except in the rare case where the child has a severe congenital defect? (In her study of African wild dogs, Jane Goodall found a "bad mother," who killed many of her own pups and some belonging to another dog. Here is a case of phylogenetic continuity!)

What if a human female nurses an animal? Can this be altruistic? No! She is doing this only to relieve the pressure of the milk in her breasts. While I exaggerate these explanations, they illustrate the biological reductionism currently found everywhere. The ultimate reduction is saying that "your genes are seeking to protect and replicate your gene pool."

What of the altruistic behavior of some animals toward the young of other species? I have seen a photograph of two elephants rescuing a baby hippo from a huge crocodile. They are standing on either side of the baby, and pulling it away from the predator. They are not lactating, The hippo has a short nose, not a long one. Yet they seem to show Christian charity in helping the helpless one, not even one of their own kind. Fundamentalists need have no fear that we will eventually be able to predict and understand all human and animal behavior. We are a long way off, and there is no end in sight.

Becker has laid the foundation for looking at death (and the striving for immortality) as one of our primary motivators, resulting in homicide and related evil. I have just carried his ideas further, to see how fear of death underlies so much of our *positive* behavior.

If death is the great evil, how are Satan (and the devil) connected to death? A church-published pamphlet gives us a modern description of Satan:

> Satan is wily, cunning, deceitful. He works deceitfully, quietly, insidiously. He knows how to arouse our curiosity, and he can play on our insecurities and fears. (Anon., 1990, p. 7)

> Satan can prey upon attitudes, moods and feelings. He is especially tuned to those negative emotions like vanity, pride, hurt feelings, revenge and lust. He is ready to fan

the embers of discontentment into flames of hatred, and is always eager to coax the
first stirring of temptation into the reality of sin. (Anon., 1990, p. 29)

The first thing we notice about Satan is that he is a trickster. Secondly,
hatred and revenge (aggression) and lust and sin (sex) are his two main fields of
expertise. This makes him very much like Loki. He even "transforms himself into
an angel of light" (Anon., 1990, p. 7, quoting Paul in Corinthians 11:14). (Loki
made himself into the Midgard serpent, and surely Satan was at work in the form
of the serpent in the Garden of Eden. Sex and carnal "knowledge" rear their
ugly, poisonous, but fascinating heads.)

The fear of death is always in the unconscious, but breaks through into consciousness from time to time. In this way, it is like repressed sexual and aggressive
content. Satan represents this sinful material, and in addition he stands for Death.
Satan rules in hell, where all but the most righteous must surely end up. Hell and
purgatory are where the dead sinners go, to suffer eternally, and we are all (or
almost all) sinners. In a strange way, hell offers a kind of horrible immortality.

Souls may burn in hell, but they are still immortal souls. The frightening
paintings of Hieronymus Bosch come to mind, with their hordes of the damned
being burned, impaled, and devoured by all manner of monsters and devils.

Death for most of us (except for suicides) is exogenous. It comes from outside, and is generally unwanted (except after prolonged pain, loss, or suffering).
Death is also sneaky, tricking us out of life when we least expect it. In this
respect, death appears to be a trickster. So an exogenous force of nature has a
characteristic that is also the mark of the unconscious (the endogenous, the
sneaky, the tricky, showing itself in dreams and jokes when we least expect it).

When we say "Get thee behind me, Satan!" (and more than 50% of U.S.
citizens still believe in hell and Satan, according to a recent poll quoted in a television news program) we are speaking about our weakly repressed feelings
about sex, aggression, and death. Satan is the trickster talking. He usually promises you money, power, or sex (as in *Faust*, or *The Devil and Daniel Webster*). But
in return, he steals your soul, and you surely will go to hell. That is the price you
pay for worldly goods and power. That is the price of your vanity (another sin).

Satan is the raw unconscious bubbling up. He is the endogenous evil inside
us. How can Satan's death aspect be both inside and outside? Very simply. The
fear of death is repressed, but reappears as Satan. Repression and denial are necessary for proper functioning. Constant thoughts of death are almost totally paralyzing. Personification of Death as Satan, or the Grim Reaper, may seem
primitive, but has less disruptive consequences than demonizing a religious or
ethnic group.

The "death" of Satan as a figure symbolizing evil is lamented in a challenging book by Andrew Delbanco (1995). He traces the history of Satan, and
finds that Satan was originally a term for the inner (endogenous) evil in man.
After centuries, he became an externalized scapegoat for evil, and this was the

start of the loss of the sense of evil. The polymorphous quality of Satan is beautifully described by Delbanco:

> Satan has no essence. He is the torturer and the flatterer, the usurer and the bearer of bribes, the satyr-like angel with the giant and multiple phallus, who knows the wantoness of women; but he can also transform himself into a lascivious temptress with silken skin. He is, in effect, a dark counterpart to Christ: an embodied contradiction, a spirit who chooses, at will, the form of his incarnation. (Delbanco, 1995, p. 27)

The ethical, political, and psychological issues that Delbanco's book raises make it a perfect springboard for exploring the relation of "Evil, Satan, and the Search for Values" in a section that follows.

The exogenous evil of death that is not man-made (not the exaggerated fear of death that occurs in narcissistic and depressed personalities) and the evil of natural catastrophes and forces seem as mysterious as endogenous evil. Why do people envy, hate, and kill each other? Similarly, why do volcanoes erupt, why does lightning strike, why do tornadoes and earthquakes kill thousands, including the innocent? Most incomprehensible of all, why should this happen to me? Why should I have to die? Why should my loved ones die? This is the cry of Job, and of all mankind.

The story of Elaine Pagels, a successful professor of religion at Princeton University who wrote on the history of early Christianity, is of interest here. Within a short time, she lost her husband due to a mountain-climbing accident, and one of her two children due to a sudden fever. She felt assaulted by (external) evil. Her life had been idyllic, and suddenly she was plunged into the depths of despair. As part of her recovery, she wrote a book on evil and demonization in early Christianity (Pagels, 1995). Her intellectual journey started with a search for external evil; the "volcano" was her metaphor. She ended up looking at internal evil in the form of demonization of groups outside the early church. She discovered that there had been a shift away from early Christian (Gnostic) concern with the internal evil in individuals toward the externalization of evil through scapegoating in later Christianity (see "The Devil Problem" in Remnick, 1995). This shift from an internal devil to an externalized (dissociated?) devil, to the projection of the devil's traits onto the stranger, minorities, slaves, or the enemy is similar to Satan's history described by Delbanco as a "loss of the sense of evil."

There is little we can do about natural evil. We have probably pushed the life span close to its limit. We have yet to conquer many viruses, cancer, and the diseases of aging. Bacteria are becoming "fast" (resistant) to the old antibiotics, threatening a resurgence of diseases we thought were part of the past, such as tuberculosis. Few people live beyond 100 years. The life expectancy for white males and females in the United States is around 80. For minorities in the United States it is much less, and for people in underdeveloped countries, it is probably half of that. "Death and taxes" are inevitable. Is it the inevitability of death that makes it so evil? Is it our helplessness, the fear of damnation or the fear of leaving loved ones? (The list of subfears making up the fear of death and dying was discussed earlier.)

What about endogenous evil, the man-made kind? What makes us think some behavior is more evil than others? I would venture that the finality and inescapability of death makes it the greatest evil, greater than man-made evil. For one thing, if man makes evil, it can perhaps be diminished by force, by law, by education. Nothing can be done about exogenous death. Yet, death after a complete life, death with family or friends by the bedside, a quiet and nonpainful death, is better (less evil) than the early death of a child, a lonely death, a protracted or painful death. These may seem minor considerations until one is dying.

The shadings of man-made evil can be even more detailed. First, an act is more evil if it is conscious, deliberate, cold-blooded. To the degree that murder is done in "the heat of passion," our legal system sees it as less evil. Premeditation, in contrast, is more evil.

Second, unprovoked aggression is more evil. Killing in revenge for a previous killing or in self-defense is less evil.

Third, if killing or another evil is done for a cause or ideology, there is a tendency to rationalize it (unless, of course, it is the enemy's ideology, which is always called spurious) as less evil. The "true believer" is usually seen as less evil. He has a belief, a motive, but if this belief doesn't coincide with our own belief system, we are likely to see the act as premeditated and unjustified.

Fourth, the size of the crime seems to affect its enormity. We use the very word "enormity" to indicate evil. A Holocaust killing 6 million people is worse than the killing of 50,000, or of one isolated murder. The killing of 168 people in the bombing of the Federal Building in Oklahoma City is more evil than 20 killed by the Unabomb letter-bomber. [There is the opposite view, expressed by Joseph Stalin, and quoted previously: "A single death is a tragedy, a million deaths is a statistic" (Seldes, 1967, p. 255). This is true when speaking of the psychological impact on the individual who hears of the killing. The law, however, does give great weight to the magnitude of the killing.]

Fifth, killing the innocent and the young is more evil than the killing of adults. One rescuer interviewed after the Oklahoma bombing said he didn't feel so badly about the adults who died, but the killing of 15 innocent children really upset him. He suggested that adults have had time to get into trouble, so they are no longer innocent, implying that maybe they deserved to die! There is also the implication that adults have had a chance to live and enjoy life, while the child who is killed had most of his life span taken away from him.

Sixth, if the "perpetrator" is also a victim, then the killing is felt to be more excusable, or less evil. Pleas for clemency have been based on the criminal having suffered childhood physical or sexual abuse. Being an orphan or an underprivileged minority member have also been grounds for clemency. Murder can be reduced to manslaughter, sentences can be minimized, because the evil-doer had less "choice."

Seventh, mental illness may mitigate or even eliminate punishment, since one must be in his "right mind" in order to commit evil. However, being in a mental hospital may be an equal or worse punishment, given the allowable intrusions upon the person in a mental hospital setting. Evil seems reduced if the evil-doer is operating under a "diminished capacity," or is unable to distinguish right from wrong.

There will never be complete agreement on degrees of evil. These are personal judgments, although the law and the culture may prescribe certain mitigating or exacerbating circumstances or conditions. Some issues are debatable. For example, I would say that for most people, their own death is more evil than that of their enemy, and even more evil than the death of their closest relative; parent, spouse, or child. Many would disagree strongly with this statement, and perhaps even be horrified by it.

That the death of others is less evil or less threatening to us than our own death is made clearer and more palatable when the death involved is that of a person far removed from "ego." An example of the thought processes involved is given by Becker (1976, p. 138). Talking of the killing of the victim of prejudice and demonization, and the motive of the killer, he says:

> He moves in to kill the sacrificial scapegoat with the wave of the crowd, not because he is carried along with the wave, but because he likes the psychological barter of another life for his own. 'You die. not me.'

We can all recognize this feeling. When even a dearly loved person dies, we may at some level experience that "You die, not me" feeling. This also goes under the title of "There, but for the grace of God, go I." Part of the sorrow at a funeral is a grieving for one's own certain death. Each death of the other is a grim reminder of our own mortality. When our age peers start to die in large numbers, this grieving for our own mortality becomes more pronounced.

So many people have tried to explain man's propensity for evil in so many different ways that we can scarcely hope to do the problem justice here. Some think that it is due to our hypothalamus, or the limbic system—some part of the brain that developed early on and is therefore "primitive." But locating a portion of the brain stem that triggers baser emotions and behavior does not solve the problem. Others think that testosterone is the villain. Much higher testosterone levels have been found in criminals, and especially in violent criminals, than in the general male population. The crime rate for men is always higher than the rate for women, especially for crimes of interpersonal violence. Crime rates for younger men are higher than those for older men, and this is another argument to support the role of testosterone.

Others, like Becker, think that fear of death is the primary factor that leads to violence. Some sociologists have talked of the subculture of violence.

(Albert Cohen, *Delinquent Boys*, 1955) and Merton ("Social Structure and Anomie", 1968b), Merton suggests that criminals have internalized the (success) goals of society, but not the socially approved means of attaining those goals (study and hard work). Numerous studies, including the longitudinal study by myself and my colleagues, have shown that violence is associated with two types of early parenting; coldness and punitiveness. Sexual abuse has also been indicted as a cause of violence. All these "causes" may make independent contributions to violent outcome variables in a multifactorial analysis. Despite this, we have yet to assign relative contributory weights to these factors over a large number of studies, so that intervention can be efficiently targeted.

Genetic explanations are confounded with the effects of social class. Twin studies may be more fruitful to test genetic hypotheses, as well as cross-adoption studies of twins (those *adopted* by violent and nonviolent parents, versus those born to violent and non-violent parents). We must also face the fact that not all violence is evil. Circumstances often transform violence into altruism or even heroism, such as killing during wars, in defense of a helpless person, in self-defense, or for a "higher cause."

In summary, we can say that fear of dying often leads to evil, but that it can just as well lead to good. A poet who hopes to write immortal lines (Shakespeare knew his verse would give immortality to those he loved), a scientist who wishes to make a discovery that will be remembered, and a mother who wants to raise children who will live after her, are all motivated in part by their own fear of death and their hope of living on in some way.

EVIL, SATAN, AND THE SEARCH FOR VALUES

Philosophers and theologians have wrestled with the problem of evil for as long as we have written records. I have referred many times to Becker's *Escape from Evil* (1976). His conclusions are essentially pessimistic, but he sees a ray of hope for diminishing evil.

> If men kill out of animal fears, then conceivably fears can always be examined and calmed; but if men kill out of lust, then butchery is a fatality for all time...
> But it is one thing to say that man is not human because he is a vicious animal, and another to say that it is because he is a frightened creature who tries to secure a victory over his limitations...
> So it is the disguise of panic that makes men live in ugliness, and not the natural animal wallowing. It seems to me that this means that evil itself is now amenable to critical analysis and, conceivably, to the sway of reason. (Becker, 1976)

This quote is in striking contradiction to Becker's statement that "... man aggresses not out of frustration and fear, but out of joy, plenitude, love of life." "*Men kill lavishly out of the sublime joy of heroic triumph over evil.*" The triumph over evil (evil that is the certainty of one's own death) is indeed based on fear—on fear of dying. Love of life and fear of death are inextricably intertwined. If one loves life enough, one fears to lose it. The "joy of killing" is based on death fear, as Becker so brilliantly argues. He cannot have his cake and eat it too. Fear, not joy, is basic to killing and evil. He even narrows his comments to "animal fear, fright, and panic" at the conclusion of his book, which I have quoted above.

In two books reviewed by Michiko Kakutani (1995) the historical and religious roots of evil are traced, rather than its psychological roots. These are *The Origin of Satan* (Pagels, 1995) and *Naming the Antichrist* (Fuller, 1995). The main message of both books is that evil is projected onto enemies and outgroups, especially in times of stress and rapid social change. Demonizing others was accomplished by viewing them as the personification of evil, as the devil or Satan himself. To know that such demonization is as old as Christianity, and that it permeates the New Testament gospels, does not help us much with the psychological origins of evil. That times of stress and social change feed massacres, pogroms, and holy crusades is well known. What makes man vulnerable to such behavior and to the leadership of demagogues who arise in such times is less understandable.

Approaching evil from the viewpoint of ethics, history, and literature, Andrew Delbanco says that the loss of Satan as a symbol of (internal) evil has led to a loss of the sense of evil in our society.

> So the work of the devil is everywhere, but no one knows where to find him. We live in the most brutal century in human history, but instead of stepping forward to take the credit, he has rendered himself invisible. Although the names by which he was once designated (in the Christian lexicon he was assigned the name Satan; Marxism substituted phrases like 'exploitative classes'; psychoanalysis preferred terms like 'repression'; and 'neurosis') have been discredited to one degree or another, nothing has come to take their place. The work of this book is therefore to think historically about the shrinking range of phenomena to which accusatory words like 'evil' and 'sin' may still be applied in contemporary life, and to think about what it means to do without them. (Delbanco, 1995, p. 9)

Delbanco seems to shy away from the use of individual psychological mechanisms to explain man's evil behavior. This seems to him to be a way of excusing evil behavior by calling it mental disorder.

> What does it mean to call these monsters (Hitler and Stalin) mentally disordered, and to engage in scholastic debate over whether their brand of madness vitiates their responsibility? Why can we no longer call them evil? (p. 4)

Although Delbanco takes many of his examples of evil from events that took place under the Nazis, there are more recent examples that may lend themselves to the particular question of evil versus illness. The insanity plea has become a battleground between those who see criminal behavior as pure intentional premeditated evil, and those who may abhor it but feel it is conditional on early experience, mental illness, or some exogenous factor in the life of the accused. A 23-year-old apprentice hairdresser killed two women and wounded five people when he attacked two abortion clinics in Brookline, Mass.

> (The defense lawyer, Mr. Carney) maintained that his client was a 'sick, sick young man' who believed that the Roman Catholic Church was being destroyed by a conspiracy involving the Ku Klux Klan, the Mafia and the Freemasons, leading him to kill to 'save the Catholic people.'
> 'In his delusional thinking' Mr. Carney said, 'Mr. Salvi came to believe that Catholic children were being injected with a jelly that made them sterile and that all of us were being monitored by bar codes. As his illness worsened … (he) also began to believe that abortion clinics were being run by the Freemasons, an international secret society whose principles are brotherliness, charity and mutual aid. 'That's why this case is not about abortion, but about insanity,' Mr. Carney said. (Butterfield, 1996, p. A14)

Granted that Salvi's ravings are clearly those of a paranoid schizophrenic, the arguments for his responsibility are several. The murders were carefully planned, and maps of the routes to the two clinics were found in his truck. He also had a newly bought assault rifle and 1000 rounds of hollow-point ammunition, which is used not to wound but to kill. As he killed one receptionist who begged for mercy, he said "That's what you get. You should pray the rosary" (Butterfield, 1996)! On March 18th, 1996, John Salvi 3d was sentenced to two life terms in prison without parole.

It can be argued endlessly that Salvi, although he planned carefully, was merely exhibiting the often striking organization of the paranoid. It is in their initial premises that these individuals are off base, but they more often than not show an uncanny ability to carry out their complex and horrible plots. I would agree with Delbanco that regardless of mental illness, the responsibility lies with the evil-doer. But does that mean he or she should be executed, imprisoned, sent to a mental hospital for life, or eventually be released from the hospital upon regaining sanity? These are the thorny questions.

Delbanco does an excellent job of tracing the history of the concept of evil, and he does it with a literary skill seldom found in such scholarly discussions. Interestingly, he sees himself as a secular liberal, but he is skating on the thin ice that covers the deadly waters of moralism and fundamentalism. It is worthwhile to see who his "enemies" are, and what he proposes as the solution for our loss of the sense of evil.

The Villains

The *ironists*: These are mainly liberals. They think that all talk of morals is "moralistic." They see evil as an illusion. In Truman Capote's book, *In Cold*

Blood, the killer is portrayed poignantly, while the victims are "unbearably wholesome." Joseph Heller's *Catch-22* and Stanley Kubrick's *Dr. Strangelove* are cited as examples of popular irony. The ironic styles of "camp" and "hip" were just new bottles for old vinegar.

The ironist sees morals as "masks for personal preference" and "the distinction between good and evil as suspect." (A recent review by David Glenn of *Irony, Trust, and Commitment in America Today,* by Jedediah Purdy, in *The New York Times,* September 12th, 1998 Book Review, takes the book to task for its right wing leanings. Purdy complains about irony and cynicism, and longs for the spread of the civic virtues and values of his parents. He seems to be another in a long line of Gemeinschaft-lovers, who bemoan today's American morals.)

The rationalists: They want proof, facts, evidence (perhaps are like scientists?) They do not have faith or belief.

"Failure of the imagination:" This is what the evil-doers lack. While this is the key phrase, it is made somewhat more explicit by further definition: "not thinking enough, not feeling enough, not loving enough." Thus the Nazis' "failure of imagination" enabled them to torture and kill without compunction. This idea is akin to Hannah Arendt's "banality of evil." To me, both concepts tend to diminish the concept of evil, and bend over backwards to avoid the psychology of the evil-doer. In using the terms "not feeling enough" and "not loving enough," Delbanco comes closer to the concept of empathy, and this is what is so clearly lacking in the killer, and all lesser degrees of evil-doers.

The fundamentalist: This is the person who demonizes others, usually in some holy cause. Evil is seen as exterior to the self. Projection is not discussed, but implied here.

Self-professed victims: Delbanco mentions the Menendez brothers, who claimed they murdered their parents because of sexual abuse. A more recent article says that:

> Erik, 25, and Lyle, 28, admit they shotgunned their mother and father to death but say they acted out of fear for their lives and because they were suffering from post-traumatic stress disorder after years of physical and sexual abuse by their father. (Anon., 1996)

On March 20th, 1996, the Menendez brothers were convicted of murder. They were sentenced to life imprisonment without parole. The judge found that their argument did not apply, because *they* had initiated the final confrontation, not their parents.

Delbanco also cites Lorena Bobbit's amputation of her husband's penis and her defense's claim that it was the "weapon of her torture." I might add that this claim to victimization has been the butt of humor for centuries. In *The Pirates of Penzance* (Gilbert and Sullivan), the pirates claim that they were all orphans, and that excuses their piracy. There is also the old platitude that a man who murdered his parents threw himself upon the mercy of the court, pleading that he was an orphan.

Self-righteousness: This is a prime characteristic of the fundamentalist. Such people are not open to the ideas of others. They are apt to be members of the Christian right wing, or militia members who would bomb the government into submission. Strangely, this villain is incompatible with another villain, the multiculturalist.

Multiculturalism: The person who fears multiculturalism may very well be self-righteous. I have mentioned Gertrude Himmelfarb and William Bennett as examples of people who know what values and morals are, and make no bones about it. The antimulticulturalist is, almost by definition, self-righteous. How can Delbanco be against both of them? Surely the "politically correct" are capable of outrageous behavior, but making room for other opinions than your own would seem to be a prerequisite for a "good" person.

Anti-universalism: This villain refuses to find absolute truths. He may be a Derrida, always looking underneath the car's hood for engine trouble. He may be a Freud, who looked into the unconscious and the denial of what might be found there. She might be an anthropologist returned from New Guinea, with a new way of looking at American culture. (This villain might be my heroine.)

Value-free attitudes and rootlessness: The avoidance of strongly held values leads to a feeling of rootlessness.

Image of hollow authority figures: "In the ironist's eye every pretender to legitimate authority becomes a Wizard of Oz, and the point is to draw aside the curtain" (as in Derrida's deconstruction).

Authority has always been suspect. How many folktales echo "The Emperor's New Clothes!" Vanity, venality, and brutality have always been associated with rulers, who are self- selected for those traits. The "benevolent despot" is a rare creature. The fall of Nixon is a fine example of the exposure of a hollow authority figure. The tapes revealed a prejudiced manipulative man out for vengeance against his "enemies." True, we tend to denigrate all our leaders now. The Clintons have barely survived the smears of the press and the Republican Party, yet they engaged in enough shady behavior to feed our hunger for scandal. The accusations of Miss Jennifer Flowers, Paula Jones, the Monica Lewinsky "bimbo eruption," and the Whitewater scandal attest again to the fact that all leaders have their Achilles' heels.

The disbelievers: Some of the individual villains in Delbanco's wax museum are Nietzsche, Freud, and anthropologists such as Margaret Mead and Ruth Benedict. They opened up the way for seeing the concept of sin as a hoax. The anthropologists laid the foundations for multiculturalism.

What I find hard to believe is that this "disbelief" is incompatible with basic human values. "Thou shalt not kill" and "Love thy neighbor as thyself" can still be guiding principles. We can draw the line at murder, torture, rape, cannibalism (now very rare), and war. The denigration of women and/or children starts to get into the shadow area, since this is so common in some African and Muslim countries, and in China (where female infanticide is apparently quite common now owing to the limits on children per family). The issue of abortion is also clouded. Is it killing, and in what month does the fetus become a human being? Respect for others' values (as long as those values do not tread on the rights of other individuals and groups in turn) would seem to be a middle ground between the two warring camps of moralists and multiculturalists.

Who are Delbanco's heroes? Of what concepts does he approve?

Heroes

Jonathan Edwards, Ralph Waldo Emerson, John Dewey, Reinhold Niebuhr, and Martin Luther King (all of whom have seen Satan "as a symbol of our own deficient love, our potential for envy and rancor toward creation"), St. Augustine ("evil as essential nothingness"), Richard Rorty, Susan Sontag, and other social critics.

The moralists, who are not afraid of drawing the line between good and evil, who are not afraid of rules, of distinctions between right and wrong. (While Delbanco does not refer to Durkheim here, this lack of socially imposed limits and law is just what Durkheim meant by "anomie.")

The *reverent* and the *believers*: This is in contrast to the rootless and non-believers, who wallow in "nothingness."

Concepts

Transcendence: Delbanco feels that we cannot have love or "imagination" (read "empathy") without transcendence. This is defined as a belief that there is much in the universe that is "not realizable in human experience" (and thus must be taken on faith). Emerson's "transcendentalism" was a "philosophy emphasizing the intuitive and spiritual above the empirical" (Flexner, 1987, p. 2009).

In a praiseful review of *The Death of Satan*, Wendy Doniger, a Professor of the History of Religions, questions the importance of transcendence.

> But can we not have transcendence without God? Can a rationalist, even an ironist, experience transcendence? I think so. (Doniger, 1995)

Imagination: The opposite of the "failure of the imagination." He sees evil as the absence of love (or "limitation," which is part of theological theory). "Sin is ignorance." If we could only imagine what our victims suffer, we would not commit such outrageous crimes against them. (This is describing a failure of empathy.) Delbanco doesn't tell us why empathy has failed, but he tells us in historical detail that it has failed, is still failing, and that it is evil.

While it is only one of many theories of the origins of evil, a failure of empathic ability can stem from excessive control of the child and early deprivation of love, both leading to an inability to love and nurture others (as in Harlow's monkeys, who had substitute mothers made of wire and cloth). Gruen's theories are especially relevant here (the child's self-betrayal — the surrender of autonomy in exchange for love and protection) (Gruen, 1992). This can lead to a rage that has no regard for the welfare of other human beings. A discussion of different theories of evil and aggression will follow later.

In sum, I agree with most of what Delbanco has to say about our losses. What he describes is so beautifully captured in Ferdinand Toennies' concepts of Gemeinschaft and Gesellschaft (Toennies, 1957, 1963). Gemeinschaft stands for "community" and Gesellschaft translates roughly as "society." The Gemeinschaft has common values, a homogeneous population, a consensus based on those common values, emphasizes belief and faith, emotional expression, love and neighborliness, the family, and so forth. The Gesellschaft needs rules, since it is not homogeneous. Owing to lack of consensus, it relies heavily on written law — it is legalistic. It is also rational rather than emotional, scientific rather than religious (facts versus belief). In modern terms it is more multicultural, more heterogeneous. Loyalty to the state is dominant over loyalty to the family.

All of us who are concerned with the current drift of our society probably long for the vanishing Gemeinschaft. How we use the rhetoric, and how we suggest the problem be solved is what separates the political right from the center and left. The "good old days" are in fact an illusion. (There's that devil "irony" again!) In her remarkable book, *A Distant Mirror*, Barbara Tuchman describes the 14th century in France and England (Tuchman, 1978). The Black Plague will kill one third of the population, and wipe out whole cities (read AIDS?) The Catholic Church, despite its high religious ideals, is grinding the peasants and nobles alike for tithes and indulgences, and acting as venal and power hungry as the nobles. The nobility, when they are not exploiting their serfs, are raping and pillaging, and holding other nobles for ransom, despite the rules of chivalry to which they have sworn oaths. When not otherwise engaged, they go on crusades, and justify their savagery and looting by demonizing the "infidels." The peasants and the bourgeoisie rise up, and are crushed by force of arms. Armed gangs roam the countryside, and are for hire by the King, the nobles, or the church.

This litany can be repeated for almost any epoch. The "old West" of Robert Altman ("McCabe and Mrs. Miller") is probably more true to life than the glorified old West of John Ford. Little old New York was the home of the Tammany Hall crooks, and at the turn of the century was rife with gangs of homeless boys who attacked by the hundreds. Nostalgia has a way of smoothing over all the horrors of the past (the repression of the unpleasant?).

What is so annoying to me is that people of obvious good will, such as Delbanco, vitiate their message by the use of misleading verbiage. Evil is not a "failure of the imagination," or "banality" (which term enraged so many critics of Hannah Arendt), or "limitation" or "privation." I think it is based on hatred, not merely on lack of love or lack of empathy. I think the killers who give the orders know that their victims will suffer.

A case in point is quoted by Delbanco. He tells of a true incident described by Primo Levi in *The Drowned and the Saved* (1986). A girl of 16 in Auschwitz who miraculously survives a mass gassing by the Nazis must be killed, because she is a living witness. Even an S. S. officer can't kill her with his own hands, and directs his underling to kill her. Delbanco sees this tale as evidence of a "poverty of imagination" on the part of the officer. Yet the officer obviously *did* understand how the girl would suffer, and that her innocent life would be ended. That is exactly why he could not kill her himself, and assigned the job to a subordinate. When describing the incident, Levi himself says that "compassion and brutality can coexist in the same individual in the same moment" (Delbanco, 1995, p. 232). This is evidence for dissociation (or splitting or doubling) discussed earlier. The compassion for the girl makes the officer turn away, but his hatred of Jews and his S. S. code of duty (his shadow side) lead him to command that she be killed by someone else. He *can* "imagine" that she will die in pain. His conduct is not "banal." He is not even the bureaucratic killer that Eichmann was. He knows what he is doing, and he even knows in one part of his consciousness that it is evil!

Real human beings are not ideal types. The totally evil psychopathic killer is an ideal type at one extreme. Real human beings must use dissociation and denial to avoid losing their self-esteem. They must use projection and demonization (or animalization) to make their victims less worthy of the gift of life. These mechanisms don't excuse evil. They are not necessarily signs of mental illness. They are common to all humans. That they are common doesn't excuse evil behavior. It does explain how compassion and brutality, or good and evil, can exist in one person at the same moment in time. This human capacity to tolerate incompatible behaviors and values within the self is basic to our understanding of man's aptitude for evil.

A recent confession by a (reformed?) modern neo-Nazi, Ingo Hasselbach, illustrates just how dissociation operates, to allow the "shadow" side to work without conflict. During an attack on a house filled with immigrant workers, Ingo and his comrades threw stones and Molotov cocktails (gasoline bombs) against and into the house.

> During the whole action, I never thought about the safety or well-being of the people in the house. They didn't exist for me. Only my friends and I existed. And the Cause, the Party. The foreigners were far away from me somehow, even though I was acting as though they were so much in my way and pasting things* on the walls of their house.* (Signs saying "Foreigners are social parasites," and "German workplaces were taken by foreign workers") (Hasselbach, 1996, p. 48)

The fact that Hasselbach eventually went on tour speaking against neo-Nazism shows that he did have the imagination to know what his victims suffered, although it was split off from the rest of his consciousness during the period of the actual attack. He even said that bombs were the ideal weapon, for they kept a "cleansing distance" between the bombers and their victims! Let no evil-doer be contaminated with the humanity of his prey. That might give rise to empathy, which would ruin everything.

What can be gleaned from this discursive discussion of evil? First, evil can be inner or outer. Inner evil is psychologically harder to deal with, and is often handled through projection onto various scapegoats. These figures must first be demonized or "animalized," so that they are more acceptable targets for aggression. Dissociation is another way of handling inner evil, since it allows one to split evil-doing off from one's basic humanistic values (if any). Some types of killing can be considered almost altruistic, but there is usually evidence of some evil (egoistic) motivation as well. The fear of death motivates much positive behavior (creativity, procreation) as well as negative behavior such as killing and suicide. That is the central theme of this book. There are several mitigators and exacerbators of evil, conditions that make us judge evil to be worse or more excusable.

There are major theories of the origins of evil and violence: neurological, hormonal, subcultural, intrafamilial (child-rearing) and genetic, in addition to fear (of death and life itself). Another theory is that the loss of symbols for evil (Satan) and changing values have allowed evil to flourish unnamed and unrecognized as such. This theory holds that ironists, rationalists, debunkers, and deconstructionists have destroyed our value system. Evil is seen as a "failure of imagination" or as "banal." This explanation falls short. It is clear that to some degree, the failure is *lack of empathic ability*. This in turn may stem from early lack of love, or excessive parental control. All of us, right, left, and center, long for some of the qualities (common values) of community (Gemeinschaft), and bemoan the characteristics of (modern, complex) society (Gesellschaft). How we propose to deal with this loss makes the political difference. Those who would bring back the spirit of community by force should be warned by the Nazi slogans of yesterday: *"Blut und Boden," "racial purity," "Aryan superiority," "ein Volk,"* "the Thousand Year Reich," *"Judenrein,"* and *"Ausländer raus"* (foreigners out).

SUMMARY AND CONCLUSIONS

Since this a summary chapter, I have taken the liberty of using a very condensed style at times. I will be making assertions that may seem like assumptions, without bothering to document them. I will not expatiate on some issues, especially those that have been discussed extensively in previous chapters. Some new material crept in, which I had not considered until the end of my writing. I hope the reader will excuse these liberties.

Life and death are inextricably intertwined. Death is an important part of life. Dying and death are by definition the end of life. Life and death are as closely linked as yang and yin. For this reason, coping with the fear of death and dying, and the struggle for survival, occupy a good deal of our efforts in living.

Death is inevitable. We all die. There is no evidence for an afterlife. All attempts to construct an afterlife are in fact part of man's elaborate system of illusion which he invokes to cope with the fear of death and dying.

Fear of dying is not instinctive. It is learned. It is clearly present in children as young as three in Western cultures. It arises from inevitable momentary periods of abandonment when parents are not immediately available to satisfy the child's needs for food and physical comfort. This fear is realistic, in view of the child's helplessness.

Fear of dying is further reinforced by experiences to which the child is exposed. These can range from the death of a pet to the death of a grandparent or parent; the loss of a parent through divorce or separation; and in many countries the immediate threat of death through war, famine, and natural catastrophes such as floods, freezing, dehydration, and the constant threat of illness. In many countries, wild animals and insects kill humans and spread disease. Painful procedures, such as male and female circumcision, clitoridectomy, and infibulation are done without the permission of children, and in the majority of cases without anesthesia or proper sterile technique. Ashes are rubbed into wounds on the face and body to produce keloid scarring. Pain, by burning or cutting, is still used to induce trance states. It was most popular among the

Plains Indians of North America. Children have been selected for sacrifice and are still sold into slavery, bondage, or prostitution in many parts of the world. Boys as young as 10 are being forcibly recruited as soldiers in several countries. Many children are subjected to sexual abuse by their parents, relatives, or (less often) by strangers. The frequent reports of torture and killing of children remind us that extreme fear of dying is not unrealistic for some children. There has been an unfortunate tendency to play down most accounts of parental sexual abuse since Freud's recanting of his initial impression that the majority of his patients were actually seduced in childhood (see Endnote).

Short of immediate physical threats to the child's life, parental behavior, especially verbal and physical punishment, lability (alternating love and rejection), and coldness can exacerbate fear of death. Extreme control and conditional love can result in the child's loss of autonomy, sacrificed in return for parental love or attention (Gruen). This loss of self results in rage, which can be alleviated only by the child's dissociation (splitting) of feeling and thought, or alterations in the levels of consciousness and changes in identity.

In the middle and upper classes of the United States and Canada, Japan, and probably most of the countries of Western Europe, children are protected from physical threats: the major ills of famine, lack of shelter and clothing, and the usual contagious diseases of childhood, against which they are inoculated. A considerable but unknown portion of these children probably have "good" parents, who do not beat them, verbally abuse them, or reject them with coldness or alternating moods.

Yet even if gross physical and parental threats and stresses are minimal, there are many stresses to which most children are exposed during the process of growing up. There are radical bodily changes, such as the loss of baby teeth, and hormonal changes. These transformations are marked by small or large rites of passage, such as hiding teeth for the "tooth fairy" or puberty rites. Often a loss is involved (teeth, circumcision, scarring) but there are rewards given to compensate (money from the tooth fairy; gifts for the confirmation, Bar or Bat Mitzvah, or graduation; permission to engage in adult activities). Soon there are the demands of school, and its discipline. Study replaces a great deal of the time formerly devoted to play. The peer group is far from consistently friendly. There is teasing, bullying, and sometimes isolation and outright rejection by schoolmates. There is pervasive competition in these cultures: in sports, in scholastic achievement, in friendships and dating, and often between siblings. There are always some viral infections against which there are no inoculations. The long series of vaccinations and pediatric examinations can in themselves be stressful. In addition, children in "advanced" societies are exposed to varying degrees of chemical environmental stresses, such as automobile exhaust, chemical water pollution, and thousands of products containing toxic compounds, such as insecticides, over-the-counter drugs, dry-cleaning fluid, and tobacco smoke.

The average parent (even the "good" parent) can do little to control what happens to her child in school or in the peer group. In general, parents can only control or change the child's nonhome environment by persistent and long-term political action. In the best of circumstances, then, children are subjected to many stresses.

These stresses, starting with early inevitable moments of being left alone and abandoned, initiate a fear of death and dying. Abandonment is clearly tantamount to death for the helpless infant, who cannot survive without a parent. Childhood fears are numerous, and can be considered substitutes or equivalents for fear of dying (fear of thunder, flushing toilets, large pets and animals, insects, dirt, germs, falling, monsters, witches, ghosts, loud noises, kidnapping, etc.) Most of these early fears are replaced by adult fears as the child matures.

Any and all devices are used to keep fear of dying to a minimum, since this fear is so strong that it is paralyzing if constantly in consciousness. These ways of coping with fear of dying fall into groups. Some are social institutions, such as religion or membership in groups. Some are broad personality styles, such as obsessive–compulsive behavior. Others are coping modes such as gambling or counterphobic behavior. Lastly, a large number are defense mechanisms, such as intellectualization, dissociation, repression, and projection.

Life is the great antidote to the inevitability of our own death. Living "fully" is the best medicine. But the "choice" of the best way to live in the face of death is not completely a free choice, and is often determined by early life experiences. Our attitude toward death and especially our choice of the way we cope with our fear of dying actually dominate our lives.

Certainly you can make choices, even in adult life. You can switch from a crippling coping mode, such as the excessive use of drugs and alcohol, or from more obviously lethal behavior such as skydiving, aggressive driving, or smoking, to more positive modes.

To be able to make good "life choices" early on, you must have experienced some love and emotional support in infancy and childhood. If you haven't had love in early life, but instead experienced primarily loss of autonomy and parental coldness, punitiveness, and lability, your coping choices will be limited. Coming from such poor early environments, your coping modes are more likely to be destructive of yourself and others.

The creative individual, the loving person, the one with a sense of humor, will all be able to cope with fear of dying and keep it "on a back burner." In contrast, the gambler, the skydiver, the potential suicide, or killer is poorly defended against fear of dying. These coping "choices" can be ranked in a rough hierarchy, from the most effective to the least effective in dealing with fear of dying, which also coincides more or less with the damage they do to the self and others.

The importance of this attempt to rank-order behaviors and societal supports is discussed in Chapter 11, in a section entitled "Coping Modes in a Moral Framework."

1. *Creativity:* Immersion in art, music, writing, science—immortality through your creations.
2. *Love:* Caring for others, especially for the stranger, lifts the individual out of himself and his fears.
3. *Humor:* Laughing at fate is life enhancing, and perhaps physiologically life-prolonging.
4. *Intellectualization:* The search for scientific or philosophical "secrets," especially the secret of death, which creates a distance from the subject, thus controlling fear.
5. *Procreation:* A way of living on, a form of immortality.
6. *Obsessive–compulsive behavior:* Striving for worldly success or a "state of grace," now often in the form of good health, productivity, and well-roundedness. Routinization of behavior is used as a method of dulling pain and fear.
7. *Living life to the hilt, living better, living longer:* Life as an orgy, or "last fling," keeps death fear away. Living better is part of "worldly asceticism," in which you work hard to achieve a state of grace. By "conspicuous consumption" you prove that you have worked hard. Possessions now stand between us and death—a special kind of obsessive behavior.
   Living longer (than those in your cohort) provides a brief period of illusory immortality.
8. *Group membership:* Belonging to a group, such as the family, state, nation, club, school, or team can give larger meaning to the life of an individual, and act as a strong bulwark against fear of dying.
9. *Religion:* Belief in the afterlife and in metamorphosis can be very effective in reducing the fear of death, and in creating the illusion of immortality.
10. *Mementos and monuments:* Family photo albums, videotapes, an autobiography, diaries, pyramids, trusts, and wills are all ways of gaining a little immortality. Such behavior can reduce fear of death, and create the illusion that the future, after one's demise, can be controlled.
11. *Counterphobic behavior:* Dangerous sports, such as hang gliding, skydiving, mountain climbing, surfing, and contact sports all involve great risk of injury and death. The counterphobe controls death fear by thinking "If I live through this, it will prove I am immortal."
12. *Gambling:* A defiance of fate (and death). While self-destructive in the long run, it preserves hope (of life, of survival) in the short term. It is a mixture of counterphobic behavior and obsessive–compulsive behavior.
13. *Dissociation:* Some people seek oblivion, because their fear of death (or a living death) is so overwhelming. Drug and alcohol use can blot out

fear of death and dying. The dissociation of schizoid thinking is another method of blotting out fear, either of external threats or fear of internal unacceptable impulses. Thus dissociation enables people to rape, torture, and kill with apparent psychological impunity. Schizophrenia, while based on a strong genetic predisposition, can be seen as a mode of coping with an overwhelming awareness of the terror of living and dying.

14. *Repression/denial*: These are closely related terms, describing the rejection from consciousness of intolerable anxiety and fear. Denial (or repression) is a mechanism used to escape the terror of death. It allows fear of dying to be put on a "back burner," so that the individual can function without constant dread and despair.

15. *Suicide*: The majority of Western suicides are a way of preempting death. They say, in effect, "You can't fire (kill) me, I quit!" Of the three wishes involved in suicide suggested by Karl Menninger (*Man Against Himself* 1938); the wish to kill, the wish to be killed, and the wish to die, the least frequent is the wish to die. Fear of a "living death," due to incapacitating illness, career failure, or loss of a loved one, can be a motive for suicide. While motives for suicide are complex, their common element is an attempt to solve a very difficult or even insoluble problem. It is one way of asserting control over the uncontrollable.

16. *Projection, killing, and the problem of evil*: Projection and killing are two mechanisms or coping modes that are closely intertwined. Killing (homicide and the killing of animals) is a special form of the mechanism of denial. The killer gains an illusory immortality by controlling the life or death of others. Thus the killer denies his own death. Projection of one's own unacceptable impulses onto others is a universal mechanism, but it is particularly dominant in the organization of the paranoid personality. The wish to kill is projected onto "the enemy," which then justifies killing him. Dissociation also enables the killer to kill with a minimum of guilt or conflict.

Awareness or consciousness of death fear varies greatly from almost total unconscious repression, through "middle knowledge" (Lifton, 1979, p. 79)* to full conscious awareness and constant obsession with death. The amount of conscious awareness of death must affect the ability of a coping mode to deal with fear of death. If the fear is too intense, no mechanism or coping mode may be able to control it.

Because conscious death fear can be so intense, people try to diminish that conscious awareness. Altering consciousness is a common way of dealing with

---

* The concept was originated by Avery Weisman. Middle knowledge of death is "partial awareness and partial denial," see p. 43 in Stephenson, 1985.

fear of death. These altered states can be induced by alcohol, drugs, religious frenzy, through prolonged dance and exposure to music (especially music with pronounced rhythm), church or other religious services that combine chanting or choral music with elaborate ritual, and meditation (as in Buddhism). These alterations avoid thoughts of death by affecting brain functioning, by focusing attention inward, or by narrowing the range of attention to an icon or a mantra. This produces a deadening or "numbing" that is often experienced as heightened (internal) awareness, but this awareness generally excludes awareness of death and the external environment.

General behavior patterns, such as obsessive–compulsive behavior, are so widespread in Western culture that we do not recognize them as modes of coping with fear of dying. This becomes clearer when we see it as "deep enculturation" (Becker). An outsider's view is also helpful. A Buddhist scholar (Sogyal Rinpoche) says:

> Western (active) laziness … consists of cramming our lives with compulsive activity, so that there is no time at all to confront the real issues. (Rinpoche, 1994, p. 19)

Constant striving, time-filling, time-killing, and time-stopping are all related modes of avoiding thoughts of death and finitude. Television addiction, which is widespread in the United States, starts early in childhood. Many pre-teens, and adults too, spend hours each day glued to the TV set. When excessive, this is probably one of the commonest time-killers of our day.

Each coping mode has its up side and down side. Even the worst choices, as judged by the outside observer, serve some function for the actor. Many behaviors, coping modes, and mechanisms appear to us at first glance as totally "self-destructive," such as gambling, drug abuse, counterphobic behavior, denial (of illness), and especially suicide and murder.

Seen from the viewpoint of the actor, however, gambling may keep up one's hopes, even though it may bring financial ruin. (It can also result in great wealth, if one is lucky in playing the stock market.) Drugs and alcohol act as anodynes to deaden the inevitable pain in life. They stop pain temporarily, but involve a high risk of job loss, marital disintegration, physical injury, or death. Suicide solves an apparently insoluble problem. It offers a choice, when there seems to be no other choice: the choice of life or death. The suicide can take an active rather than a passive role in "solving" his problems. Murder, as Becker pointed out, gives the illusion of immortality. The power to decide whether someone else lives or dies supports a grandiose delusion that the same power is transferable to one's own life.

The circumstances in which a defense mechanism is used can determine whether it is adaptive (and perhaps aids in survival) or is not adaptive. For example, denial in the event of terminal illness may ease the emotional turmoil of facing an often painful death. However, denial in the early stages of lethal cancers may lead to death. The timing of defenses can determine whether they are adaptive or maladaptive.

Even the most positive coping modes come at a price. For example, creativity often demands long periods of solitude and isolation from society. Social relationships may have to be sacrificed for a person to become productive and innovative. Distancing from ordinary society is necessary for the inventive genius, who must avoid total enculturation in order to be innovative—to see things in a new way.

Dissociation and projection underlie those behaviors that are most destructive of others. Wars, torture, racial and religious discrimination, political manipulation, and exploitation of the public are all abetted and enabled by these two modes. Dissociation and projection may protect the actor's (the individual's) self-esteem, for he is not really faced with the evil that he is perpetrating, or with the hatred he bears others. Guilt feelings are diminished or absent. While the actor is protected, these defense mechanisms often spell injury or death for the targets of his anger.

It is common knowledge that when fear is extreme, people are unable to "think straight." As noted before, all life is a struggle for survival, although it is less obvious in developed countries. We were built to fight against death. While most of us no longer fear being eaten by wild animals, our arousal system stems from this early experience of constant danger from both man and animals. This system is archaic, and is often turned against the self. The limbic system, particularly the amygdala and hypothalamus, is the seat of our arousal system, governing emotions, sexuality, and smell. The cerebral cortex, with its two hemispheres, is concerned with functions such as language, visual pattern recognition, perception of melody, and planning of action. The limbic system often overrides the "higher" cognitive processes of thinking and planning. Controlling the arousal system, which is often working overtime when fear of death and dying are involved, is crucial to our emotional and even our physical survival. This control has been characterized by Goleman as the main factor in "emotional intelligence" (Goleman, 1996). Programs that teach children and teenagers to talk rather than attack when they are "dissed" (disrespected or insulted) is an attempt to teach control of the arousal system.

If cognition can triumph over arousal, or at least achieve a balance with it, then fear of dying in general can be reduced. The lethal modes of coping with death, such as suicide and homicide, can be reduced by early training programs of this type. Making children aware of their sexual and aggressive impulses, so that they can control them, is part of this growing education of the emotions.

Fear of (the process of) dying is more common in the elderly ill, who anticipate prolonged pain before death. There is a movement in the medical world to increase the use of pain-killing drugs during terminal illness, even if this runs the risk of addicting the dying. (The U.S. government has made it hazardous for doctors to give adequate pain medication in these cases. The idea of protecting a dying person from drug addiction seems absurd on its face.) The dying elderly may also fear more than younger people for the protection of the dependents they will leave behind, and for the physical deterioration of their bodies.

Fear of death itself, of nonbeing, or loss of the self, may occur at all ages. In a recent Gallup poll (Anonymous, 1997) 42% of a U.S. national sample said that "when they thought about dying, they worried 'a great deal' that God would not forgive them." This indicates the heavy load of guilt feelings that our society engenders. Regrets about tasks not completed in life are also common elements in the fear of death. Fear of death and dying is a complex of fears that varies between individuals and by demographic characteristics. The same Gallup survey found that 72% of the respondents believed in heaven, and four out of five of those who believed said their chances of getting there were excellent or good. Only 56% believed in hell, and only 4% of that group thought they would probably go there. This shows a remarkable optimism, given the current state of our morality.

Some of the defense mechanisms can affect our entire system of government. For example, the greater the dissociation of our leaders, the less democracy we will have. If our leaders dissociate (or if they just alternate between dissociation and just plain lying) then the bond between the leaders and the people is broken. Politicians were probably always unpopular, especially in developed democracies, but nowadays they have lost a great deal of their charisma. The average man becomes cynical when politicians promise one thing and deliver another.

Dissociation is a skill that is often adaptive. It may be a necessary skill for someone who, in the course of leadership, must make many enemies. Our leaders are certainly different from the average man. Presidential candidates usually campaign for years before they can run for national office. Their dedication to that goal is great, and involves unusual sacrifice for them and their families. If dissociation springs from early traumas in those with multiple personality disorder, then there might also be a tendency for preselecting presidential timber from people who have suffered or struggled in early life.

Theodore Roosevelt was in frail health during his early years, and overcame this through macho behavior, such as big game hunting and leading the charge at San Juan Hill during the Spanish–American War. Franklin Roosevelt was transformed by his paralysis due to poliomyelitis in his young adulthood. Many biographers believe that he would never have become president were it not for his need to overcome his illness. Nixon was reported to have suffered poverty when a boy. During his teens Clinton had to protect his mother from his stepfather's violence. I am guessing that the ability to dissociate may stem from some of these early economic and emotional hardships, and that this particular ability serves a president or any politician very well.

The cure for this split between the public and the leaders is to shift as much as we are able from a representative democracy to a participatory democracy.

What has this book, *Choices for Living: Coping with Fear of Dying*, been all about? Can it be of help to all of us who must struggle with our finitude—our existential angst? While I have said that the choices are limited by early experience, this is a time of "protean process." We may have a second, third or fourth chance to "reinvent the self," a phrase we hear ad nauseam nowadays. We may get several chances to make use of coping mechanisms that are less self-destructive, and less destructive of others.

Who will read this book, and perhaps profit by seeing an array of choices for thought and behavior? The homicidal maniac and the psychopath certainly won't read this book.

The creative genius, at the other end of my moral-adaptive hierarchy, is too busy with his own projects to read. In between these extremes there may be readers who will enjoy this book, and benefit from its review of life-paths and coping choices.

Will reading this book reduce fear of dying? That depends on the reader. I hope this book provides insight for readers of various ages—not just those who are closer to death because of aging, but also those just embarking on their adult life journeys. They still have time to make some choices.

Those choices involve the basic contradictions in our values and our culture: family life and enculturation versus isolated creativity, obsession and tunnel vision versus the open mind, repetition versus originality, selfishness versus generosity, gambling and risk-taking versus cautious no-risk living, denial of danger versus "realistic" fear of death and a dangerous world, the social cohesion of the in-group versus multicultural openness with its risk of loss of central values, and so on.

There are strains in our culture, there are built-in value conflicts, there are dilemmas built into our biology (such as sexual and aggressive drives that must be tamed or at least redirected if we are to have a society at all). The individual coping modes are directed and channeled by society, at first through parental practices, then through the peer group, schools, mass media, advertising, and later in the workplace and in organized groups such as churches or informal and voluntary groups of all kinds, such as 4H, Scouts, street gangs, and so on. These agents of society mold the coping choices, so that the "choice" is often not totally voluntary. For example, the Army molds coping behavior by strenuous training, so that the recruit is able to respond to threat with violence and killing. I remember the message "Kill or be killed" being drummed into us by lecture, film, and in bayonet practice during my basic training during World War II. Even further, my officer's training involved a strict code of honor, sacrifice, and endurance of hardship, which was supposed to turn an enlisted man into an "officer and a gentleman." The rapid socialization processes of "total institutions," such as the armed services, hospitals, and police schools, as described by Erving Goffman (1962) may be able to change coping modes temporarily, but recruiting for the armed forces *during peacetime*, and for police and firemen and the clergy has been shown to be more a function of preexisting values than of indoctrination, which merely reinforces those values.

Occupational choice, except when there is a wartime draft, is based more on preselection than on indoctrination or socialization of adults.

For these reasons, choices for living have to be made wider from early childhood on. Parenting has to be taught in school. Avoidance of harsh practices especially must be taught to teenagers who are about to become parents. The suicides and homicides, gambling, drug abuse, and racial violence are often products of early training and modeling on neglectful or violent parents.

This book tries to see coping—even that which is destructive to self and others—as an attempt to go on living, to adapt. This is not to excuse murder or suicide or aggression or oppression. People who make these coping choices must be studied. Since serial killers, multiple personality disorders, suicides, and other pathological behavioral types are rare, studies that seek to define their etiology need a large population base to start with. My belief is that only with very large longitudinal studies and better record keeping can we trace the development of the destructive life paths that plague our society. At the present time, not a great deal is known about the differential early influences leading to psychopathy, dissociational disorders, and depression. More is known about the etiology of schizophrenia and manic–depression, but these disorders are relatively rare compared with psychopathy and depression.

I want to preempt the argument that we so often hear from the right wing in politics, that "these people are not sick. They are just lazy, vicious, bestial, and stupid." The purpose of such longitudinal studies is not to claim victim status for people who behave badly, so that they can use early parental abuse as an excuse for murder. It is to point the way to changes in early experience that will aid in primary prevention. Evil is evil, and the etiology of evil does not excuse it. If it was found that the genesis of the German Holocaust or the slaughter of the Armenians was due in part to extremely rigid and punitive child-rearing practices, it might help to avert another such tragedy. Childhood is not the only period for study. Political factors in genocide must not be overlooked. Who are the killers? The young men among the Hutus, who slaughtered the Tutsis in Rwanda? The bureaucrats who direct them (as suggested by Hannah Arendt's "banality of evil" used in describing Eichmann's role in the German Holocaust)? What is the background of the leaders, such as Hitler or Stalin? Are these factors a necessary but not sufficient condition for genocide?

Not everyone would like to stop the killing, the torture, the deprivation. Those who want to stop it might profit by studies that lay bare its origins. These are complex problems ("multifactorial," in the language of social science). Only massive long-term research and remedial efforts will stem the tide of blood. It may never be eliminated, but it can be reduced. Homicide and crimes of violence dropped as the teenage population of the United States decreased.

Hundreds of early education programs have been started, and some of them have succeeded in reducing dropouts, who usually end up in trouble.

The explanations for evil (see Chapter 18) are legion. A short summary of some of these explanations is given below.*

Some Hypotheses About the Conditions That Enable Humans to Harm or Kill Others (One Definition of Extreme Evil)

1. If a child is raised in an authoritarian family, the father's orders (especially) must be obeyed. This obedience is easily transferred to political leaders or military leaders who order the killing.
2. An ability to dissociate easily enhances the ability to kill or harm. There is a loss of consciousness of the evil act, or a temporary "numbing."
3. Loss of autonomy in order to gain parental love in one's early childhood can lead to rage over the loss of the self. This rage is then directed not against the parents, but against minorities, strangers, and so forth (see Gruen)
4. Manipulation of the more suggestible part of the population by leaders. Historical myths are elaborated [Roman glory by Mussolini, Aryan myths by Hitler, Serbian myths of the ancient battle against the Muslim Turks]. A "paranoid group" is created (see Richard Brickner's *Is Germany Incurable?*) exhibiting retrospective falsification and projection.
5. Animalization: The dehumanization of the victim through the use of language. These labels facilitate killing, since humans aren't being killed, only animals.
6. The use of "shame" in a culture, as opposed to "guilt," as a means of social control. Some authors have felt that the absence of a strongly internalized superego or conscience allows for killing. (Ruth Benedict's "The Chrysanthemum and the Sword" suggested this hypothesis.) I feel that neither guilt nor shame stops killing.
7. The Gustave Ichheiser hypothesis: The killer projects his repressed impulses directly onto the victim. The target is seen as a sexual beast, as aggressive, stingy, lazy, and cunning. These are actually qualities of the unconscious itself, which is sneaky and uncontrollable. The authoritarian parent has suppressed these impulses, which are then repressed by the child.
8. Ernest Becker: There is a joy in killing which is the result of ego expansion. This is related to the instinct for survival. The joy comes from the

---

* I had originally placed these hypotheses in a long footnote, but then realized that they deserve a central place in this chapter. Since killing is at the bottom of the moral hierarchy of coping modes (most damaging), the motivation for this behavior remains as one of the foremost unsolved problems in the world.

conquering of the killer's own fear of death. Becker calls this the killer's triumph over evil (the "evil" being his own death). Goldhagen describes S. S. troops dancing with joy after killing a group of Jews. Killing is also seen here as offering an illusion of immortality: "I have the power of life and death."

9. Killing thrives in a subculture of violence: Where killing is encouraged and rewarded, it will thrive. This is true in the armed forces, which teach killing. It is also true in violent street gangs and in the Mafia, where violence brings monetary and interpersonal rewards. Models for this type of indoctrination are described in Albert Cohen's *Delinquent Boys* and in Whyte's *Street Corner Society*, although these deal with delinquent rather than homicidal subcultural norms. Male bonding plays a large role.

10. Early exposure to killing, as in prolonged wars or minority ghetto violence. Children 10 years of age and up in Somalia and in the Sudan (some of them kidnapped into service) carry automatic weapons, and use them readily. Young boys and teenagers were heavily involved in the fighting in Rwanda, and have been witness to or engaged in much slaughter.

This list of hypotheses only scratches the surface. There are neo-Lombrosian theories. Genetics and chemistry have been invoked (the XYY chromosomes supposedly found in serial killers such as Richard Speck, and high levels of testosterone).

A most interesting explanation that has received widespread publicity is that of Jonah Goldhagen, a historian. His expertly documented thesis is that Germany had a long tradition of anti- Semitism. After the addition of a racist ideology to the historical anti-Semitism, it became virulent. The only solution to the "Jewish problem" was to kill the Jews. Conversion to Christianity was no longer an option, since racial traits cannot be changed!

Goldhagen's thesis is rightly criticized by Istvan Deák:

> The reasons why ordinary people torture and kill innocents must be sought elsewhere than in the simplistic argument of national tradition ... The behavior of 'ordinary' people in extreme situations remains as inexplicable and as saddening as ever. (Deak, 1997, pp. 40, 42)

While Deák does not offer any single explanation, he raises complex issues such as non-German Europeans' responsibility for the death of Jews, and the differences between German traditions and the traditions of Austria and Hungary. Jews achieved high status in both countries, but gentiles of Austria became active anti-Semites after 1918 and Hungarian attitudes changed sharply after the German Army occupation in 1944.

My conclusion is that we really understand very little about the origins of killing, violence, and the exertion of power over others. Becker's explanation (Becker, 1973, although certainly containing a great deal of truth, does not leave us with many alternatives for stopping killing. His idea that "men kill lavishly out of the sublime joy of heroic triumph over evil" is discussed in Chapter 18. It is his belief that men live in fear of death, dying, and being killed (evil), and that the joy of killing others comes not from instinctive lust, but from fear. If so, he thinks reason may mitigate fear.

Many thinkers are convinced that the *autonomous* individual does not kill, and cannot be persuaded to kill by any vicious tradition. How are we to breed this autonomy, and still maintain a cohesive society? Are these two goals incompatible?

Gruen (1992) seems to speak to this same notion of the autonomous individual. He thinks that children give up their autonomy, (their self) to win and maintain their parents' (conditional) love. In the process, they give up so much of their inner self that they develop a lasting rage. This rage is ready to be called up by an incident, a slight, or a demagogue. Thus killing is a function of a sacrifice of the self to obtain and maintain love and protection against abandonment (see Bowlby, 1973).

I feel that these thinkers (Bowlby and Gruen) have gotten closer than most others to the causal factors in killing. I don't think that children are born with rage, although there are differences in temperament. Essentially this is an optimistic view, since parenting can be changed, and parental substitutes, such as teachers, can be trained to develop or give back each child's individuality and autonomy.

Of course, education and legislation must continue to be used to curb racism and hatred of out- groups. There has been a wave of anger against immigrants in the United States and in some European countries. Jobs have to be created so that the immigrant is not seen as cheap labor stealing native-born jobs. Fair employment practices and anti-discrimination in housing and promotions must be reinforced. Racist, ageist, sexist, homophobic, and other hatreds have to be controlled through education and laws. Values of tolerance, acceptance, and inclusion have to be taught, rather than those of exclusion and hatred. These values are not a standard part of the school curriculum now.

Most crucially, corporations have to be rewarded with tax breaks for keeping jobs within their countries, rather than exporting them to countries with cheaper labor. This was proposed by our former Secretary of Labor, Robert Reich, but was ignored by both Congress and the Administration. Organized labor and various environmental groups view globalization as a threat to jobs at home and to the world environment. The angry demonstrations against the World Bank and International Monetary Fund have been put down by mass arrests and the use of police force. This is only a dress-rehearsal for the hatreds that will be engendered by the quickening pace of globalization.

The task for society is to make available the less damaging coping modes to its members. Love, creativity, and humor can thrive best in a protected environment. Only exceptional individuals can love others, be creative, or retain a sense of humor under conditions of war, poverty, and pestilence. The worldwide reduction of poverty, support for physical and mental health of families, and training in parenting and interpersonal relations as part of the normal grade and high school curriculum are just some of the steps that can be taken to reduce fear of dying. These steps, in turn, might even reduce the possibility of war. Open discussion of death and dying, still a tabooed subject in the United States, is slowly growing. Grants by George Soros through his Open Society Institute, and by the Robert Wood Johnson Foundation, seek to change American attitudes toward death and dying, and to improve the care given to people at the end of life (Miller, 1997).

For most of us, and for many generations after us, the fear of death will still be around. Living life as fully as you can; giving as much love as you are capable of to your family, co-workers, and neighbors; and being as creative as you can be within the limits of your abilities is the final answer to dying without fear, and living without fear of death. Fulfillment leaves few regrets.

Ignace Lepp, who was a psychotherapist as well as a priest, has stated the case so simply and beautifully that it is a fitting end to this book:

> It is my conviction that an intense love of life is the best and perhaps the only effective antidote against the fear of death. There is no need to repress fear or forget that we are mortal. But we can realize that we might die at any moment and yet live as though we were never going to die. I know many men, both men of action and intellectuals, who have honestly succeeded in living this apparent contradiction. They succeed because they do not repress their life instincts. (Lepp, 1968, No. 231, p. 76)*

ENDNOTE

There is not room here for a complete discussion of this basic problem in psychology and in science in general. When is reporting accurate, and when is it heavily influenced by the subject reporting, or by the observer? A newpaper article raises the issue of the reality of reporting about early childhood. Sarah Boxer ("Analysts Get Together for a Synthesis," *The New York Times*, 3/14/98, pp. B9 and B11) says, "In 1896 Freud said he found the key to hysteria: all hysterics were seduced as children. The next year he took it back. He decided that the key to hysteria was not the actual seduction of children but their sexual fantasies. It is not physical reality but psychic reality that counts." Boxer mentions Jeffrey Masson's book, *Assault on Truth*, which says that Freud abandoned the sexually abused children who do exist, and excused their oppressors.

* Lepp summarizes the views of the existentialists Heidegger and Sartre. He notes that the "lucid and courageous acceptance of death and the fear of death" recommended by this philosophy has not even helped Sartre to overcome his "overwhelming anxiety … when he reflects upon man's mortal condition" (pp. 74–75).

It is time we refrained from "Freud-bashing," at which Masson is an expert, and looked at the circumstances of this "flip-flop." In a lecture by Ernest Jones, which I attended, he described Freud as having an open, receptive, almost naive mind. He accepted his patients' reports of seduction without question for a while. His more sophisticated Viennese colleagues would have regarded these reports as nonsense. Freud was an outsider, and no doubt worried that he and his theories about the unconscious and the whole psychoanalytic movement would be made a laughing stock if he persisted in treating the seduction reports as "real." He posited the "psychic reality" of the unconscious, and seduction reports were to be considered psychic, but not physical, reality. He warned that, "If we had before us the unconscious wishes, brought to their final and truest expression, we should still do well to remember that psychic reality is a special form of existence which must not be confounded with material reality." (S. Freud, "The Psychology of the Dream Processes," in *The Basic Writings of Sigmund Freud*, The Modern Library, Random House, New York, 1938, p. 548.)

Boxer quotes Dr. Robert Michaels, an analyst, speaking at a meeting to discuss seduction, reality, and fantasy at Mt. Sinai Hospital in Manhattan. "We are experts not in helping patients learn facts but in helping them construct useful myths. We are fantasy doctors, not reality doctors." Another analyst, Jody Davies, said "The discussion of true versus false is a false issue." Now this attitude toward physical reality may be fine in the context of the analysts's office. She or he is treating an individual who is less likely than most others to have been sexually or physically abused in childhood, Preselection of higher social class patients for the expensive process of psychoanalysis or any form of protracted psychotherapy suggests a lower rate of early abuse. (It certainly does not exclude the possibility of real physical abuse.)

In the real world, outside the analyst's office, the attitude of the analysts toward reality took hold in situations where it did not apply. Reports of widespread child physical and sexual abuse were played down, minimized, or ignored. They were treated as "psychic reality." They were not real. This basically conservative attitude toward abuse fits in with a national trend toward political conservatism, which ignores or plays down the problems of children, women and minorities.

During the last 20 years, there was a sudden reversal in attitude, not in the psychoanalytic establishment, but in a motley crew of therapists, some of them trained as police interrogators. These people, most of them on the fringe of the profession, encouraged their patients to report memories of Satanic cults, gang rapes, and various forms of seduction involving the participation of their parents. Lawsuits by children or their "protectors" against parents (and teachers) became a cottage industry. Therapists testified that these events must have really happened. They were no longer constrained by Freud's warning about the difference between physical and psychic reality. Then a third reversal came during the last few years, when lawsuits were brought against therapists for eliciting reports of seduction from the plaintiffs. In one case, a large award with punitive damages was won by a father against a therapist who had elicited a report of Satanic gang rape from this man's teenage daughter. The father lost his job (as a policeman), his wife, and his two daughters. He was even convinced for a while that he had actually been an abuser.

The pendulum has swung from Freud's belief to his disbelief, to belief, and finally to disbelief (inspired by fear of lawsuits) in reports of childhood sexual abuse and recovered memories. The hysteria over the "he said–she said" facts or "factoids" in the lawsuit of Paula Corbin Jones lawsuit against President Bill Clinton should tell us about the low reliability of reporting in adult (adulterous?) life. In this age of deconstruction, everything is subject to varying interpretations. There are revisionists everywhere. We are encouraged to look under the hood to see what makes the car go, just as Freud did 100 years ago. Real abuse is rampant. Abuse of children is a subject crucial to the creation of a better world for all of us, offering possible reduction of hostility and war, and greater individual happiness. Its study should not be limited to psychoanalytic reports of wealthy patients, nor to psychiatry, social workers, or anthropologists, nor to those organizations seeking to protect children. These groups often do not speak to each other. There is good reason for this; they usually don't even speak the same language. They should pool their skills.

REFERENCES

Abbott, L. K. (1996, 4/9/96). Death rattle. *The New York Times Book Review*, p. 11.

Adler, A. (1927 Original publ, reprinted 1994). *Understanding Human Nature*. Oxford, England. Oneworld Publications.

Allen, W. (1971). *Getting Even*. New York: Random House.

Allen, W. (1993). *The Illustrated Woody Allen Reader*. New York: Alfred A. Knopf.

Alvarez, A. (1973, Bantam Books, original 1971). *The Savage God* (seventh ed.). New York: Bantam (originally Weidenfeld & Nicholson, London).

Angier, N. (1995, 8/29/95). New view of family: Unstable but wealth helps. *The New York Times*, pp. C1, C5.

Anon. (1990). The spirit world: Enlightenment or hidden dangers? (ARBN USA 010 019 986): *Wordwide Church of God*.

Anon. (1994, 8/2/94). Odd disorder of brain may offer new clues to basis of language. *The New York Times*, p. C6.

Anon. (1996, 2/19/96). Closing arguments in Menendez trial. *NY Times*.

Anon. (1996, 7/10/96). Above all, don't dress up as a cow. *The New York Times*, p. A3.

Anon. (1997, 12/6/97). Poll looks at innermost feelings about life's end. *The New York Times*, Religion Journal.

Apter, M. J. (1992). *The Dangerous Edge: The Psychology of Excitement*. New York: The Free Press.

Arensberg, C. and Kimball, S. K. (1940). *Family and Community in Ireland*. Cambridge, MA: Harvard University Press.

Atlas, J. (1996, 5/12/96). The age of the literary memoir is now. *The New York Times Magazine*, pp. 25–28.

Barber, B. R. (1996, 11/4/96). A civics lesson. *The Nation*.

Bartlett, J. (1995). *Bartlett's Familiar Quotations* (16th ed.). Boston: Little, Brown.

Becker, E. (1962,1971). *The Birth and Death of Meaning*. New York: The Free Press.

Becker, E. (1964). *Revolution in Psychiatry* (1974 paperback ed.). New York: The Free Press of Glencoe.

Becker, E. (1973). *The Denial of Death*. New York: The Free Press.

Becker, E. (1976). *Escape from Evil* (EFE). New York: The Free Press.

Belluck, P. (1996, 3/16/96). Man expected to go to prison for helping wife kill herself. *The New York Times*, pp. 23 and 28.

289

Blau, T. H. (1980). *The Lure of the Deep: Scuba Diving as a High-Risk Sport*. In Farberow, Ed., The Many Faces of Suicide, New York, McGraw-Hill.

Borch-Jacobsen, M. (1997, 4/24/97). Sybil: The making of a disease. *The New York Review of Books, XLIV*, pp. 61–64.

Botsford, G. (1997, 4/13/97). Dispatches. *The New York Times Book Review*, p. 6.

Bowlby, J. (1973). *Separation: Anxiety and Anger*, Vol. II. New York: Basic Books.

Boxer, S. (1995, 9/10/95). Derailing the train of thought. *The New York Times Book Review*, p. 40.

Boyer, P. J. (1995, Sept. 11, 1995). Life after Vince. *The New Yorker*, p. 62.

Bradshaw, J. (1992). *Creating Love*. New York: Bantam Books.

Brahms, J. (1968). *Songs, Selections, Lieder for Voice and Piano*. Melville, NY: Belwin Mills.

Branden, N. (1981). *The Psychology of Romantic Love*. New York: Bantam Books (originally Tarcher,1980).

Brickner, R. (1943). *Is Germany Incurable?* Philadelphia: J. B. Lippincott.

Broad, W. J. (1996, 5/14/96). El Popo's rumblings draw volcanologists to the edge of danger. *The New York Times*, pp. C1 and C6.

Brockway, W., and Weinstock, H. (1939). *Men of Music*. New York: Simon & Schuster.

Brody, J. E. (1997, 11/4/97). Girls and puberty: The crisis years. *The New York Times*, p. F9.

Brooke, J. (1996, 2/7/96). Abundance of snowfall and daring proves deadly. *The New York Times*, p. A13.

Brown, N. O. (1959). *Life Against Death*. Middletown, CT: Wesleyan University Press.

Browne, M. W. (1997, 2/11/97). Young astronomers scan night sky and Help Wanted ads. *The New York Times*, p. C7.

Burke, K. (1954). *Permanence and Change: An Anatomy of Purpose* (2nd rev. ed.). Los Alos, CA: Hermes.

Burns, J. F. (1996, 5/14/96). Everest takes worst toll, refusing to become stylish. *The New York Times*, p. A1 and A3.

Butterfield, F. (1996, 2/15/96). Insanity drove a man to kill at two clinics, jury is told. *The New York Times*, p. A14.

Cannon, W. B. (1919, 1963). *Bodily Changes in Pain, Hunger, Fear and Rage* (2nd ed. 1963, Harper Torch Books). New York: Harper & Row.

Carroll, L. p. o. C. L. D. (1865 original publication). *Alice's Adventures in Wonderland (and Through the looking Glass)* (1996 printing). New York: Grosset & Dunlap.

Clinton, H. R. (1996). *It Takes A Village and Other Lessons Children Teach Us*. New York: Simon & Schuster.

Cohen, A. K. (1955). *Delinquent Boys: The Culture of the Gang*. Glencoe, IL: Free Press.

Cohen, D. (1996). Alter Egos: Multiple Personalities. London: Constable.

Cohen, J. M. C. M. J. (1978). *The Penguin Dictionary of Quotations*. New York: Penguin Books.

Conrad, J. (1962). *Joseph Conrad's Secret Sharer and the Critics*. Belmont, CA: Wadsworth.

Cooper, M. (1995, 12.25.95). Boy's mother is charged with abuse. *The New York Times*, p. 43.

Cousins, N. (1979). *Anatomy of An Illness*. New York: W. W. Norton.

Croce, A. (1995, Jan 2,1995). Discussing the undiscussable. *The New Yorker*.

Daley, S. (1997, 11/9/97). Apartheid torturer testifies as evil shows its banal face. *The New York Times*, pp. 1 and 12.

Deak, I. (1997, 6/26/97). Memories of hell. *The New York Review of Books*, XLIV, pp. 38–43.

Delbanco, A. (1995). *The Death of Satan: How Americans Have Lost the Sense of Evil*. New York: Farrar, Strauss and Giroux.

Delk, J. L. (1980). High risk sports as indirect self-destructive behavior. In N. L. Farberow (Ed.), *The Many Faces of Suicide*. New York: McGraw-Hill, pp. 393–409.

Demause, L. (1974). Book review: The denial of death. *History of childhood quarterly*, 2(2), 281–283.

Dempsey, D. (1996, 10/6/96). The long joy ride. *The New York Times Magazine*, p. 82.

Doniger, W. (1995, 10/22/95). Giving the devil his due. *The New York Times Book Review*, p. 45.

Durkheim, E. (1897). *Le Suicide, Etude de Sociologie* (J. Spaulding and G. Simpson, Trans.) (also English translation, New York, Free Press, 1951 ed.). Paris: Alcan.

Durkheim, E. (1915). *The Elementary Forms of the Religious Life* (Joseph Ward Swain, Trans.). London: Allen & Unwin.

Eisenberg, J. G. e. a. (1975). Differences in the behavior of Welfare and non-Welfare children in relation to parental characteristics. *Journal of Community Psychology, Monograph Supplement* No. 48 (October 1975), 33 pp.

Eisenberg, J. G. e. a. (1976). A behavioral classification of welfare children from survey data. *American Journal of Orthopsychiatry*, 46(3), 447–463.

Eissler, K. R. (1955). *The Psychiatrist and the Dying Patient*. New York: International Universities Press.

Engel, G. L. (1975). The death of a twin: Mourning and anniversary reactions. Fragments of 10 years of self-analysis. *International Journal of Psycho-Analysis*, 56, 23–40.

Erickson, E. H. (1968). *Identity: Youth and Crisis*. New York: W.W. Norton.

Fagin, D. M. L. (1996). *Toxic Deception*. Secaucus, NJ: Carol Publishing Group (Birch Lane Press).

Farberow, N. L. (Ed.) (1980). *The Many Faces of Suicide*. New York: McGraw-Hill.

Feifel, H. (1959). Attitudes toward death in some normal and mentally ill populations. In H. Feifel (Ed.), *The Meaning of Death*. New York: McGraw-Hill, pp. 114–130; see p. 126.

Feifel, H. (Ed.) (1959). *The Meaning of Death*. New York: McGraw-Hill.

Fenichel, O. (1939). The counter-phobic attitude. *International Journal of Psycho-Analysis*, 20, 263–274.

Ferenczi, S. e. J. D. (1988). *The Clinical Diary of Sandor Ferenczi*. Cambridge, MA: Harvard University Press.

Fjerkenstad, J. (1990). Who are the criminals? In Zweig, C. and Abrams, Z. (Eds.) *Meeting the Shadow*. New York: Jeremy P. Tarcher/Putnam.

Flexner, S. B. (Ed.) (1987). *The Random House Dictionary of the English Language* (2nd ed.). New York: Random House.

Foxe, A. N. (1939). *The Life and Death Instincts*. New York: The Monograph Editions.

Fraser, J. (1923). *The Golden Bough (The Scapegoat)*. New York: Macmillan.

Freud, S. (1916, 1917). *Wit and Its Relation to the Unconscious* (A. A. Brill, Trans.). New York: Moffat and Yard.

Freud, S. (1920). *Beyond the Pleasure Principle*, Vol. 18 (Standard Edition) London: Hogarth, pp. 3–64.

Freud, S. (1929). *Civilization and Its Discontents* (1953 ed.), Vol. 4, *Civilization, War and Death*. London: The Hogarth Press.

Freud, S. (1957). *The Future of an Illusion*. New York: Doubleday Anchor Books.

Fromm, E. (1955). *The Art of Loving*. New York: Harper & Brothers.

Fromm, E. (1959). *Sigmund Freud's Mission: An Analysis of His Personality and Influence*. London: G. Allen & Unwin.

Fukuyama, F. (1994, 4/10/94). The war of all against all (a review of *Blood and Belonging* by Michael Ignatieff, New York, Farrar, Strauss & Giroux, 1994). *The New York Times Book Review*, p. 7.

Fuller, R. (1995). *Naming the Antichrist*. New York: Oxford University Press.

Fulton, R. (1970). *Death and Identity*. (Revised edition, 1976). Bowie, MD: The Charles Press.

Furse, J. (1996, 6/8/96). Kin can make difference, docs say. *Daily News*.

Gersten, J. C. e. a. (1974). Child behavior and life events. In B. S. D. a. B. P. Dohrenwend (Ed.), *Stressful Life Events*. New York: John Wiley & Sons, pp. 159–170.

Gersten, J. C. e. a. (1976). Stability and change in types of behavioral disturbance of children and adolescents. *Journal of Abnormal Child Psychology*, 4(2), 111–127.

Gilbert, S. (1996, 6/27/96). Emotional ills tied to stunted growth in girls. *The New York Times*.

Gladwell, M. (1996, 9/30/96). The new age of man. *The New Yorker*, pp. 56–67.

Glass, J. M. (1993). *Shattered Selves: Multiple Personality in a Postmodern World*. Ithaca, NY: Cornell University Press.

Goffman, E. (1952). On cooling the mark out. *Psychiatry*, 5, 451–464.

Goffman, E. (1962). *Asylums: Essays on the Social Situation of Mental Patients and Other Inmates*. Chicago: Aldine.

Goldberg, J. G. (1993). *The Dark Side of Love*. New York: Jeremy P. Tarcher/Putnam.

Goldberg, G. (1995, 12/15/95). Suicide's husband is indicted. *The New York Times*.

Goldstein, R. (1998, 3/15/98). Adrian Marks, 81, war pilot, is dead. *The New York Times*, p. 43.

Goleman, D. (1995, 1/4/95). Religious faith and social activity help to heal, new research finds. *The New York Times*.

Goleman, D. (1996). *Emotional Intelligence*. New York: Bantam.

Goodman, W. (1997, 3/10/97). Time for reassurance and disaster. *The New York Times*, p. B12.

Gould, S. J. (October 1944). Jove's thunderbolts. *Natural History*, 103, 6–13.

Greene, E. L. e. a. (1973). Some methods of evaluating behavioral variations in children six to eighteen. *Journal of the American Academy of Child Psychiatry*, XII, 3 (July).

Gruen, A. (1992). *The Insanity of Normality* (Hildegarde & Hunter Hannum, Trans.). New York: Grove Weidenfeld (Grove Press).

Haberman, C. (1995, 12/26/95). The spirit of a little girl haunts a day. *New York Times*, p. B1.

Hamlin, S. (1995, 8/9/95). Health letters scratch out a niche. *The New York Times*, p. C1 and C2.

Hasselbach, I., with Tom Reiss. (1996, 1/8/96). How Nazis are made. *The New Yorker*, pp. 36–56.

Hendin, H. (1965). *Suicide and Scandinavia* (Anchor Books 1965, paperback ed.). New York: Anchor Books (originally published by Grune & Stratton, 1964).

Herbert, B. (1997, 3/10/97). The artful dodger. *The New York Times*, p. A15 (Op Ed page).

Hirshey, G. (1994, 7/17/94). Gambling nation. *The New York Times Magazine* p. 36f.

Holloway, L. (1995, Sept 17, 1995). Gunman in Queens kills 3 in family and himself. *The New York Times*, p. 43–44.

Ichheiser, G. (1944). Fear of violence and fear of fraud; with some remarks on the social psychology of antisemitism. *Sociometry, 7,* 376–383.

Iserson, K. V. (1994). *Death to Dust: What Happens to Dead Bodies?* Tucson, AZ: Galen Press.

James, G. (1995, 12/28/95). Papers tell of a wife's suicide plan. *The New York Times*, p. B5.

James, J. (1995, 3/19/95). He no longer has to make points. He just makes them. *The New York Times*, pp. 31 and 46.

Jamison, K. R. (1995). *An Unquiet Mind* (Vintage Books, first edition, 1996). New York: Random House (originally Knopf hard cover).

Janofsky, M. (1995, 5/31/95). Demons and conspiracies haunt a "patriot" world. *The New York Times*, p. A18.

Jefferson, M. (1996, 10/6/96). Mirror, mirror. *The New York Times Book Review*, p. 109.

Josephson, E. a. M. (Ed.) (1962). *Man Alone: Alienation in Modern Society.* New York: Dell.

Josephson, E. (1985). Smoking, alcohol and substance abuse. In E. A. Donald F. Tapley (Ed.), *The Columbia University College of Physicians and Surgeons: Complete Home Medical Guide.* New York: Crown, pp. 340–359.

Kakutani, M. (1994, 6/22/94). Critics notebook: With reality reeling, pity the poor realist. *The New York Times*, pp. C13 and C18.

Kakutani, M. (1994, 11/8/94). Of time, loss and death: The Vista is lengthening. *The New York Times*, Section C, p. 17.

Kakutani, M. (1995, 6/15/95). Seeking Satan, bogeyman and balm. *The New York Times*, p. C18.

Kardiner, A. (1945). *The Psychological Frontiers of Society.* New York: Columbia University Press.

Keats, J. (1988). *The Complete Poems* (3rd ed.) New York Penguin Books.

Kendrick, W. (1995, 9/10/95). The child who wasn't there. *The New York Times Book Review*, 34.

Kenny, M. G. (1986). *The Passion of Ansel Bourne.* Washington D.C.: Smithsonian Institution Press.

Klausner, S. Z. (1980). The Societal Stake in Stress-Seeking. In N. L. Farberow (Ed.), *The Many Faces of Suicide.* New York: McGraw-Hill, pp. 375–392.

Kluft, R. P. C. G. F. (Ed.) (1993). Clinical Perspectives on Multiple Personality Disorder. Washington, D.C.: American Psychiatric Press.

Kristof, N. D. (1996, 6/10/96). In Japan, deflating a poisonous pufferfish legend. *The New York Times*, p. A4.

Kubler-Ross, E. (1969). *On Death and Dying.* New York: Collier Books (MacMillan).

Kübler-Ross, E. (1975). *Death: The Final Stage of Growth* (Touchstone Edition, 1986 ed.). New York: Simon & Schuster.

Labaton, S. (1997, 10/11/97). A report of his suicide draws a portrait of a depressed Vincent Foster. *The New York Times*, pp. A1 and A8.

Laird, C. G. (1985 revised edition), *Webster's New World Thesaurus*. New York: Simon & Schuster.

Lang, A. (Ed.) (1966 reprinted). *The Blue Fairy Book* (First edition circa 1889. Hardcover edition 1966 of Dover Publications edition of 1965 paperback ed.). New York: McGraw-Hill.

Langner, T. S. , S. T. M. (1963). *Life Stress and Mental Health*, Vol. II. New York: Free Press.

Langner, T. S. e. a. (1969). Psychiatric impairment in Welfare and nonWelfare children. *Welfare in Review*, 7, 10–21.

Langner, T. S. e. a. (1970) Children of the city: Affluence, poverty and mental health. In V. L. Allen (Ed.), *Psychological Factors in Poverty*. Chicago: Markham.

Langner, T. S. e. a. (1974). Treatment of psychological disorders among urban children. *Journal of Consulting and Clinical Psychology*, 42, 170–179.

Langner, T. S. e. a. (1974). Approaches to measurement and definition in the epidemiology of behavior disorders: Ethnic background and child behavior. *International Journal of Health Services*, 4, 483–501.

Langner, T. S. e. a. (1976). A screening inventory for assessing psychiatric impairment in children six to eighteen. *Journal of Consulting and Clinical Psychology*, 44, 286–296.

Lasch, C. (1979). *The Culture of Narcissism* (Warner Books ed.). New York: W. W. Norton.

Leary, W. E. (1994, 12/27/94). To save more lives, doctors urge making even cheaper defibrillators. *The New York Times*, p. C3.

Lepp, I. (1968). *Death and Its Mysteries* (Bernard Murchland, Trans.). (First published in France by Editions Bernard Grasset, as *La Mort et Ses Mysteries*. Paperback 1969 and hardcover ed.). New York: MacMillan.

Levey, J. S. a. A. G. (Ed.) (1983). *The Concise Columbia Encyclopedia*. New York: Columbia University Press.

Levin, M. (1962). Political Alienation In E. A. M. Josephson (Ed.), *Man Alone: Alienation in Modern Society*. New York: Dell.

Lewis, C. S. (1960). *The Four Loves*. New York: Harcourt, Brace & World.

Lichtenstein, H. (1977, 1983). *The Dilemma of Human Identity*. New York: Jason Aronson.

Lifton, R. J. (1971). Protean Man. *Archives of General Psychiatry*, 24, 298–304.

Lifton, R. J. (1979). *The Broken Connection*. New York: Simon & Schuster.

Lifton, R. J. (1986). Doubling and the Nazi Doctors. In Zweig (Ed.), *Meeting the Shadow*. New York: Jeremy P. Tarcher/Putnam.

Long, K. A. T. R. (1985). *Fatal Facts* (1986 ed.). New York: Arlington House.

Lothane, Z. (1992). *In Defense of Schreber: Soul Murder and Psychiatry*. Hillsdale, NJ: The Analytic Press.

Malcolm, J. (1983). *In the Freud Archives*. New York: Knopf.

Marshall, S. E. (Ed.) (1967). *A Young American's Treasury of English Poetry*. New York: Washington Square Press.

Marshall, W. H. (Ed.) (1966). *The Major English Romantic Poets*. New York: Washington Square Press.

Martin, D. (1996, 10/18/96). The choreography of desire: Former Ziegfeld girl recalls the glory days. *The New York Times*, p. B17.

McCarthy, E. D. e. a. (1975). The effects of television on children and adolescents: Violence and behavior disorders. *Journal of Communication*, 25, 71–85.

McCullough, D. (1992). *Truman*. New York: Simon & Schuster.

McFadden, R. D. (1996, 9/2/96). Girl, 4, is dead in Manhattan. *The New York Times*, pp. 1 and 24.

McQuiston, J. T. (1995, 8/22/95). A new and deadly fad comes riding into town. *The New York Times*, p. B5.

Mead, G. H. (1962). *Mind, Self and Society*. Chicago: University of Chicago Press.

Meerloo, J. A. M. (1962). *Suicide and Mass Suicide*. New York: Grune & Stratton.

Menninger, K. A. (1938). *Man Against Himself*. New York: Harcourt, Brace & World.

Menninger, K. (1963). *The Vital Balance: The Life Process in Mental Health and Illness*. New York: Viking.

Merton, R. K. (1968a). *Social Theory and Social Structure*. New York: The Free Press.

Merton, R. K. (1968b). Social structure and anomie, In *Social Theory and Social Structure* (see p. 140). New York: The Free Press.

Miles, R. (1991). *Love, Sex, Death and the Making of the Male*. New York, London: Summit Books (Simon & Schuster).

Millay, E. S. V. (1941). *Collected Sonnets of Edna St. Vincent Millay*. New York, Evanston, London: Harper & Row.

Miller, J. (1997, 11/22/97). When foundations chime in, the issue of dying comes to life. *The New York Times*, pp. B7 and B9.

Mumford, L. (1934). The Mechanical Routine. In E. M. Josephson (Ed.), *Man Alone: Alienation in Modern Society*. New York: Dell.

Nagy, M. H. (1959). The child's view of death. In H. Feifel (Ed.) *The Meaning of Death*, New York: McGraw-Hill, p. 97.

Nieburg, H. A. A. F. (1982). *Pet Loss*. New York: Harper & Row.

Norman, M. (1996, 1/14/96). Living too long. *The New York Times Magazine*, pp. 36–38.

Nuland, S. B. (1993). *How We Die*. New York: Alfred A. Knopf.

Pagels, E. (1995). *The Origin of Satan*. New York: Random House.

Pear, R. (1997, 3/16/97). Ex-official criticizes Clinton on Welfare. *The New York Times*, p. 39.

Percy, T. B. (1905). *The Boy's Percy*. New York: Charles Scribner's Sons.

Phillips, L. a. J. C. S. (1953). *Rorschach Interpretation Advanced Technique*. New York: Grune & Stratton.

Prince, M. (1906). *The Dissociation of a Personality* (2nd ed, 1969 is reprint of 1906 original ed.). Westport, CT: Greenwood Press.

Rank, O. (1932, reprinted 1989). *Art and Artist*. New York: originally Alfred A Knopf, W. W. Norton (Norton Paperback).

Rank, O. (1958) (originally printed 1941). *Beyond Psychology*. New York: Dover.

Reed, W. L. a. B., M. J. (Eds) (1993). *National Anthems of the World* (8th ed., 1993. First edition 1960). London: Cassell.

Remnick, D. (1995, 4/3/95). The Devil Problem. *The New Yorker*, pp. 54–65.

Reston, J. J. (1995, 9/10/95). The Monument Glut. *The New York Times Magazine*, pp. 48–49.

Rich, F. (1994, 6/23/94). Addicted to O. J.: From celebrity to cold turkey. *The New York Times*, Op Ed section.

Rieber, R. W. (1997). *Manufacturing Social Distress: Psychopathy in Everyday Life*. New York: Plenum.

Riesman, D. (1950). *The Lonely Crowd*. New Haven: Yale University Press.

Rinpoche, S. (1994). *The Tibetan Book of Living and Dying* (paperback ed.). New York: HarperSanFrancisco (HarperCollins).

Rosenbaum, R. (1995, 5/1/95). Explaining Hitler. *The New Yorker*, pp. 50–73.

Rue, L. (1994). *By the Grace of Guile: The Role of Deception in Natural History and Human Affairs*. New York: Oxford University Press.

Schaar, J. H. (1961). *Escape from Authority: The Perspectives of Erich Fromm*. New York: Basic Books.

Schonberg, H. C. (1981). *Facing the Music*. New York: Simon & Schuster (Summit Books).

Schreiber, F. R. (1973). *Sybil* (Also published by Warner Books, and by Allen Lane, division of Penguin Books, London, 1973 ed.). Chicago: H. Regnery.

Schwartz, H. (1996). *The Culture of the Copy*. New York: Zone Books.

Seldes, G. (Ed.) (1967). *The Great Quotations*. New York: Pocket Books (Simon and Schuster).

Shakespeare, W. *As You Like It* (Oxford single volume ed.).

Shakespeare, W. *MacBeth* (Oxford ed.).

Shakespeare, W. *Measure for Measure*. New York: Pocket Books (Simon & Schuster, Washington Square Press).

Shneidman, E. (1985). *Definition of Suicide*. New York: John Wiley & Sons.

Shneidman, E. S. (1993). Suicide as psychache. In J. B. Williamson (Ed.), *Death: Current Perspectives* (4th ed.). Mountain View, CA: Mayfield, pp. 369–374.

Siebert, C. (1996, 7/7/96). The cuts that go deeper *The New York Times Magazine*, pp. 20–34.

Siegel, B. S. (1986). *Love, Medicine & Miracles*. New York: Harper & Row.

Sietsma, R. (1997, 3/25/97). Sashimi to die for. *The Village Voice*, pp. 46–47.

Sims, C. (1995, 3/13/95). Argentine tells of the dumping of captives at sea. *The New York Times*, pp. A1 and A8.

Singer, J. L. (Ed.) (1990). *Repression and Dissociation* (paperback edition 1995). Chicago: The University of Chicago Press.

Soble, A. (1990). The Structure of Love. New Haven and London: Yale University Press.

Sontag, S. (1977). *On Photography* (editions in 1973 and 1974). New York: Farrar, Strauss & Giroux.

Speare, M. E. (Ed.) (1940). *The Pocket Book of Verse*. New York: Pocket Books.

Spiegel, D. (1993). Multiple posttraumatic personality disorder. In R. P. Kluft (Ed.), *Clinical Perspectives on Multiple Personality Disorder* (*see Kluft*, pp. 87–99).

Spiegel, H. (1963). The dissociation–association continuum. *Journal of Nervous and Mental Disease* 136, 374–378.

Spitz, R. A. i. c. w. W. G. C. (1965). *The First Year of Life: A Psychoanalytic Study of Normal and Deviant Development of Object Relations*. New York: International Universities Press.

Srole, L., Langner, T., Michael, S., Opler, M, and Rennie, T. A. C. (1962). *Mental Health in the Metropolis*, Vol. I. New York: McGraw-Hill.

Starr, K. W. (1997). Excerpt from *Independent Counsel's Report on Foster's Death*. Washington, D.C.: U.S. Court of Appeals, Wash. D.C.

Stauffer, S. e. a. (1949–1950). *The American Soldier: Studies in Social Psychology in World War II*. Princeton, NJ: Princeton University Press.

Steiner, W. (1995, 9/24/95). Hannah Arendt, Martin Heidegger (Review of a book by Elzbieta Ettinger). *The New York Times Book Review*, 41.

Stendhal. (1949, first published in 1822). *On Love* (*De L'Amour*) (Translated by the author under the supervision of C.K. Scott-Moncrieff, Trans.). New York: Liveright.

Stephens, M. (1994, 1/23/94). Jacques Derrida. *The New York Times Magazine*, pp. 22–25.

Stephenson, J. S. (1985). *Death, Grief, and Mourning*. New York: The Free Press.

Sternberg, R. J. (1986). A triangular theory of love. *Psych. Review*, 93, 119–138.

Sternberg, R. J. a. M. L. B. (Ed.) (1988). *The Psychology of Love*. New Haven: Yale University Press.

Stevens, W. K. (1979, 10/4/97). Computers model world's climate, but how well? *The New York Times*, pp. F1 and F6.

Storr, A. (1988). *Solitude*. New York. The Free Press.

Thigpen, C. H. C., & Hervey M. (1957). *The Three Faces of Eve*. New York: McGraw-Hill.

Thomas, D. (1957). *Collected Poems*. New York: New Directions.

Toennies, F. (1957, 1963). *Gemeinschaft and Gesellschaft* (*Community and Society*) (Charles P. Loomis, Trans. and editor) New York: Harper & Row.

Train, J. (1993). *Love*. New York: HarperCollins.

Tuchman, B. W. (1978). *A Distant Mirror: The Calamitous 14th Century*. New York: Alfred A. Knopf.

Twain, M. (1962). *Letters from the Earth*. New York: Harper & Row.

Updike, J. (1994). *The Afterlife and Other Stories*. New York: Knopf.

Van Gennep, A. (1960). *The Rites of Passage* (Monika B. Vizedom and Gabrielle L. Caffee, Trans.) (7th impression, 1975 ed.). Chicago: The University of Chicago Press.

Wade, N. (1996, 8/20/95). Decline and conquer. *The New York Times Magazine*, p. 22.

Wahl, C. W. (1959). The fear of death. In H. Feifel (Ed.), *The Meaning of Death*. New York: McGraw-Hill, p. 19.

Wald, M. L. (1995, 7/26/95). Undetonated nuclear arms can destroy, study says. *The New York Times*, p. A12.

Waldman, R. O. (1971) *Humanistic Psychiatry*. New Brunswick: Rutgers Univ. Press. pp. 123–124.

Weisman, A. (1986). *The Coping Capacity: On the Nature of Being Mortal* (paperback 1986 ed.). New York: Human Sciences Press.

White, J. (1988). *A Practical Guide to Death and Dying*. Wheaton, IL: The Theosophical Publishing House.

Whitmont, E. C. (1991). The Evolution of a Shadow. In Zweig (Ed.), *Meeting the Shadow*. New York: Jeremy P. Tarcher/Putnam.

Whyte, W. F. (1955). *Street Corner Society: The Social Structure of an Italian Slum*. Chicago: University of Chicago Press.

Wyschogrod, E. (Ed.) (1973). *The Phenomenon of Death* (paperback after hardcover edition). New York: Harper & Row (Harper Colophon Books).

Zakaria, F. (1996, 8/13/95). Trust (a review of *The Social Virtues and the Creation of Prosperity*, by Francis Fukuyama, The Free Press, 1995). *The New York Times Book Review*, pp. 1 and 25.

Zilboorg, G. (1943). Fear of death. *Psychoanalytic Quarterly*, 12, 468–471.

Zweig, C. and Abrams, Z. J. (Ed.) (1991). *Meeting the Shadow*. New York: Jeremy P. Tarcher/Putnam.

INDEX